WHAT YOU EAT R
MAKE A DIFFERENCE!

In DOCTOR, WHAT SHOULD I EAT?, Dr. Rosenfeld offers nutrition prescriptions—many as surprising as they are effective—to help you prevent or recover from a variety of ailments including:

- **Parkinson's disease:** when "good" food and healthy multivitamins can harm you!

- **Infertility:** the right foods could conceivably help you get pregnant

- **Heart disease:** can a glass of wine really protect you?

- **Premenstrual syndrome:** a doctor gives you his blessing to eat chocolate!

- **Diet and sex:** can what you eat rev up your love life?

- **Jet lag:** fly first class, eat economy

- **Hyperactivity:** the sugar myth

- **Multiple sclerosis:** a high-fat diet may actually be good for you!

Dr. Rosenfeld's sound, accessible advice on these and many other ailments will help you and your doctor work together more effectively for your good health.

Doctor, What Should I Eat?

Nutrition Prescriptions for Ailments
in Which Diet Can Really
Make a Difference

Isadore Rosenfeld, M.D.

WARNER BOOKS

A Time Warner Company

Warner Books Edition
Copyright © 1995 by Isadore Rosenfeld, M.D.

This Warner Books edition is published by arrangement with Random House, Inc., New York

Warner Books, Inc., 1271 Avenue of the Americas, New York, NY 10020

⦿ A Time Warner Company

Printed in the United States of America

First Warner Books Printing: April 1996

10 9 8 7 6 5 4 3 2 1

Library of Congress Cataloging-in-Publication Data
Rosenfeld, Isadore.
      Doctor, what should I eat? : nutrition prescriptions for ailments in which diet can really make a difference / Isadore Rosenfeld.
        p. cm.
      Previously published : New York : Random House, 1995.
      Includes index.
      ISBN 0-446-67261-0 (trade paper)
      1. Diet therapy—Popular works. 2. Nutrition—Popular works.
      3. Diet therapy. 4. Nutrition. I. Title.
      RM216.R833   1996
      618.8 ' 54—dc20   95-41965
                                              CIP

Jacket design by Jennifer Eisenpresser
Jacket photograph by Claire Yaffa

TO THE NEWEST WOMAN IN MY LIFE, REBECCA,

BORN MAY 18, 1992, AND ALREADY EATING "RIGHT"

ACKNOWLEDGMENTS

I never read the acknowledgments in a book unless I have thoroughly enjoyed it. I don't particularly care to know who was involved in creating a work that I did not appreciate. If you find what I have written useful, understandable, and worthwhile, you should know who helped me with it.

There were many times when I was frustrated by my superb and unflappable editor, Ms. Betsy Rapoport. (This will come as a complete surprise to her because I never let on!) She is probably the most sophisticated medical editor in the country—knowledgeable, meticulous, dispassionate about the material at hand— and at the same time, has great compassion for the harried author. She has edited many other doctor-written books and knows her stuff. Why she doesn't go to medical school just to round out the few areas she hasn't yet addressed is beyond me. I am grateful to her for her help, skill, patience, and I apologize again, Betsy, for the countless revisions with which I burdened you.

Most acknowledgments offer thanks to all kinds of people for their "support and encouragement." I'm not always sure what that means. In my own case, however, I am very grateful to Alberto Vitale, chairman of Random House, and Harold Evans, its publisher, for their continued expressions of confidence in my ability to complete this work—long after I promised I would deliver it!

I have referred to Ms. Sandra Pressman in the text. She's a cracker-jack nutritionist—experienced and practical. We spent many hours discussing the impact of nutrition on health and disease. I have incorporated much of what I learned from her in these pages. I should also give credit to her tireless and patient answering machine, which never failed to transmit to her all the urgent messages about calories and RDAs I felt I had to send her—at night when she was asleep, or on weekends, and holidays when she was away. She always had something to come home to!

You would have had a tough time reading this book had it been printed in my handwriting! (Have you ever tried to decipher a prescription?) Elaine Glaser, who has typed the manuscripts of most of my books, did this one too. She deserves an honorary M.D. degree, or at least an R.D. She types more quickly than most people speak—and far more accurately.

This book is a testament to modern communication. In most of my earlier works, I spent countless hours at the Cornell Medical Library retrieving references and researching the literature. This time, however, I sat at my computer and accessed the files of the National Library of Medicine, which had every medical journal containing the information I needed—just by the push of a button! What a wonderful way to learn—and to write a volume such as this. So I am grateful to the countless authors and researchers the fruit of whose work is embodied in these pages.

After I completed a particular section or chapter, I asked one or more of my colleagues whose expertise I respect to review it for accuracy and completeness. I have accepted most of their valuable suggestions and corrections. If you disagree with anything I have written, it's probably because I did not always heed their advice! These are the doctors—all special friends—who gave of their time and expertise:

Denise Barbut, M.D., M.R.C.P., Attending Neurologist
Associate Professor of Neurology
Director, Stroke Center
New York Hospital–Cornell Medical Center

Myron I. Buchman, M.D., F.A.C.S., F.A.C.O.G.
Clinical Associate Professor
Cornell University Medical School
Attending, The New York Hospital
Associate, Lenox Hill Hospital

Harry Bush, M.D.
Associate Professor of Surgery
Cornell University Medical College

Armand F. Cortese, M.D.
Clinical Associate Professor of Surgery
Associate Attending Surgeon
The New York Hospital–Cornell Medical Center

Murray Dworetsky, M.D.
Clinical Professor of Medicine
Attending Physician
The New York Hospital–Cornell Medical Center

Philip Felig, M.D.
Attending Physician
Senior Medical Staff
Lenox Hill Hospital

Howard Goldin, M.D.
Clinical Professor of Medicine (Gastroenterology)
The New York Hospital–Cornell Medical Center
Consultant, Hospital of Rockefeller University

Robert A. Greenberg, M.D.
Clinical Assistant Professor
Ronald O. Perlman Department of Dermatology
New York University Medical Center
Attending Physician
Lenox Hill Hospital

Barry Jay Hartman, M.D.
Clinical Associate Professor of Medicine
Division of Infectious Diseases
Cornell University Medical Center

Lawrence J. Kagen, M.D.
Professor of Medicine
Cornell University Medical College
Attending Physician
Hospital for Special Surgery
Attending Physician
The New York Hospital

Marilyn G. Karmason, M.D.
Associate Clinical Professor of Psychiatry
The New York Hospital–Cornell Medical Center

John H. Laragh, M.D.
Hilda Altschul Master Professor of Medicine
Director of Cardiovascular Center and Hypertension Center
Chief, Cardiology Division, Department of Medicine
The New York Hospital–Cornell Medical Center

Bruce Lerman, M.D.
Professor of Medicine, Cornell University Medical College
Director, Cardiac Electrophysiology Laboratory
The New York Hospital–Cornell Medical Center

Daniel M. Libby, M.D.
Clinical Associate Professor of Medicine (Pulmonary and Critical Care)
Cornell University Medical College
Associate Attending Physician
The New York Hospital

James P. McCarron, Jr., M.D.
Assistant Clinical Professor of Urology
Attending Urologist
The New York Hospital–Cornell Medical Center

Paul F. Miskovitz, M.D.
Clinical Associate Professor of Medicine
Cornell University Medical College
Associate Attending Physician
The New York Hospital–Cornell Medical Center

Mark Pasmantier, M.D.
Clinical Associate Professor of Medicine
The New York Hospital–Cornell Medical Center

Stephen Scheidt, M.D.
Professor of Clinical Medicine and Director
Cardiology Training Program
The New York Hospital–Cornell Medical Center

Michael Schmerin, M.D.
Clinical Assistant Professor of Medicine
New York Hospital–Cornell Medical Center

Samuel H. Selesnick, M.D.
Assistant Professor, Department of Otorhinolaryngology
Cornell University Medical College

Raymond L. Sherman, M.D.
Clinical Professor of Medicine
Cornell University Medical College

Meyer N. Solny, M.D., F.A.C.G.
Clinical Instructor in Medicine
New York Hospital–Cornell Medical Center

Michael A. Weinstein, M.D.
Associate Attending Surgery
Lenox Hill Hospital

Marc E. Weksler, M.D.
Wright Professor of Medicine
Director, Division of Geriatrics and Gerontology
Cornell University Medical College

David J. Wolf, M.D.
Clinical Associate Professor of Medicine
Cornell University Medical College
Assistant Attending Physician
The New York Hospital

When these colleagues had completed their medical review, I asked one of the most distinguished medical nutritionists in this country, Dr.

Richard Rivlin, Professor of Medicine at Cornell University Medical College, Chief of the Division of Nutrition at The New York Hospital and Memorial Sloan-Kettering hospital, and President of the American Society of Nutrition, to review the entire manuscript. He responded to this imposition on our friendship with diligence, good humor, patience, and skill. I am very much in his debt for spending so many hours making sure that my explanations and advice are reasonable and correct.

Finally, a word about my wife, to whom I have referred many times in these pages, and to whom I have dedicated earlier books—for good reason. (She relinquished her proprietary rights to this one to our first grandchild.) Any of my readers who have themselves written a book know the time and stress involved in doing so, even when it's a full-time pursuit. In my case, I undertook this project in my "spare time," because I wanted to continue practicing medicine and teaching. That "spare time" came from the moments Camilla and I would otherwise have spent together—on vacations, in the evenings, when we might otherwise have gone out or just sat together at home. Many pleasures were deferred so that I could write this book. She never complained. (Well, *never* may be a bit strong.) Camilla, darling, I promise to make up for our lost time together—with a vengeance. Thank you for your patience, understanding, and love.

PREFACE

WHY THIS IS NOT THE USUAL "DIET BOOK"

When is the last time your doctor said to you, "Here, let me give you a list of the foods that will help you feel better," or "C'mon, let's go to the supermarket. I'll show you which foods to buy and how to read their labels"? When did he or she last look in your grocery cart to see how you're feeding your family? Probably never, unless, of course, you're married to your doctor or are catering his or her next party. But does your doctor give you prescriptions to bring to your pharmacist specifying what *drugs* you need and how to take them? You bet! That's what doctors do best. They give you medication—and they should—because many drugs are lifesaving. But that's not enough. Proper medical care should also include advice about the right foods to eat to help you prevent illness as well as to help cure it. There should be no contest or confrontation between diet and medication; it is not a matter of either/or. Too many nutrition enthusiasts and holistic practitioners decry the use of pharmacologic agents, while "traditional" doctors don't pay enough attention to the importance of your diet. Yet almost every major medical condition you can think of is either caused or affected in some way by what you eat. Ulcers, kidney or liver malfunction, anemia, asthma, heart disease, hemorrhoids, diverticulitis, diabetes—you name it—for these and other conditions the right diet can help, and the wrong one can hurt.

Everybody pays lip service to the importance of food in the prevention and management of disease. But in the real world, when you're sick, you're on your own as far as nutrition is concerned. Chances are you don't ask the question "Doctor, what should I eat?" often enough, and when you do, it's rarely answered.

Why don't more doctors pay enough attention to nutrition? Because they're not comfortable with it. They almost certainly never studied it in medical school. Your own physician probably never took a *single course in nutrition*! Even today, nutrition is a required course in only 25 percent of medical schools. It is still an elective in the rest, and that's not enough to really get into the subject or to impress future doctors with its importance. So over the years, the medical establishment has left the matter of diet to health food enthusiasts, many of whom they view as "nuts."

Even doctors who *are* trained to give you nutritional guidance don't provide it nearly often enough because the "system" punishes them for doing so. Insurance companies, for some reason, are more interested in what a doctor *does* than what he or she *says*! Removing a cinder from your eye or lancing a boil, both of which take only a few moments, are generously reimbursed. But you won't even find a place on your insurance claim form to record the *time* spent by your doctor explaining the importance of lifestyle, exercise, weight loss, alcohol and substance abuse, birth control—and nutrition. These are only some of the reasons why you are likely to receive either a vague answer or no answer at all when you ask, "Doctor, what should I eat?"

Most patients don't hound their doctors for nutritional guidance, either. Most of us would just as soon not restrict our diet in any way. It's a relief to leave your doctor's office *without* having been told to forgo a favorite food. Who wouldn't rather take a pill and eat whatever he or she likes than follow *any* diet, whether it's to lose weight or to lower cholesterol? Unfortunately, no such pill exists, and, in any event, in every medicine there's a little poison. And, let's face it. Nutrition can be boring! It conjures up words and phrases like *milligrams, deciliters, percentage of total calories,* as well as charts, exchange tables, food scales—all of which are Greek to most people. Who wants to sit down to dinner with a calculator?

When people can't get simple, direct nutritional information from their doctor, they turn elsewhere. Unfortunately, it's not always to trained dieticians or nutritionists (who tend to turn people off with the mechanics of nutrition), but rather to self-styled "authorities" whose credentials are wanting or nonexistent. Dispensing bad nutritional advice can be as harmful as prescribing the wrong drug, but unlike medication, which cannot be sold until the Food and Drug Administration checks it out for safety and efficacy, food is not regulated.

I am an "establishment" physician, and I use every effective medication at my disposal to treat the sick. That was the subject of my last book, *The Best Treatment*. In this volume, I focus on nutrition—to help you work with your doctor, with a nutritionist if necessary, and maybe even with your grocer, to make sure that what you eat is good for you.

This book spells out specifically what you should and should not eat for more than seventy common disorders in which nutrition can really make a difference. In each one, I have explained the nature of the disease, how it develops, as well as *how* and *why* the food you consume can affect its outcome. (I have also indicated which medications are called for, because combining the right diet and drugs produces the best results.) The diseases and symptoms I have selected are those I have come across most often in my own practice. I have omitted some that are either very uncommon, or in which the role of diet has not been clearly and scientifically established. If your doctor won't go food shopping with you, take this book along instead. It's the next best thing!

I want to be very clear on one point: This book is *not* a substitute for a doctor's care. No book is. Your doctor knows you best, and you should consult him or her about any medical condition—before you put the advice in this or any other health book to work. This is especially important because, as I just mentioned, for many of the conditions I describe here, eating the right foods is most effective when combined with taking the right medications—which only your doctor can prescribe. For every one of my books for the general public, my goal has been to help patients communicate better with their doctors. I hope you'll use this book together to make you healthier and happier.

Ms. Sandra Pressman, a registered dietician with a master's degree in nutrition, is an experienced, practicing dietician with whom I have worked closely for some time. (To find an R.D. near you, contact the American Dietetic Association for a recommendation.) Sandy has verified, amplified, and translated my medical advice into *practical* dietary terms. I hope you find the book useful and enjoyable. The guidelines are no more complicated than selecting "one from column A, two from column B" in your favorite Chinese restaurant. Sandy and I are not ascetics; we love good food and have kept in mind on every single page how much pleasure a great meal can bring. So, good health, hearty appetite, and enjoy.

CONTENTS

Doctor, What Should I Eat?

ACNE

WHEN DOCTORS

AND PATIENTS DISAGREE

I was a pimply teenager. So were most of my friends. The unlucky ones had pimples on their faces; the rest had them mostly on their backs and chests. We called them "zits"; the doctors called it acne. None of us ever went to see a dermatologist because, as far as we were concerned, adolescents were expected to have zits—zits came with the turf and with all the "fun food" we were eating. (This generation calls it "junk food.") Our pimples came and went for no apparent reason and often flared up at the worst times, like just before the junior prom. However, by the time I was in my early twenties, my skin was as clean and pure as the driven snow.

Your genes have a lot to do with whether or not you have acne, but the kind of skin you have and the kind of glands it contains are important too. Still, if both your parents have or had acne, chances are good that you will develop it as well. Acne usually appears at puberty coincident with the normal, expected, and hoped-for increased production in men *and* women of the male hormone testosterone. (Women also produce this male hormone.) Male hormones (androgens) act on several organs in the body in addition to those that come to mind, including the skin. A specific enzyme converts testosterone to a more active form called 5 alpha dihydrotestosterone (DHT). Men and women with acne have as much as thirty times the usual amount of DHT on their skin—and it's the DHT that causes acne. (Males who have been castrated never have acne.)

Tiny glands, most of which are located in the skin of the face, back, and upper chest, produce a waxy material called sebum that is carried to the skin surface via little ducts. DHT alters the cells lining these ducts so that they stick together and interfere with the free flow of sebum out of the gland and onto the skin. The sebum accumulates in the glands, distending or enlarging them to form small lumps called *comedones*. These comedones become infected by the bacteria that normally inhabit the skin. As long as the comedones remain beneath the skin, they are called *whiteheads*; those that make it to the skin surface are *blackheads,* whose dark color is not from dirt, but due to a pigment called melanin (the stuff that makes you tan). All the soap and water in the world will never turn a blackhead into a whitehead.

Most acne is mild, and only one youngster in six or seven ever needs treatment from a doctor. However, sometimes acne can be severe and disfiguring. The eruptions are usually worse in boys because they make ten times as much testosterone as do girls. (Females with acne produce more male hormone than do their girlfriends with clear skins.) The disorder peaks in the late teens and early twenties and usually disappears by age thirty (although I have sometimes seen it persist into the sixties and even seventies). The contraceptive pill improves acne in some women, and aggravates it in others. Pimples tend to flare up with the onset of a woman's monthly period, or during unusual stress. Certain medications can cause the skin to break out—e.g., dilantin (for the treatment of epilepsy), anti-TB drugs, lithium (for manic-depressive disorders), and anabolic steroids (abused by some athletes to build up their muscles).

Acne can be either the inflammatory or the noninflammatory variety. The latter is by far the more common of the two and is also easier to treat. Its hallmarks are whiteheads and blackheads—appearing mostly on the face. In inflammatory acne, they extend deeply into the skin and ultimately end up as infected cysts that may cause pitting and scarring.

Although there is no cure for acne, there are many ways to improve it. The best treatment for you depends on how bad the condition is and how disturbing you find it. Some people tolerate and accept their pimples with greater equanimity than do others. Topical over-the-counter salicylic acid or benzoyl peroxide creams may be all you need. If you do not respond to them, you may be helped by antibiotics (either taken by mouth or applied directly to the skin); Retin-A cream (tretinoin); sanding or other surgical procedures if there are scars or pockmarks on your face; or glycolic acid, currently very popular with some dermatologists. Accutane (isotretoin) taken orally is extremely effective for acne, but it should never be used within three months of a planned pregnancy (about 50 percent of pregnancies in the United States are unplanned) because of the fetal abnormalities it so frequently causes. I never recommend it to my own female patients in whom there is *any* chance that they will become pregnant. The same precautions apply to vitamin A itself.

Does what you eat play any role in the formation of acne pimples and pustules? Doctors used to think so and prescribed an "acne diet" for youngsters with this skin problem. Teenagers were encouraged to eat lots of vegetables, cereals, and fruits and to avoid sweets, fried and fatty foods, nuts, chocolate, cola drinks, and dairy products. But most physicians have abandoned the dietary approach to acne. Still, some of my patients insist that what they eat *does* affect their skin, and that certain foods such as chocolate or other sweets, milk and milk products, cola drinks, fatty foods, nuts, and peanut butter predictably worsen their acne. It's one of those strange phenomena that doctors encounter now and then when a patient will insist that something he or she is doing helps or exacerbates a particular symptom or condition, even though scientists are unable to prove it.

In a recent experiment designed to determine who's right about diet and acne, the kids or the "experts," forty-five youngsters with acne underwent dietary testing for three months. They were divided into three groups: The first ate whatever they wished; the second were given a diet that they believed aggravated their acne; the third group avoided all food to which they had previously skin-tested positive (meaning they were allergic), regardless of its impact on their acne. When the test subjects were reexamined after three months, doctors found *no difference* in the severity of the acne among all three groups. They concluded that there is no reason for anyone to follow an "acne diet." I remember another experiment years ago that I believe was run by the Hershey's chocolate company. Volunteers with acne and those with normal skin consumed a pound of chocolate every day for weeks. The subjects may have gained weight, but the chocolate had no impact whatsoever on their skin.

I'm not sure that these and other experiments tell the whole story because there have been other observations that suggest diet *is* important. For example, young blacks in Africa have much less acne than do African-Americans, with whom they share a similar genetic constitution. Zulus in the Hedra land of South Africa are acne-free until they leave the countryside and move to the city, where they drastically change their eating habits. The most striking observation, however, was made in Canadian Eskimos, in whom acne was rare before World War II. After the war, the children of those families who moved from their igloos to city apartments and altered their dietary habits developed acne. Although stress (which has been shown time and time again to worsen acne) almost certainly played an important role in all these migrations, I believe that dietary changes had something to do with it too. So the position of the medical profession notwithstanding, I continue to recommend to everyone, including acne-plagued teenagers, that they reduce their intake of fat, salt, and sugar and focus on the fruits, vegetables, and fiber prescribed by dermatologists of yesteryear. Over the long term, that kind of diet will reduce their vulnerability to clogged arteries, mutated genes, cancer, diverticulosis, diabetes, dental caries, and all the other modern killer diseases—and may even leave their skin looking better too. If you are convinced that your acne is aggravated by any particular food, you should avoid it by all means. You are a better judge of that than any "expert" or statistician.

ACTINIC KERATOSES

NO FUN IN THE SUN

If you spend a great deal of time in the sun, you may well have some little skin tumors called "actinic keratoses," which manifest themselves in a variety of ways. For example, they may be rough patches more easily felt than seen, or they may appear as pink, flat, or slightly scaly blemishes ranging in size from less than a millimeter to one or two centimeters (two and a half centimeters equals one inch). These are the most common tumors in the body, and unfortunately, anywhere from 1 to 25 percent of them become malignant—sometimes not for ten years or more after their appearance. These keratoses are the most important complication of sun–induced skin damage. How can you prevent them? The obvious answer is to stay out of the sun, use sunblock, or wear a hat, long sleeves, and long pants. In addition, however, if you already have actinic keratoses, or a previous history of skin cancer, you should also follow a low–fat diet. In a recent study, people with actinic keratoses who cut their fat consumption to 20 percent or less of their total daily caloric intake had two-thirds fewer new actinic keratoses!

See "Your Heart" on page 182 and "When You're Overweight" on page 317, for how to best reduce the fat in your diet. When you do, you'll enjoy not only clearer skin, but a healthier heart and a lower risk of many kinds of cancer. It's a change well worth making.

AGING

NO ONE LIVES FOREVER—

BUT IT'S WORTH A TRY

Some five hundred years ago a Spanish sailor-explorer named Juan Ponce de León heard rumors about a land whose springs gushed with rejuvenating tonic waters. He set sail in search of this fountain of youth—and found Florida instead! Although there are some who are convinced that Florida *is* the fountain of youth, people the world over are spending billions of dollars on "life-extending" vitamins, exotic herbs, and a host of other chemicals and foods in the ongoing quest for eternal youthfulness. Multimillion-dollar cosmetics and plastic surgery industries promise and often deliver tighter and trimmer buttocks, firmer breasts, and younger-looking faces. But the real question remains: Can the aging process itself really be slowed?

Do not confuse *life span* with *life expectancy*. The former is the genetic limit of survival. It differs from species to species and has not changed throughout recorded history. For example, rats and your pet gerbil are old at three; your dog at fifteen; houseflies live some thirty days (although I am sure the same one has been dive-bombing me at home for at least twice that long!); horses survive twenty-five years; humans are considered old at eighty. Practically speaking, no person lives beyond 110. *Life expectancy,* on the other hand, is the actual average survival for any given population. Life expectancy has increased thanks to social, economic, and medical advances that have made it possible for more of us to approach our potential life span. Thus, the average woman in America now lives to eighty (men die a little earlier) in contrast to forty-five years in the early part of this century. The downside of all this is that the many who now head into their seventies, eighties, and nineties have become vulnerable to "degenerative" diseases that were rarely a problem when people died younger.

Why are some individuals old at sixty while others gallivant, make love, play tennis, and even run marathons at eighty-plus? Although the main reason is genetics (the stuff you inherited from your parents and their parents before them), a new and growing awareness of the importance of lifestyle and nutrition, as well as a focus on "wellness" and prevention, are contributing to increasing longevity and a better quality of life.

As we get older, many of the cells in our body begin to wear out and the organs of which they are composed don't work as well as they once did. The immune system, which protects us against infection and cancer, becomes less efficient, so that older people are more vulnerable to cancer, pneumonia, and other illnesses. Sex hormones, both male and female, are now produced in smaller quantities; women become menopausal and testosterone levels begin to drop in men; sex is often no longer what it used to be—and who cares anyway; our hair becomes gray, our skin wrinkled, our bones thin, and our muscles skimpy. No one fully understands exactly how or why all of this happens.

The National Institute on Aging has come up with a series of guidelines to help slow down the aging process. Their basic advice is: (1) stop smoking; (2) get regular exercise; (3) have routine "wellness" exams to nip any disease or malfunction in the bud; (4) stay involved with family and friends and don't retire any earlier than necessary; (5) maintain an active social life and an ongoing search for new friends; (6) get lots of sleep, rest, and relaxation; (7) eat and drink in "moderation"; (8) avoid overexposure to sun, heat, and cold; (9) practice good safety habits at home, work, and play (including wearing seat belts in the car); (10) plan for financial security so that you don't have to worry where your next meal is coming from and so that you can afford a vacation when you need or want one; (11) maintain a positive outlook on life; and finally, and perhaps most important, (12) do what makes you happy at work or at play.

We spend our adult lives preoccupied with calories, our cholesterol level, and our weight. But when we enter "old age" (the definition of which is vague and largely one of self-image), some of us feel that maybe we should be less stringent in our dieting. Although many doctors recommend continuing the vigil as far as calcium, cholesterol, and salt are concerned, others are aware that too many senior citizens are undernourished for a variety of reasons—they may not be able to chew well because their teeth are missing, loose, or decayed, or because their dentures don't fit; they may not have the money to buy the right foods; they may be afraid to go shopping because of crime on the streets; many are prone to depression; their appetite may be diminished by some medication they're taking or by an underlying illness. Their zest for food may also be curtailed by a decrease in the acuity of their senses. Smell is affected most, taste to a lesser degree. They appreciate less even the most tempting foods. For all these reasons, as well as the fact that their organs shrink and can no longer replenish themselves, older persons usually lose weight.

So should they eat more, and will doing so retard the aging process in any way? The answers are by no means in, but there is considerable evidence that more is *not* better. Research in laboratory animals has consistently demonstrated that slashing their caloric intake by 40 percent makes them healthier. They have less heart disease, cancer, kidney trouble, and fewer cataracts than do animals maintained on the usual laboratory diet. What's more, these nutritionally "deprived" rodents also live longer. Similar observations have been made in humans. On the island of Okinawa, whose population is genetically Japanese, there are many more centenarians than in Japan itself. Presumably it's because Okinawans consume 30 percent fewer calories than do the Japanese. This theory is now being tested in primates (rhesus and squirrel monkeys) being fed calorie-restricted diets. Preliminary observations suggest that the monkeys receiving fewer calories are healthier than their "normally" fed counterparts. But monkeys are not flies with a thirty-day life span; they live between twenty and forty years. So we are going to have to wait awhile to know for sure whether these dietary restrictions really do prolong life.

Analysis of the effects of these diets in rodents, monkeys, and humans suggests that the biological benefits observed are mostly due to reducing their *total* caloric intake, although protein restriction is favored by some researchers.

It's interesting to speculate how fewer calories might benefit the elderly. An analogy with the automobile comes to mind. Like a car, the human "machine" generates waste from its biological processes, but our exhaust mechanisms are not nearly as efficient as those of our car. (No one I know has two tailpipes.) We are unable to eliminate enough of the toxic by-products of metabolism in the urine, stool, and sweat. These substances, the best known of which are *oxygen-free radicals,* are harmful, but can be reduced by cutting down the amount of "fuel" (food) you consume; the less you eat, the less "exhaust" is generated.

According to a popular theory (but still not a proven fact), these free radicals accelerate the aging process, promote the development of cancer, high blood pressure, and senility, and reduce resistance to disease and infection. Unless quickly neutralized or destroyed, they accumulate to toxic levels. Experimental animals with low levels of oxygen-free radicals live longer, enjoy enhanced resistance, and have fewer cancers. A low-calorie, low-fat diet rich in *natural* antioxidants (vitamin E, beta-carotene, vitamin C, and selenium) may lower the concentration of free radicals. Adding these antioxidants to the diet in supplement form has not, in most cases, been shown to be effective. Indeed, in the largest study to date, supplemental beta-carotene actually increased the incidence of lung cancer by 18 percent among cigarette smokers. By contrast, in another study of nonsmokers, those who had consumed the largest amount of *raw* fruits and vegetables over the years had the lowest incidence of this malignancy. So you should obtain these nutrients in your food, because the foods may contain some other beneficial substances not present in the pill or capsule processed by man.

Some scientists think that as we grow older, we consume not only too many calories, but an excessive amount of *protein* as well. They believe that less protein available for cell biological processes reduces the likelihood that it will cause cell abnormalities. So they advise reducing your *protein* consumption after age fifty, with an RDA for men of 63 grams a day, and 50 grams for women. They also recommend a parallel decrease in *calories* after age fifty and advise that men eat 600 fewer calories every day and women 300 less. According to this theory, then, the ideal diet for older folks is one that generates the fewest harmful free radicals and is lower in calories, high in complex carbohydrates, and low in both fat and protein. In addition, in order to stave off osteoporosis (see page 335), it's very important for post-menopausal women to have at least 1,000 milligrams of calcium a day if they are receiving estrogen-replacement therapy, and 1,500 milligrams if they are not. Men should consume 800 milligrams daily. The table on pages 342–43 lists the calcium content of various foods and how many calories they contain per serving.

If you're following recommendations to reduce your protein intake, your diet must contain all the *essential amino acids*. I have found that many of my patients do not fully understand the difference between essential and nonessential amino acids. The term *nonessential* is not pejorative. All the amino acids, of which there are twenty-two, are important. Here is the difference among them. Amino acids are the smaller, simpler building blocks that make up proteins, and they combine in many different ways in different foods. As a result, the protein in eggs, for example, is not the same as that in wheat or rice. Nine of the amino acids are essential, which means that they cannot be put together by the body from any combination of amino acids, and must come from food. Unless all nine are present in your diet, your body will lack the variety of proteins required to make all your complex hormones, enzymes, and other substances. *Nonessential amino acids* can be synthesized within the body, and are no less important than the *essential* ones. Foods such as milk, eggs, cheese, meat, fish, and fowl in which essential amino acids are plentiful are designated as being of "high biological value," and their proteins of "high quality." Plant foods, cereals, vegetables, and fruits do not contain a significant amount of essential amino acids and are therefore referred to as being of "low biological value" and their proteins of "low quality." That is not to say they are not good for you, but as far as protein balance is concerned, none of them alone fills the need. However, you can combine a variety of nonessential amino acids, as, for example, those present in legumes, with other amino acids in grains or cereals to obtain a complete protein. If you are a strict vegan and concerned that you may not be consuming enough protein, the book *Diet for a Small Planet,* by Frances Moore Lappé (Ballantine Books, 1982), will show you what foods to eat for optimal protein balance.

As in so many other fields of medicine, there is no unanimity of opinion on whether these low-calorie, low-protein diets can slow down the aging process. Dr. Ruben Andrus, the clinical director of the National Institute on Aging, believes, based on *his* interpretation of the data, that we need more, not less, nutrition and that we should *increase* our weight as we get older (he recommends gaining one pound a year after age thirty). According to his reasoning, as we grow older we absorb many nutrients less effectively and our metabolism slows.

Who's right? My own interpretation of the evidence leads me to favor a calorie-restricted, low-fat diet that contains less protein for the *healthy* elderly. Which nutrients to cut back on, and by how much, must be determined on an individual basis, based on your age, height, weight, body frame, and overall health. However, generally speaking, after age fifty, I recommend a protein limit of 60 grams a day for healthy men and 50 grams for healthy women, a reduction of your previous calorie intake by some 25 percent, and fat consumption below 25 percent of total calories. (See the sample menus at the end of this chapter.)

I have serious doubts about the value of most of the various "life-extending" products so slickly promoted. For example, I do not recommend super oxide dismutase (SOD), dehydroandrosterone (DHEA), and megavitamins. However, oil made from *black currant seeds* contains a combination of fatty acids that may strengthen and/or protect the cardiovascular and immune systems. These fatty acids are said to reduce the amount of prostaglandins in the body in much the same way as does aspirin. (Prostaglandins are naturally occurring chemicals that *promote* inflammation and impair the function of the immune system.) The right dosage of this black currant extract is yet to be determined, but when it is, it may confer many of the beneficial effects of aspirin without the latter's complications. (Flaxseed oil, on the other hand, has not been shown to offer the same benefits.)

Zinc (see page 147) has recently come into prominence as a potential booster of the immune system in older persons. Most of the enzymes needed to maintain normal function of the cells of the immune system require zinc. Think of zinc deficiency in any older person who does not have access to an adequate diet (as well as in chronic alcoholics and persons with kidney disease or malabsorption—see pages 18, 277, and 307—and sickle-cell anemia); does not heal normally; has frequent infections; and complains of a loss of taste and smell. The RDA of zinc is 15 milligrams a day, which can easily be obtained by eating a variety of zinc-rich foods such as meat, fish, and poultry, as listed on page 151. I much prefer these natural sources to the supplements. There is also a substance produced by the thymus gland in the neck that is essential for normal immune function. (Do not confuse the thymus with the thyroid gland. You can see and feel the latter, whereas the small thymus is buried more deeply in the same general area.) As we grow older, the supply of this thymus factor drops sharply, and so does the competence of the immune system. But when zinc is added to the diet, the levels of thymus factor increase—and so does our immune "resistance."

What should you be eating after your fiftieth birthday so that one day you'll reach your hundredth (assuming, of course, that you've wisely chosen your ancestors)? Unless you're in perfect health or very much overweight, do not embark on a crash weight-loss program. Reduce your intake of fat to between 20 and 25 percent of your total calories (use no more than 1 tablespoon of olive oil for cooking); limit your consumption of animal protein to 4 ounces of chicken or meat twice a week; have the same portions of fish three other days in the week; drink 1 or 2 cups of skim milk a day (unless you are lactose intolerant); and have at least two vegetarian entrees per week, such as bean soup, whole-grain dishes, or pasta and beans. Also make sure you eat five or more servings of fruit and fresh or steamed vegetables daily. How much bread or other grains you eat will depend on your overall caloric target. Women who adhere to this diet may not satisfy their calcium requirements, and so should be sure to take 1,000 milligrams worth of calcium in supplement form.

Below are two sample menus that incorporate these guidelines: a 1,500-calorie menu for older women and an 1,800-calorie menu for older men. I consider such menus optimal for older people in terms of their fat, fiber, and protein composition.

SAMPLE MENU FOR OLDER WOMEN
(ABOUT 1,500 CALORIES)

	PORTION	CALORIES
Breakfast		
All-Bran cereal (Kellogg's)	⅓ cup	70
Skim milk	1 cup	86
Banana, sliced	1 medium	105
Coffee or tea	8 ounces	5
Sugar	1 teaspoon	16
Lunch		
Nonfat plain yogurt	1 cup	110
Fruit cup:		
cantaloupe, cubed	⅓ medium	60
strawberries, sliced	1¼ cups	60
Bibb lettuce	4 leaves	4
Fat-free salad dressing	2 tablespoons	20
Jelly sandwich:		
whole-wheat bread	2 slices	160
jelly	1 tablespoon	48
Sparkling water	8 ounces	0
Snack		
Popcorn, air-popped	3 cups	75
Caffeine-free diet cola	12 ounces	0
Dinner		
Grilled swordfish with herbs	4 ounces	176
Olive oil for fish	1 tablespoon	125
Succotash:		
corn kernels and lima beans	½ cup each	128
Steamed broccoli and cauliflower	1 cup	37
Salad greens	2 cups	14
Olive oil for dressing	1 tablespoon	125
Vinegar for dressing	2 tablespoons	4
Lemon juice for dressing	2 tablespoons	0
Fresh peach	1 medium	60
Herb tea	8 ounces	0
Sorbet	½ cup	124

SAMPLE MENU FOR OLDER MEN
(ABOUT 1,800 CALORIES)

	PORTION	CALORIES
Breakfast		
Branflakes (Kellogg's)	¾ cup	90
Skim milk	1 cup	86
Raisins for cereal	2 tablespoons	60
Cantaloupe	⅓ medium	60
Coffee or tea	1 cup	5
Sugar	1 teaspoon	16
Lunch		
Tuna salad sandwich:		
tuna packed in water	2 ounces	70
reduced-calorie mayonnaise	1 tablespoon	50
diced celery and onion	2 tablespoons	7
whole wheat bread	2 slices	160
Salad:		
romaine lettuce	½ cup	4
tomato	½ small	14
olive oil	1 tablespoon	125
vinegar	2 tablespoons	4
lemon juice	2 tablespoons	0
Fresh peach	1	60
Caffeine-free diet cola	12 ounces	0
Snack		
Nonfat sugar-free yogurt (Dannon Lite)	8 ounces	100
Fresh blueberries	¾ cup	60
Dinner		
Grilled chicken breast, skinless	4 ounces	222
Potato baked with skin	1 large	220
Steamed broccoli	½ cup	22
Steamed carrots	½ cup	35
Salad greens	2 cups	14
Olive oil for dressing	1 tablespoon	125
Vinegar for dressing	2 tablespoons	4
Lemon juice for dressing	2 tablespoons	0
Herb tea	8 ounces	0
Sugar for tea	1 teaspoon	16

SAMPLE MENU FOR OLDER MEN *(Continued)*

	PORTION	CALORIES
Dinner *(cont.)*		
Fat-free, cholesterol-free frozen dessert	4 ounces	100
Fresh grapefruit	½ medium	60
Snack		
Popcorn, air-popped	3 cups	75

ALCOHOL

PLEASURE, POISON,

AND EMPTY CALORIES

The terms *alcoholic* and *drinking problem* conjure up different images. *Alcoholic* is likely to bring to mind a derelict on skid row whose habit has destroyed his or her personal life. Someone with a "drinking problem" is more commonly viewed as a source of social embarrassment. But however you define it, alcohol in excess is a threat to everyone, and not always recognized as such. The CAGE test below can help identify a drinking problem by means of four simple questions:

1. Have you ever felt the need to *C*ut down the quantity of your drinking?
2. Do you get *A*ngry when someone tells you that you drink too much?
3. Do you feel *G*uilty after drinking?
4. Do you need an *E*ye-opener to get you started in the morning?

One "yes" answer is borderline; two or more indicate a problem with alcohol. To confirm it, answer the MAST (Michigan Alcoholism Screening Test) questionnaire developed by Drs. Pokorny and Kaplan. Answer the ten questions, then total the points:

1. Do you feel you are a normal drinker?   Y (0) N (2)
2. Do friends or relatives think you are a normal drinker?
Y (0) N (2)
3. Have you ever attended a meeting of AA?   Y (5) N (0)
4. Have you ever lost friends or girlfriends/boyfriends because of drinking?   Y (2) N (0)
5. Have you ever gotten into trouble at work because of drinking?
Y (2) N (0)
6. Have you ever neglected your obligations, your family, or your work for two or more days in a row because you were drinking?
Y (2) N (0)
7. Have you ever had delirium tremens or severe shaking, heard voices, or seen things that weren't there after heavy drinking?
Y (2) N (0)
8. Have you ever gone to anyone for help about your drinking?
Y (5) N (0)
9. Have you ever been in a hospital because of drinking?
Y (5) N (0)
10. Have you ever been arrested for drunk driving or driving after drinking?   Y (2) N (0)

A score of 6 or more will identify 95 percent of problem drinkers.

The tolls of excess alcohol consumption are well known. Alcohol is a major cause of automobile fatalities; it can produce abnormalities in the fetuses of mothers who drink even small amounts; it leads to cirrhosis, a potentially fatal liver disorder; it contributes to cancer and stomach problems; it is bad for diabetics and for those with high blood pressure. And these are just the tip of the iceberg! You're lucky if you can handle the alcohol you drink; many people can't. Medical texts vary in their recommendations as to how much alcohol is "permissible." Most advise not exceeding two drinks a day. The truth is that how you react will depend on your age, sex, nutritional state, whether or not you have any underlying disease (such as ulcers or liver trouble), and your genetic makeup (some people can't take even a sip without becoming dependent on the booze). The type of alcohol you drink is also important. Some individuals can tolerate wine or beer, and not, for example, vodka. In my own experience, anyone who takes more than three or four drinks a day is likely to run into the kind of trouble described below (if you're older than seventy, make that one or two), and it goes without saying that no one should drive or operate any machinery after drinking.

You should be aware of the direct effects—bad and good—of alcohol on your physical and mental health, regardless of how well (or poorly) you think you're tolerating it. Alcohol irritates the lining of the stomach, especially when it's empty, but its greatest damage is to the liver. Among the myriad functions of this organ, one of the most important is its storage of sugar in the form of glycogen. When extra energy is needed, glycogen is converted back to sugar and released into the bloodstream. Alcoholics who eat poorly do not have that sugar reserve, and even if they do, their damaged liver may not be able to handle it. Because they do not have this energy backup, their blood sugar often falls too low. During these attacks of hypoglycemia, they feel weak and dizzy and have cold sweats and heart palpitations.

Although alcohol is calorie dense and satisfies the definition of a "nutrient," it is not a good food. An ounce and a half of 86-proof whiskey contains 105 "empty" calories, that is, they are without any protein, vitamins, and minerals whatsoever. These empty calories add extra pounds, so if you're having trouble losing weight, cut back on the booze.

Chronic alcoholics are often thin and wasted because of poor nutrition, which leaves them lacking in essential minerals such as zinc, calcium, magnesium, selenium, and potassium, as well as vitamin deficiency. This deprivation also aggravates any coexisting health disorders.

Whenever I suspect that someone drinks too much (patients do not always admit it to their doctors), I make sure he or she gets extra B-complex, vitamin C, vitamin E, calcium, zinc, and iron—in amounts greater than five to ten times their RDAs, depending on the state of their nutrition. If there is not yet any evidence of chronic liver disease, I also prescribe at least 75 grams of protein a day (some doctors recommend even more), with the remaining calories provided by fresh fruit, vegetables, complex carbohydrates, and fat. "Serious" drinkers need extra protein because their malnutrition deprives vital organs of the building blocks necessary for their growth and function. To get enough protein without adding too much fat, I advise two or three servings of skim milk and a maximum of 10 ounces of animal protein from such relatively low-fat sources as skinless chicken and turkey and/or fish daily. The sample menu at the end of this chapter provides about 75 grams of protein and 2,000 calories.

After one or more bouts of sustained heavy drinking, your liver may become inflamed. This condition, called acute alcoholic hepatitis, occurs in 10 to 35 percent of heavy drinkers and causes pain, swelling, and tenderness in the upper-right-hand side of the abdomen. These attacks can often be reversed by total abstinence from alcohol and a diet containing no less than 3,000 to 3,500 calories per day. Doctors no longer restrict protein intake in such people because we now realize that most of them have protein malnutrition. If you develop acute alcoholic hepatitis, you should eat about a half gram of protein per pound of body weight every day. You are apt to tolerate vegetable- and milk-based proteins better than those present in meat. The onset of "encephalopathy"—tremor, confusion, and drowsiness—indicates that your liver isn't able to process the protein you're eating. At this point, your doctor will recommend reducing your protein by about half (to a quarter gram per pound of body weight). This protein allotment should come from equal measures of high-quality animal protein, nonfat dairy products, and vegetables. You could, for example, have a 3-ounce serving of meat or fish, 1 or 2 cups of skim milk or nonfat milk, and two or three servings of vegetables per day. To compensate for this decrease in your dietary protein, your physician will decide whether you need a daily supplement of 15 to 30 milligrams of a special protein in the form of branched-chain amino acids, commercially available as Travasorb Hepatic and Hepatic-Aid. Since your appetite is not likely to be ravenous when you have alcoholic hepatitis, you'll probably tolerate four or five smaller feedings a day and a snack about two hours before you go to bed better than you would three evenly spaced meals.

Chronic heavy drinking almost always causes fat to be deposited in the liver, and raises the level of a fat called triglyceride in the blood. Elevated triglycerides are an independent risk factor for arteriosclerosis—another good reason to stop drinking. If you have high triglycerides, eliminate fruit juices and concentrated sweets from your diet and eat no more than two servings a day of fresh fruit because the sugar they contain raises the triglyceride level even further.

One of the major objectives (and difficulties) in treating someone with an alcohol problem is controlling his or her craving for booze. No one understands why alcoholics have such an intense need to drink, but it may be nature's way of correcting a low blood sugar. Alcoholics with impaired liver function are prone to attacks of low blood sugar because their bodies cannot store enough glycogen in that organ for conversion to sugar when needed. Laboratory animals respond to an artificially induced low blood sugar by increasing their alcohol intake. When fed a diet that maintains normal sugar levels, their craving for booze is diminished. So if you are trying to get on the wagon, do not fast for long periods of time, and eat frequent small meals rich in protein and complex carbohydrates to keep your blood sugar normal. Since hypoglycemia is associated with low serotonin levels in the brain, which may cause depression (see page 396), that's yet another reason to observe such a diet. You are also better off limiting your coffee intake to two cups a day, for two reasons: Caffeine is a gastric irritant and alcohol has already probably wreaked havoc with your stomach lining, and coffee also stimulates the desire for alcohol.

Repeated bingeing and recurrent episodes of acute alcoholic hepatitis over the years lead to permanent liver damage and *cirrhosis* in 8 to 20 percent of cases. When this occurs, liver cells are replaced by tough scar tissue that interferes with the return of blood from the lower body through that organ en route to the lungs and heart. Blood then backs up into the legs and abdomen, which become swollen. At this late stage of liver disease, treatment is aimed at making the individual more comfortable. The accumulated fluid is removed by diuretics and a very-low-salt diet, containing no more than a gram of sodium per day. This severe restriction is neither easy nor fun to follow. To adhere to it you will obviously need to shun all frankly salty foods such as pickles, bacon, cold cuts, frankfurters, soy sauces, sauerkraut, tomato and V8 juices, and bouillon. The table on page 248 lists some high-sodium foods you *must* avoid. What you *drink* may also contain sodium. The table on page 247 identifies several such beverages and their salt content. How much sodium a given food has may depend on the manner in which it has been prepared—something you should be very careful about. For example, a cup of fresh corn has only traces of salt, but once it's canned, it contains 496 milligrams of sodium; a cup of raw cabbage has only 14 milligrams of sodium, but after it's been made into sauerkraut, that same cup contains almost 1,600 milligrams, very much more than your entire daily allowance! On such a very-low-salt diet, you will have to depend largely on fruits and vegetables (except for celery), most of which have only negligible amounts of salt.

Cirrhosis also causes the veins in the gullet to become engorged, very much like varicose veins in the legs. When these rupture, as they sometimes do, the individual may hemorrhage to death. Persons with these "esophageal varices" should therefore be restricted to a soft diet—custards, purées, and liquids—and avoid hard, crusty foods that can tear open the distended veins. (To avoid bacterial contamination, do not keep puréed food in the refrigerator for more than twenty-four hours.) Some doctors doubt that altering the texture of the diet makes any difference in such cases, but I would rather be safe than sorry and I continue to recommend it. I also have these patients avoid irritating acidic liquids such as citrus and tomato juice and caffeine-containing beverages, and I encourage them to drink preformulated supplements such as Ensure or Sustacal between meals. (Incidentally, since *estrogen* is detoxified by the normal liver, it too accumulates as liver function becomes more deranged by alcohol. That's why men with cirrhosis have large breasts and small testicles, lose their sex drive, and need to shave only once daily or every second day. So much for the macho image of the "guy who can hold his liquor"!)

Alcohol also inflames the pancreas, a condition called acute alcoholic pancreatitis. Attacks are accompanied by fever and very severe pain in the mid-upper part of the abdomen. If you continue to drink despite these recurring episodes, they will permanently damage your pancreas (chronic pancreatitis) so that many of its functions are impaired. When your pancreas can no longer make enough of the enzymes needed to digest the fat you eat, "malabsorption" results. This means that your food cannot be digested because the enzymes required to break it down into constituents that can penetrate the intestinal lining are missing.

There are many causes of intestinal malabsorption (see page 307), in which the bowel does not assimilate or absorb dietary nutrients. Almost 10 percent of all such cases are due to alcohol—either as a result of its direct toxic action on the gut or, more commonly, after it has damaged the pancreas or liver. If you have malabsorption from alcohol excess, there are three steps you must take: (1) get on the wagon *now*; (2) replace the missing pancreatic enzymes available by prescription from your doctor, who should be monitoring their effectiveness. The dosage range is usually at least three capsules with each meal and often more, depending on how badly the pancreas has been damaged; (3) take daily vitamin supplements, especially A (1,000 RE), D (400 IU), and E (400 IU), the fat-soluble ones that are lost in the diarrhea. I also recommend 1,000 micrograms of vitamin B_{12} for good measure.

Heavy drinking over the long term also seriously hurts the brain. We used to think that the personality changes and memory loss in some alcoholics were due to damage or destruction of brain cells. That's apparently not the case. It's the pathways *connecting* the cells that are primarily affected, and not the cells themselves. When that happens, signals or messages to and from different parts of the brain never get transmitted, and that's what accounts for the neurological symptoms of alcoholism. The good news is that while brain cells once destroyed cannot be restored, damage to the connecting pathways is, to some extent, reversible—if you stop drinking. So, as with tobacco, it's never too late to quit.

There are signs at most bars and restaurants warning pregnant women not to drink. That's because alcohol crosses the placenta and enters the fetal circulation. As little as 1 ounce a day can result in an infant of low birthweight. Larger amounts of alcohol, and there are no precise figures because the response varies from woman to woman, may cause a miscarriage. Almost every doctor advises *total* abstinence during pregnancy because no one knows what amount of alcohol will not cause birth defects. We do know that a woman who drinks 5 ounces a day while pregnant has a one-in-three chance of giving birth to an infant with fetal alcohol syndrome (FAS)—deformities of the face and head, poor growth, severe mental retardation, abnormalities of the nervous system, and congenital deformities in the heart. If you are planning a family and suspect that you may have an alcohol problem, take the CAGE and MAST tests described above. If they are positive, get help with your drinking *before* you conceive.

Can anything you eat or drink "cure" a drinking problem? So far there's no such miracle nutrient, but there is a plant extract now being studied at Harvard Medical School and elsewhere. For centuries, the Chinese and Japanese have been treating alcoholism with an extract from the kudzu weed. (Kudzu, a "nuisance weed" that often chokes trees, was imported into the United States in the early 1900s as a possible source of animal fodder. It did not turn out to be suitable for that purpose, but once here, it spread very quickly, and is now an agricultural pest.) When the active ingredient in kudzu, called daidzin, is injected into booze-loving Syrian golden hamsters, they drastically curtail their drinking, but continue to have a normal appetite. In Asia, kudzu extract can be bought either as a tablet or as a tea.

This chapter would not be complete if I failed to tell you about the *protective* effects of wine. Taken in moderation, meaning a limit of two drinks a day (no more than 2 ounces in each), or a couple of glasses of wine (red *or* white), alcohol appears to reduce the risk of a heart attack by as much as 50 percent! There are several theories as to why this is so. According to one, red wine sipped slowly with food "thins" the blood just enough to prevent clotting; another suggests that it raises the level of HDL by 15 percent (that's the "good" cholesterol that prevents the buildup of plaques in the coronary arteries of the heart).

Alcohol can provide pleasure and relaxation. Everyone has his or her own biological tolerance level and limit. It is extremely important to find yours, and not to exceed it—for all the reasons mentioned above.

SAMPLE MEAL PLAN FOR HEAVY DRINKERS
(75 GRAMS PROTEIN, 2,000 CALORIES)

	PORTION	PROTEIN (gm)	CALORIES
Breakfast			
Poached egg	1	6.3	77
Whole wheat toast	2 slices	4.8	160
Tub margarine	2 teaspoons	0	90
Fresh grapefruit	½ medium	0	60
Coffee or tea	1 cup	0	5
Sugar	1 teaspoon	0	16

SAMPLE MEAL PLAN FOR HEAVY DRINKERS *(Continued)*

	PORTION	PROTEIN (gm)	CALORIES
Lunch			
Turkey sandwich:			
white meat turkey	2 ounces	14	100
rye bread	2 slices	4.2	160
lettuce	2 leaves	0	3
tomato, sliced	½ small	0	14
mayonnaise	1 tablespoon	0	100
Apple juice	8 ounces	0	116
Fruit cocktail, packed in water	½ cup	0	40
Snack			
Nonfat sugar-free flavored yogurt	1 cup	8	100
Dinner			
Grilled flounder with lemon and herbs	6 ounces	32	156
Baked potato with skin	1 large	4.7	220
Tub margarine	2 teaspoons	0	90
Salad:			
romaine lettuce	1 cup	0	8
sliced cucumber	½ cup	0	7
olive oil and vinegar	1 tablespoon each	0	127
Steamed broccoli	½ cup	2.3	22
Regular ginger ale	12 ounces	0	124
Rum	1 ounce	0	36
Snack			
Fruit ice	8 ounces	0	168
		76.3	1,999

ALZHEIMER'S
DISEASE
WHAT'S COOKING WHERE

Alzheimer's disease is the greatest health concern among my patients pushing sixty (and sometimes even younger than that)—and for good reason. This is not one of those rare conditions you hear about but never actually come across. It is the most common form of dementia and affects 5 percent of people over sixty-five. That means there are at least four million Americans with Alzheimer's, and their number is increasing as the population ages. What agony it is to witness the gradual intellectual and physical deterioration of a loved one whose life is destined to end in a state of vegetation. If your parents or one of your siblings has Alzheimer's, there is at least one chance in five that you will too. (Should you live to be ninety, that probability jumps to 50 percent.)

In my other books, I have emphasized several critical caveats about Alzheimer's that bear repeating here. It is *not* part of the natural aging process; it is a *disease*. It is *not* due to hardening of the arteries in the brain; most people with vascular disease who have suffered a stroke, even a serious one, remain mentally alert. *Never* assume that an older person has Alzheimer's just because he or she has developed personality changes—withdrawal, depression, inattention, inappropriate behavior, or a failing memory. These symptoms may be due to loneliness or boredom; malnutrition; taking the wrong medicine or the right one in the wrong dosage; or having a bad reaction to a sleeping pill, sedative, or tranquilizer. An older person may "act funny" because of some underlying condition that has gone undiagnosed and un-treated—anemia, a malfunctioning thyroid, kidney trouble, liver problems, a hidden malignancy, a stroke, even a brain tumor. Older individuals who have sustained a minor blow to the head to which they paid no attention at the time may later develop a clot under the skull that presses on the brain (subdural hematoma) and causes a variety of behavioral changes. So before you decide that anyone, including yourself, has Alzheimer's, first make sure that a competent internist and/or neurologist has excluded all these other conditions, most of which are either curable or at least treatable. There's no longer any excuse for a wrong or missed diagnosis, given today's sophisticated neurological tests, such as the CT scan, PET scan, and MRI.

Unfortunately, there is as yet no proven prevention, treatment, or cure for Alzheimer's disease, although there are several interesting and promising approaches now being investigated. For example, it appears that postmenopausal women taking estrogen replacement therapy (ERT) may reduce their risk of Alzheimer's by as much as 40 percent, and if they do get it, the condition is apt to be milder and progress more slowly. (Similar studies have not been done in males, who, as a rule, do not take estrogen supplements!) The potential benefit of this hormone appears to be dose related—the more you take and the longer you do so, the greater the protection. It has also been suggested that the NSAIDs (nonsteroidal anti-inflammatory drugs, such as ibu-profen) may also protect women against the ravages of Alzheimer's.

Until these and other theories are confirmed, is there anything you can do for someone with Alzheimer's, in addition to providing lots of support, care, and love? Is there some nutritional approach that will prevent, delay, or modify the course of this disorder? To answer these questions, you need to know something about Alzheimer's.

In Alzheimer's disease there is a gradual shrinking of the outer layer of the brain and a deficiency of *acetylcholine,* a substance whose func-tion is to speed the transmission of nerve impulses. No one knows why acetylcholine is lacking, but there is no way to replace it in the brain. Pay no attention to advertisements for special diets and food supplements (lecithin and choline are the most popular) purporting to provide you with the missing acetylcholine. Virtually all of them are, in my experience, ineffective. The one possible exception is a tea brewed with a type of club moss *(Huperzia serrata)*, which over the centuries has been used by Chinese folk doctors to improve memory. American scientists, who traditionally do not take most herbal claims seriously, are now looking into this substance, and their *initial* observations suggest that it does raise the acetylcholine level in the brain. There is a naturally occurring enzyme in the brain that breaks down acetylcholine, something we do not want to happen in anyone with Alzheimer's. This herbal tea apparently neutralizes that enzyme, perhaps even more effectively than does tacrine (THA), which is currently being used in the management of Alzheimer's. The active ingredient in club moss is now being tested humans, but I would not rush out to buy this tea until its evaluation has been completed. You are better off, in my opinion, with tacrine whose potential benefits, limitations, and side effects are known.

There is a theory about aluminum that has been around for some thirty years that is worth bearing in mind. When we look under the microscope at brain tissue from someone who has died with Alzheimer's, we see areas in which the nerve fibers are all tangled up. When stained with special dyes, these tangles are seen to contain abnormal amounts of *aluminum*. There are doctors who believe that this aluminum has something to do with the development of the disease, although precisely how remains a mystery. Other neurologists disagree, and are of the opinion that the aluminum is simply a contaminant, or that it's sucked in by tissue that was previously damaged by another disease process and is not, in fact, a cause of Alzheimer's.

The credibility of this "aluminum hypothesis" was enhanced by the findings of Dr. Donald McLachlan, a neurologist at the University of Toronto. He has been giving his Alzheimer's patients a chelating agent called desferrioxamine, which binds to aluminum and then eliminates it from the body. He claims that it has measurably slowed down the progress of the disease in these individuals. A chelating agent or *chelate,* derived from the Greek word for claw, attaches itself to certain metals and holds on to them until they are excreted together from the body. Chelates are widely and successfully used to treat poisoning by such heavy metals as mercury and copper. (Whether or not they also improve arteriosclerosis, as claimed by some, remains in dispute.)

I think Dr. McLachlan's theory and observations to date warrant your avoiding aluminum wherever possible. Even if they don't turn out to be valid, what will you have lost?

So the aluminum theory has been neither proved nor disproved, but according to the director of the office of Alzheimer's research at the National Institute on Aging in Bethesda, it's still an open question. The chief of neuropathology at Mount Sinai School of Medicine in New York feels even more strongly. According to him, aluminum plays a pivotal role in causing Alzheimer's. A recent report in the British medical literature also implicates aluminum. Patients receiving kidney dialysis who were given compounds rich in aluminum to control high phosphate levels in their blood were found to have increased amounts of an abnormal protein found in the brains of Alzheimer's patients—additional circumstantial evidence.

Several doctors I know are decreasing their own exposure to aluminum—just in case. The reaction of many physicians to this theory is very much like what it is to multivitamins. Ask most M.D.s *in their professional capacity* whether such supplements have been proven to be effective, and you'll get either an "I'm not sure" or a frank "no" for an answer. But if you were a fly on your doctor's bathroom wall, you might very well see him or her taking a multivitamin every morning. Here is one doctor's reaction to the aluminum theory. Recently I was in a stuffy and overheated conference room sitting next to a physician who was a perfect stranger. We were listening to a discussion of laser therapy for clogged coronary arteries—which has nothing whatsoever to do with Alzheimer's. I turned to him and said, "You believe that aluminum causes Alzheimer's, don't you?" He was stunned. "How on earth did you know—and what made you ask now?" What made me ask was his body odor! He was obviously *not* using an underarm deodorant, most of which contain aluminum!

Aluminum confers no health benefits, so why not consume as little as possible? That's easier said than done because there's so much of it around. Aluminum is everywhere—in our food, in the soil, and in the air we breathe. And it is a substance that is stored in the body, not excreted. Several studies have even correlated the incidence of Alzheimer's disease with the aluminum level in the drinking water, especially when that water is acidic. You are exposed to aluminum when you drink regular, nonherbal tea, swallow an antacid for your ulcer, take a buffered aspirin for your headache, use a nondairy creamer, eat pickles or processed cheeses, or bake your cakes and cookies with baking powder to make them rise. Whenever you coat your underarm with a roll-on, cream, or spray deodorant, some aluminum enters your body. (If that worries you and you can't decide which is worse, Alzheimer's or offensive body odors, you can buy aluminum-free deodorants at the herbal counters in most cosmetic departments or at health food stores.) Natural aluminum cookware is yet another source of aluminum, since it is shed easily when you prepare or store acidic or salty foods in it, including tomatoes, oil, beans, flour, and grains.

Almost all the sources I have listed above really expose you to trivial amounts of aluminum. Frankly, I find it impractical to worry about the aluminum content of every food or liquid I consume, or to avoid soft drink cans and aluminum foil. Moreover, I think the concern about aluminum cookware is exaggerated. The most you can absorb from these pots and pans, even if you cook three meals a day in them, is less than 4 milligrams a day. Compare that to the 10 to 20 milligrams in just one buffered aspirin, or the 50 milligrams in the usual antacid you chew to relieve the burning in your stomach. If you have ulcers or gastritis and pop antacid pills all day, you might ingest as much as 1,000 milligrams a day—or more. Still, because it's so easy to do, I have neurotically replaced all our natural aluminum cookware at home with the anodized variety, which has a hard coating to prevent any aluminum from getting into the food. You can prepare anything in these pots and pans, acidic or salty, without worrying about aluminum contamination. But I doubt that any harm will befall you if you stay with your present cookware!

I do, however, avoid antacids when possible and I take enteric-coated, not buffered, aspirin because I think it's easier on the gut. My wife insists, however, that I continue to use aluminum-containing roll-on deodorants because she doesn't think the aluminum-free herbal products are as effective—at least not for me!

The evidence implicating aluminum in Alzheimer's disease is not overwhelming, but neither is the possibility far-fetched. Although I am much more excited by the promise of some of the new drugs now being developed to prevent or reverse this disease, until these are available, avoiding large amounts of aluminum, where practical, certainly can't hurt.

One final thought on how to help a loved one with Alzheimer's. There is no question in my mind that nutrition makes a difference in the rate of progression of their disease. Because of its very nature, those who suffer from Alzheimer's are not always aware whether they have eaten, when they did so, and what their meals consisted of. So if such an individual is living at home, you must monitor his or her daily food intake. Serve meals on a regular schedule, and try to slip in some extra snacks just in case he or she forgets to eat! It is also not unusual for someone with Alzheimer's to favor one food to the exclusion of most others, which can cause nutritional imbalances. Many people with Alzheimer's tend to pace. In so doing, they may expend 1,000 to 1,500 extra calories a day—energy that must be replaced. If there is any question about the adequacy of your loved one's diet, feed him or her nutritional supplements such as Ensure or Sustacal, which provide balanced, concentrated energy sources in small (8-ounce) servings.

The manner in which their meals are served and prepared is also important to many people with Alzheimer's who may be unable to sit at the table, or cut or chew their food. Finger foods such as small sandwiches cut into quarters can make things much easier for everybody. Beverages should be served in containers with a tight lid and hole for a straw to prevent spilling. Common sense dictates that you should offer these individuals foods that are easy to eat, such as cottage cheese, sliced fruit, mashed potatoes, and puréed vegetables—always supplemented with a liquid daily multivitamin. And no matter how you prepare any dish for someone with Alzheimer's, if you know what his or her favorite foods are, try to provide them whenever possible.

WHEN YOU'RE ANEMIC

IS YOUR BLOOD REALLY "TIRED"?

Some TV announcers must either be medical students or moonlighting doctors. Otherwise, why would they so often ask us if we lack energy, ambition, and pizzazz, or suggest that we might feel cold, listless, moody, and that we look pale? And how can they so confidently attribute it all to "tired blood" or iron-deficiency anemia (without even a doctor's exam or a blood test)? To top it off, they even have a cure for it, and it's the same one for everybody—iron. Just take this brand or that for whatever ails you and, in no time at all, you'll have pep to spare! Don't you believe it! Before rushing off to buy that miracle tonic, check with your doctor. The TV announcer may well be wrong, and as you will read below, extra iron that you don't need can hurt you.

Anemia is not a disease, it's a laboratory finding. When you're anemic, your blood does not contain enough oxygen to supply all the tissues and organs in your body. There are many different kinds of anemia, of which iron-deficiency is only one (albeit the most common). Being told you are "anemic" is akin to saying that you have pain. You should know what kind you have and *why* you have it.

Oxygen is transported throughout the body by the red blood cells, which contain a molecule called *hemoglobin*. Hemoglobin consists of two parts: heme (iron) and globin, a protein. You may be anemic with a low hemoglobin level because you're lacking in heme or iron. But then again, you may have plenty of iron, and still be anemic because you're making too few red blood cells to transport it. Other conditions that can cause anemia despite *normal* amounts of iron include folic acid deficiency, a lack of vitamin B_{12} (which may be due to a disorder called "pernicious anemia," or in some Vegans because of their diet) or copper deficiency if you have a malabsorption disorder (see page 307). The anemia that occurs when red blood cells are destroyed by an autoimmune reaction, by certain medications, and even by foods (e.g., fava beans) does not leave you iron deficient, because when the red blood cells disintegrate, the iron they contain remains in the blood and is recirculated. Several diseases and chemical agents can hurt the *bone marrow* so that it is unable to make red blood cells, even though there is plenty of iron around.

So if you are found to be anemic, do not rush to take iron before your doctor determines that you need it. In any of the above circumstances, iron supplements are not only unnecessary, but potentially harmful. Too much iron can settle in your liver, heart, and other organs and interfere with their normal function. There is also a suspicion that excessive iron may contribute to heart attacks and even cancer. A current theory holds that the anemia so often present in infections is a defensive, adaptive reaction by the body and should not be corrected. According to the proponents of this theory, harmful bacteria must have enough iron in order to multiply and do their dirty work. The body responds by rendering you anemic and depriving them of that iron. You can apparently withstand the impact of the anemia better than the nasty little bugs can. It's very much like fever, which we used to rush to reduce until we realized that the increased body temperature kills many invading organisms, and that unless the temperature is so high it's making you sick, you should leave it alone.

Anemia due to almost any cause triggers a series of complicated signals and responses in the body. The first organ to react is the kidney. It produces a hormone called erythropoietin that stimulates the bone marrow to make more red blood cells. But the marrow can respond only if it has all the ingredients, including iron, necessary to make the red cells.

It's ironic (no pun intended) that iron deficiency is so common, given that iron is one of the most abundant metals on earth. Twenty-five percent of American infants, 30 percent of pregnant women, 15 percent of menstruating females, and 6 percent of growing children do not have enough of it. (Anemia in men and postmenopausal women is not usually due to a relative deficiency of iron in the diet, but more commonly to subtle, ongoing blood loss from the intestinal tract.)

There are several different ways you can become iron deficient. You may not be consuming enough, as can happen if you're on a fad diet, are a strict vegan, have an intestinal problem that interferes with the absorption of iron, or take large amounts of antacids which also prevent its getting through the intestinal lining. Red meat is the richest dietary source of iron, but because we worry so much (and with good reason) about all the fat and cholesterol it contains, we are eating less of it than ever before. The increased refining and processing of food have also resulted in the decreased availability of dietary iron.

You can also develop iron-deficiency anemia because of blood loss, suddenly and in large amounts due to a hemorrhage, or gradually over time—from heavy menstrual flow, repeated nosebleeds, chronic oozing from hemorrhoids, bleeding ulcers, or continuing blood loss from the intestinal tract irritated by long-term aspirin or NSAID (nonsteroidal anti-inflammatory drugs, such as ibuprofen) therapy. You may also become anemic if you require more iron than you're getting in your diet, as, occurs for example, in pregnant women and growing children.

At what point should you take extra iron? Below what number are you truly anemic? You should suspect iron-deficiency anemia if you tire more easily than usual, look pale, or feel cold, or your heart seems to beat faster, perhaps even to pound, while you're resting or when you exert yourself only slightly. Frankly, I believe doctors are much too liberal in diagnosing anemia, and as in the case of height-weight tables, we need to reconsider the criteria we use. It makes no sense to use the same values for an adult male or postmenopausal female, neither of whom normally loses any blood and has no increased iron needs, as we do for a growing child or a menstruating woman. In our zeal to "cure" iron-deficiency anemia when it doesn't really exist, we may be doing more harm than good. Researchers have suspected for some time that excessive body iron may trigger the formation of free radicals, the end-products of normal energy processes that can cause all sorts of bad things—from cancer to premature aging. Free radicals also convert the "bad" cholesterol (LDL) circulating in the blood-stream into plaques on the arterial walls that obstruct blood flow. Women are apparently protected before menopause by monthly loss of iron with their periods. In yet another recent study it was reported that men with 10 percent or higher iron content in their bodies are at greater risk of having cancer, particularly of the colon and liver. You're better off donating blood if you are too iron rich than to continue consuming iron supplements or eating iron-fortified foods! While these hypotheses are being further evaluated, it seems prudent to avoid iron supplements if you don't need them. You should, however, continue to eat a diet adequate in iron to prevent a real anemia.

If your body iron level does need to be replenished, there are several ways to do it. If you're "bled out" from an injury and it's an emergency, you will need a blood transfusion. The risk of AIDS, hepatitis, and other complications from such transfusions, though real, is low. If there is a "hurry," but not an emergency, you can be given iron by injection, either into a vein or a muscle. That will correct the anemia in a matter of days. If the deficiency needs to be corrected but there is no real rush, then 50 to 60 milligrams a day of iron supplements taken orally will restore normal levels within two weeks and replenish your depleted body stores of iron in three months. (Don't panic when your stool turns as black as shoe polish. It's the iron—not blood!) For most persons, however, the key to getting enough iron is eating the right diet, not taking supplements.

The body needs about 1 milligram of iron a day, but you have to get ten times that amount in your food because an average of only 10 percent of the iron in a mixed diet is actually absorbed. That's why the RDA for iron is 10 milligrams for men and 15 milligrams for women. Some foods yield more than others, so when calculating your iron intake, consider its source. Twenty to 30 percent of the iron in meat is absorbed, as is 20 percent from soybeans, but only 15 percent is absorbed from fish. The typical American diet contains between 10 and 30 milligrams daily, so most of us do get enough. But infants, growing kids, and women who are pregnant, lactating, or menstruating need more. (If you are on a weight-reduction program and limiting your calories to between 1,200 and 1,500 daily, you are probably getting only 6 to 9 milligrams of iron per day.)

The table on page 40 lists the iron content of various foods. The most iron is present in organ meats such as liver and kidney, beef, chicken, seafood (notably cooked clams), dried peas and beans, dried fruits, dark green leafy vegetables, molasses, wheat bran and wheat germ, oatmeal, and soybean flour. Eggs, milk, and cereals contain some iron, but not impressive amounts, which is why kids should have iron-fortified cereals. Infants who drink cow's milk may become anemic because it is not an especially good source of iron. (Ask your pediatrician whether your child needs a vitamin supplement with iron.) If you're not a meat eater, you can get your iron from chicken and fish. Popeye was no nutritionist, and he was wrong about the powers of spinach! While there is iron in spinach and lentils, relatively little of it is absorbed from the intestine because these vegetables contain phytate (also present in wheat flour and bran), which blocks its absorption from the gut. On the other hand, vegetables with an abundance of vitamin C, such as tomatoes, cauliflower, broccoli, potatoes, cabbage, and even sauerkraut, all enhance the absorption of iron.

There are two kinds of dietary iron: nonheme and heme. The absorption of nonheme iron, which is found in fruits, vegetables, and grains, is enhanced by consuming it together with vitamin C. If you drink a glass of fruit juice or take a 100-milligram tablet of vitamin C *with* each meal, you will increase the absorption of iron from nonheme foods by as much as four times. Adding even small amounts of animal protein, as little as 1 or 2 ounces, to your vegetable salad, can also enhance iron absorption. There are also foods that *reduce* nonheme iron absorption: Large amounts of bran, calcium, tea, excessive amounts of zinc supplements, and phytate (found in unleavened bread, unrefined cereals, and soybeans) all block the entry of iron from the gut into the body. So a very-high-fiber diet can decrease the absorption of nonheme iron. Antacids will too, so if you have an ulcer and are taking something to neutralize your stomach acid, be sure to do so *between* meals. The same is true for tea and coffee, because of the tannin they contain. Tea with your meal can reduce the amount of iron you absorb by as much as 60 percent, while coffee will drop it by

40 percent. Heme iron, which is present in meat, fish, and poultry is not potentiated by vitamin C. How much iron you absorb is also dependent on the amount present in your body stores—the more pronounced the anemia and the more you need, the greater will be the absorption.

Another common nutritional anemia is that due to a deficiency of *folic acid,* a vitamin present in greatest amounts in animal organs such as kidney and liver (rich sources), green leafy vegetables (spinach, collards, asparagus, and broccoli), orange juice (which provides much more folic acid than a whole orange), whole wheat products, beets, peas, and beans. The table on page 42 lists the folic acid content of various foods. As is the case with iron, how much of the folic acid you eat is actually absorbed depends on its source. There is very little from an orange, but approximately 80 percent from a banana. So there's more to it than just determining the folate *content* of a food; you must also be familiar with its absorption characteristics. However, since in the real world you can't go through life with your pockets or purse filled with equivalency charts, just assume that an average of 25 to 50 percent of what you consume will make it past the stomach.

The RDA for folic acid is 180 micrograms for women (but if you're pregnant or lactating, you'll need 400 micrograms) and 200 micrograms for men. (If you're planning to become pregnant, begin taking your folic acid supplements *beforehand* to prevent neural tube defects in your child.) The average intake in the typical American diet easily satisfies the RDA. One cup of boiled red kidney beans contains 230 micrograms; six spears of boiled asparagus have 132 micrograms; ½ cup of boiled spinach contains 131 micrograms; and there are 109 micrograms in 8 ounces of orange juice. Fat, oils, and sugar contain none. Overcooking vegetables causes as much as 50 percent of their folic acid content to be lost. Also, if you leave any raw vegetables sitting around at room temperature for two or three days, they'll lose up to 70 percent of their folic acid. Although less is destroyed in the fridge, it's best to eat vegetables fresh. Remember too, that antacids may decrease the efficiency of folate absorption from your diet.

Chronic alcoholics are prime candidates for folic acid anemia because alcohol damages both the intestine and the liver, so that folic acid is less well absorbed and processed. Poorly nourished older persons may also be folic acid deficient, as are one-third of all pregnant women. You may lack it if you are taking oral contraceptives, or if you have an overactive thyroid gland, chronic diarrhea, sprue (see page 308), or are taking drugs like Dilantin or certain anticancer preparations.

You should suspect folic acid deficiency if you are anemic, if your tongue is red, smooth, and sore, and you have chronic diarrhea. If your child's growth and development seem to be impaired, or he or she has a learning disability, review his or her diet with your pediatrician. It may be due to a lack of folic acid.

Symptoms of folic acid deficiency will usually clear up promptly with supplementation of 1 *milligram* a day (there are 1000 micrograms in one milligram). Once the deficiency has been corrected, try to maintain adequate amounts of folic acid intake in your diet. But never, never take folic acid supplements to cure any anemia without first consulting your doctor. A deficiency of vitamin B_{12} causes an anemia indistinguishable from that due to a lack of folic acid. If you take folic acid without vitamin B_{12}, you may improve the anemia, but will make the nerve disorder caused by lack of B_{12} much worse.

In summary, you may feel tired even when your blood is not. Don't self-diagnose anemia on the basis of advertising hype for iron-containing tonics or vitamins. There are many different types of anemia, of which iron-deficiency is only one. Taking iron supplements when you don't need them may cause iron deposits that damage the heart, liver, and other organs, and may even increase the risk of heart disease and cancer. Most Americans consume enough iron in their diet, but growing children, pregnant and lactating women, people who are chronically losing blood from their hemorrhoids, ulcers, or heavy periods, people who hemorrhage for any reason, or those who are following fad diets need more—in their food, in supplements, by injection, and finally, via blood transfusion. Another important cause of nutritional anemia is due to lack of folate. This is especially likely to occur in pregnant and lactating women, alcoholics, fad dieters, elderly people, and those suffering from chronic illness. Folic acid is found in a wide variety of foods, including liver, kidney, and a host of fruits and vegetables.

IRON CONTENT OF FOODS

FOOD	PORTION	IRON (mg)	CALORIES
Beans/legumes			
black-eyed peas, canned	1 cup	2.34	184
green peas, cooked	1 cup	2.48	134
lentils, cooked	1 cup	6.59	231
lima, cooked	1 cup	4.50	217
navy, cooked	1 cup	4.51	259
red kidney, cooked	1 cup	5.20	225
split peas, cooked	1 cup	2.52	231
Beef			
flank, choice	3.5 ounces	3.47	237
ground, lean	3.5 ounces	2.09	268
kidney	3.5 ounces	7.31	144
liver	3.5 ounces	6.77	161
Bread/flour			
soybean flour, defatted	1 cup	9.24	327
wheat bran, toasted (Kretschmer)	⅓ cup	3.63	57
wheat bread	1 slice	0.84	61
wheat germ, toasted (Kretschmer)	¼ cup	2.30	103
white bread	1 slice	0.68	64
whole-grain 100% wheat bread	1 slice	1.30	66
Cereals			
All-Bran (Kellogg's)	⅓ cup	4.50	70
oatmeal, regular	1 cup	1.59	145
Quaker Extra Fortified Oatmeal	1 ounce (packet)	18.00	95
Special K	1⅓ cups	4.50	110
Total	1 cup	18.00	100
Wheaties	1 cup	4.45	100
Chicken			
dark meat, skinless	3.5 ounces	1.33	205
light meat, skinless	3.5 ounces	1.06	173

IRON CONTENT OF FOODS *(Continued)*

FOOD	PORTION	IRON (mg)	CALORIES
Dried fruits			
apricots	10	1.65	83
figs	10	4.18	477
prunes	10	2.08	201
raisins	⅔ cup	2.08	300
Egg, poached	1 large	0.72	74
Fish/shellfish			
clams, cooked or canned	3 ounces	23.76	126
clams, raw	4 large	11.88	63
gefilte fish	1 piece	1.04	35
mussels, blue	3 ounces	5.71	147
oysters, Eastern, raw	6 medium	5.63	58
oysters, Pacific, raw	3 ounces	4.34	69
salmon, Chinook, raw	3 ounces	0.60	153
shrimp, cooked	3 ounces	2.62	84
tuna, white, canned in water	3 ounces	0.51	116
tuna, yellowfin, raw	3 ounces	0.62	92
Molasses			
blackstrap	1 tablespoon	3.5	47
regular	1 tablespoon	0.94	53
Vegetables			
broccoli, cooked	1 cup	1.30	44
kale, cooked	1 cup	1.18	42
potato, baked with skin	1 medium	2.75	220
spinach, cooked	1 cup	6.40	42

FOLIC ACID CONTENT OF FOODS

FOOD	PORTION	FOLIC ACID (mcg)	CALORIES
Asparagus, cooked	6 spears	132	22
Beans/legumes			
black, cooked	1 cup	256	227
chickpeas, cooked	1 cup	282	269
green peas, cooked	1 cup	102	134
lentils, cooked	1 cup	358	231
lima, cooked	1 cup	156	217
navy, cooked	1 cup	255	259
soybeans, cooked	1 cup	93	298
split peas, cooked	1 cup	127	231
Beef			
flank, choice	3.5 ounces	9	237
ground, lean	3.5 ounces	9	268
kidney	3.5 ounces	98	144
liver	3.5 ounces	217	161
Beets, cooked	1 cup	90	52
Bread, whole wheat	1 slice	14	61
Brewer's yeast	1 tablespoon	313	40
Broccoli, cooked	1 cup	78	44
Collard greens, frozen, cooked	1 cup	130	62
Orange	1 medium	47	65
Orange juice, frozen, from concentrate	1 cup	109	112
Potato, baked with skin	1 medium	22	220
Spinach, cooked	1 cup	262	42
Sweet potato, baked with skin	1 small	26	118
Wheat bran, toasted (Kretschmer)	⅓ cup	49	65
Wheat germ (Quaker Honey Crunch)	¼ cup	82	105

ANXIETY, PANIC ATTACKS, AND FOOD

ANGST-FREE FOODS

Anxiety and panic attacks are an appropriate human response to danger. If you're on a plane and the pilot announces that there is a serious engine malfunction and the possibility of a crash landing, you *should* be anxious! If your job is in jeopardy, anxiety or panic is also understandable. But when the threat ends, so should the emotional response to it. Feelings of panic and anxiety that continue indefinitely for no *apparent* reason are not "normal" behavior.

Recurring panic attacks, whether purely psychiatric or rooted in some physical disorder (they often plague persons with mitral valve prolapse), frequently require medication (psychotropic drugs). Ideally, however, efforts to discover and remove the cause of the attacks, whatever their origin, should be continued even as these drugs are prescribed. For example, you and your doctor may find that your "nervousness" and jitters are due to the caffeine in the six cups of black coffee you've been drinking every day. That's the obvious (and richest) source of *caffeine,* with 103 milligrams in every 6 ounces brewed. Remember, however, that it's also present in carbonated cola drinks (a 12-ounce can, regular or sugar-free, contains 46 milligrams of caffeine), in tea (there are 36 milligrams in 6 ounces), chocolate, and cocoa. See page 45 for a list of caffeine-containing foods. You may also find caffeine where you wouldn't normally expect it. For example, if you have a cold and decide to take an over-the-counter preparation to relieve your cough or nasal stuffiness, chances are it will contain two unnecessary ingredients—an antihistamine and caffeine. Most antihistamines make you sleepy, so the caffeine is added to help keep you awake. Antihistamines are great for allergic symptoms, but the common cold is a viral infection, against which they are useless (see page 102). If you determine that caffeine is indeed the cause of your symptoms, don't go cold turkey with it. As with so many other drugs, abrupt withdrawal can also give you emotional "jitters."

Alcohol, which is normally a sedative, can also cause anxiety, depression, paranoia, and a host of other psychiatric symptoms, both while you're drinking and after abrupt withdrawal. I remember one of my patients with a drinking problem who knew that alcohol was bad for him, so he would promise, in good faith, to have only one drink just to nip his anxiety and jitters in the bud. The one drink, however, invariably depressed him, and he needed more—enough, in fact, to drink himself into oblivion.

Nicotine can also induce anxiety and panic, and, like alcohol, its use leads to a vicious cycle. Heavy smoking can make you feel nervous, so that you smoke even more to "quiet" your nerves. And that makes matters even worse—a Catch-22 situation.

Cocaine can also produce emotional ups and downs, as can *appetite suppressants*. Several different drugs, including cold preparations, that contain stimulants such as phenylpropanolamine and ephedrine derivatives, *painkillers,* and even *sedatives* can all make you nervous and anxious. Chronic *lack of sleep* and *stopping an exercise routine* abruptly can also leave you "stressed." Some researchers are convinced that prolonged exposure to fluorescent lighting during office hours can also make you anxious. But don't change your job yet for that reason. This observation is still controversial. In this era of fad diets and obsession with weight control, there is always the risk of *low blood sugar*. Skipping breakfast can drop your sugar to levels that will leave you feeling anxious and tremulous. If you are prone to such crises, a high-complex-carbohydrate breakfast will prevent hypoglycemia later in the day. Such a breakfast might consist of a serving of fresh fruit, one or two eggs (use only the whites if you are on a low-cholesterol diet), and one or two slices of whole-grain toast with nonfat cottage cheese. If you prefer, you may have a high-fiber cereal with 1 cup of nonfat milk.

Before the Miltown-Valium era, physicians often recommended the amino acid tryptophan to help soothe your nerves. But tryptophan in capsule form has been banned in the United States because of contamination in the manufacturing process. You can find naturally occurring tryptophan in milk and turkey. Some of my anxious patients still drink a glass of warm milk at bedtime to calm them down and help them sleep, but, quite frankly, I haven't been able to persuade any of them to eat turkey sandwiches and drink milk throughout the day. They prefer to go to the drugstore and buy a tranquilizer!

Don't look for a quick fix of your panic and anxiety attacks with a tranquilizer "borrowed" from a friend. Discuss your symptoms with your doctor. Review your lifestyle together, especially your use (or abuse) of substances such as coffee, alcohol, tobacco, and medication. A thorough medical exam may reveal a curable, or at least treatable, cause such as mitral valve prolapse or an overactive thyroid gland. Let your doctor decide whether you really need a tranquilizer.

CAFFEINE CONTENT OF FOODS

FOOD	PORTION	CAFFEINE (mg)
Candy bars		
Hershey's Krackel	1.6 ounces	9
Milky Way	2.1 ounces	11
Nestlé Crunch	1.4 ounces	10
Chocolate		
baking, unsweetened	1 ounce	58
chocolate chips, semisweet	¼ cup	14
German sweet, Baker's	1 ounce	8
Hershey's special dark	1.4 ounces	31
milk chocolate	1.6 ounces	11
semisweet, Baker's	1 ounce	13
Chocolate fudge topping	2 tablespoons	4
Chocolate pudding, instant	½ cup	5
Cocoa		
hot cocoa mix	1 ounce	5
cocoa powder, unsweetened	1 tablespoon	12

CAFFEINE CONTENT OF FOODS *(Continued)*

FOOD	PORTION	CAFFEINE (mg)
Coffee		
brewed	6 ounces	103 to 164
brewed decaf	6 ounces	2 to 5
General Foods Amaretto Coffee	6 ounces	60
General Foods Irish Creme	6 ounces	53
instant	1 teaspoon	57
instant decaf	1 teaspoon	2
Devil's food cake mix	$1/12$ package	9
Double fudge brownie mix	$1/24$ package	5
Soft drinks		
Cherry Coke	12 ounces	46
Coca-Cola	12 ounces	46
Diet Cherry Coke	12 ounces	46
Diet Coke	12 ounces	46
Diet Pepsi	12 ounces	36
Dr Pepper	12 ounces	41
Pepsi-Cola	12 ounces	38
Tea		
brewed for 3 minutes	6 ounces	36
instant	1 teaspoon	31

ARTHRITIS
(OSTEO- AND RHEUMATOID)
NIGHTSHADES AND ALL

At least 36 million people of all ages in the United States have some form of "arthritis." It is responsible for a great deal of pain and suffering, as well as for countless millions of dollars spent on medication, doctors' bills, and lost wages.

Arthritis does not refer to a specific diagnosis, any more than do the words *fever, pain,* or *cough.* The term means inflammation of a joint, for which there are at least a hundred different causes—everything from a simple injury (traumatic arthritis) to some disturbance of body metabolism (gouty arthritis) to several infections, including sexually transmitted diseases (gonococcal arthritis), hepatitis B, and even influenza. But the arthritis that most people have is either osteoarthritis or rheumatoid arthritis.

Osteoarthritis, the most common form of arthritis, is a degenerative process, a wear-and-tear phenomenon that begins during adult life and gets worse as you grow older. By age forty, routine X rays of your back, knees, or hip are likely to show evidence of osteoarthritis even if you have no symptoms. By the time we're seventy, we all feel our osteoarthritis somewhere—a creaky joint here, an ache there, mild stiffness in the hands or the back, or a hip so painful it needs to be replaced. In most people, these symptoms respond to over-the-counter analgesics such as aspirin, acetaminophen, and NSAIDs (nonsteroidal anti-inflammatory drugs) like ibuprofen; others benefit from physical therapy; many obese persons feel better after losing weight (probably the most effective thing you can do for any kind of arthritis, because it helps relieve the stress on the joints).

I have some osteoarthritis myself. When I sit at my desk for several hours, pen in hand, writing page after page of my books (I never did learn to type), my fingers begin to hurt. When they ache a little and feel stiff in the morning, I take a couple of aspirin tablets or one of the NSAIDs (depending on what samples the pharmaceutical detail representatives left me this week), and the discomfort disappears. Recently, however, I developed a bad back, which I get from time to time when I sit at my desk too long. My wife persuaded me to see a physiatrist who examined me, took some X rays, and diagnosed "just a little osteoarthritis—the same thing you have in your fingers." "Is there anything I can do to stop it from getting worse and creeping up on me insidiously in another finger, then maybe a knee, or a hip?" I asked. He looked me over carefully from head to toe with his discerning physiatric eyes, which finally came to rest on my paunch (not apparent on the cover photograph of this book). That searching glance delivered his message loud and clear! "Weight loss—and exercise," he said. "For my fingers?" "No, just for your back. The best way to control osteoarthritis is to lose weight, exercise regularly, and get some good physiotherapy." "What about diet?" I asked, because so many of my own patients had regaled me with stories of how their arthritis was "cured" by a wide variety of foods, ranging from honey-laced apple cider vinegar to some herb or other food purchased in a local health food store. "Do you have any food allergies?" he asked. "None that I know of," I responded. "Then there is no diet that will help your osteoarthritis."

That's what the Arthritis Foundation says too. I also checked the latest *Merck Manual* (sixteenth edition) under "osteoarthritis." The only headings I found there were Incidence, Phylogeny, Classification, Etiology, Pathophysiology, Signs and Symptoms, Diagnosis, Prognosis and Treatment, and Surgery. Nary a word about any wonder foods. So no shortcuts for me. Time to cut more fat out of my diet and work out more often on that treadmill.

Rheumatoid arthritis (RA), which is more disabling and crippling than osteoarthritis, appears to be a disorder of the immune system. I expect that this disease will be more successfully treated in the near future than it currently is. At least seven million people in this country alone have rheumatoid arthritis, whose adverse effects, unlike those of osteoarthritis, are not limited to the joints, but involve several other organs such as the lungs, heart, and skin. When it is active (the disease tends to wax and wane), you'll experience fever, anemia, fatigue, weight loss, lack of appetite, and general malaise. Your joints will become painful, warm, stiff, swollen, and, after repeated acute bouts, often deformed. However, the serious crippling most people associate with this disease occurs less frequently than is popularly supposed.

In addition to medication, physiotherapy, exercise, and corrective surgery, there are a variety of drugs that can be used to manage rheumatoid arthritis. These include gold, penicillamine, antimalarial agents such as Plaquenil and chloroquine, certain anticancer drugs such as methotrexate that interfere with the immune system, and steroid hormones.

Can what you eat help your rheumatoid arthritis? As with osteoarthritis, I could not find a single "establishment" textbook of medicine that recommends any dietary changes that may have a benefit for this disease. So at this point, I was sorely tempted to abort this chapter since this book deals with conditions in which nutrition is important. But then, I came across a paper in the prestigious *Annals of Internal Medicine* (the official publication of the American College of Physicians) reporting that a fatty acid extracted from seed oil made from evening primrose and borage herbs can benefit people with rheumatoid arthritis. The oil, which contains gammalin olenic acid, was put in capsules and given to patients with rheumatoid arthritis. When taken daily for six months, there was significant reduction of inflammation, pain, and swelling in the affected joints. Borage is a plant widely cultivated in gardens. Extracts from its leaves have been used as an intestinal antispasmodic, and some people apply it topically to inflamed areas of their skin. Evening primrose is an edible plant found in the United States and Canada, whose shoots and leaves can be added to salads or stews, or made into tea. For years it has been touted, but never really proven to be effective in the prevention of premenstrual syndrome. This paper may be the first scientifically evaluated claim for evening primrose oil. You can be sure that it will generate renewed interest in this plant, not only for its use in rheumatoid arthritis, but in other disorders as well. But don't rush to your health food store yet to stock up on evening primrose oil. The doses used in this study were fairly large and should only be administered by a doctor—if and when the claims are substantiated.

Given this impetus, I decided to look a little further into any possible link between diet and arthritis that I might have missed in my reading. I was further motivated to do so because of the many anecdotal accounts of improvement from my own patients and the widespread belief in our culture that there *must* be some relationship between food and arthritis—the experts notwithstanding. In reviewing the medical literature, I did find some dietary leads for both osteoarthritis and rheumatoid arthritis of which you should be aware.

For example, there were several studies suggesting that a deficiency of certain vitamins or minerals, notably vitamin B_6 (pyridoxine), vitamin B_3 (pantothenic acid), zinc, folic acid, vitamin E, and selenium, can sometimes result in arthritis. Frankly, the evidence was underwhelming. So don't rush to take these supplements. They *may* help only if, after analyzing your blood, your doctor finds you deficient in them. Unless you are on a fad diet or deliberately starving yourself to lose weight, the likelihood of such a deficiency is not great. Supplements can be expensive, and too much of them, especially B_6, can be toxic. In order to prevent vitamin B_6 deficiency, your diet should contain at least 2 milligrams per day. That's the RDA for men; for women it's 1.6 milligrams. Because vitamin B_6 is so plentiful, most deficiencies occur in malnourished infants, not in adults. The richest natural sources of B_6 are liver, kidney, lean beef, chicken, avocado, potatoes, bananas, brewer's yeast, wheat germ, wheat bran, oatmeal, whole-grain cereals, legumes, sunflower seeds, soybeans, and rice (see page 364 for a more complete listing.) Vegetables and fruits have only small amounts, and there is virtually none in milk and cheese. Seventy-five percent of the B_6 in wheat is lost in the process of milling white flour, and as much as 50 percent is leached out in cooking. Alcohol, oral contraceptives, and certain medications such as isoniazid also interfere with B_6 metabolism and can leave you deficient in it. In the unlikely event that you are, review your diet carefully with your doctor. The quickest and best way to correct a lack of B_6 is with supplements. You should suspect a deficiency of B_6 if you have skin rashes (especially on the tip of the nose), kidney stones, nausea and vomiting, depression, convulsions, and confusion.

You've really got to try hard to become deficient in *pantothenic acid* (vitamin B$_3$), which like B$_6$, is very widely distributed in food. So if your diet contains organ meats such as liver, egg yolk, yeast, salmon, chicken, and wheat germ, you are not likely to lack it. There is very little in milk and butter. The RDA for vitamin B$_3$ is between 4 and 7 milligrams. Most multivitamin supplements contain much more than the RDA.

Zinc is present throughout the body—in your hair, skin, bones, nails, eyes, and, perhaps most important for men of a certain age, the prostate gland. Oysters are the richest dietary source, but zinc is also found in lesser amounts in liver, beef, wheat bran, wheat germ, nuts, and poultry (see page 145 for other sources). If you're eating a varied diet, you'll be getting all you need (15 milligrams a day). Suspect a deficiency if you see white spots under your nails.

Unlike B$_6$, B$_3$, and zinc, *folic acid* deficiency is not at all uncommon. Its RDA is 180 micrograms a day for women and 200 micrograms for men. Its richest natural sources (see page 42) are brewer's yeast, leafy green vegetables such as spinach, asparagus, collards, and broccoli, liver, kidney, lentils, and beans. There's lots in whole wheat products and orange juice too, but you won't find much in most meats, milk, and eggs. Folic acid deficiency can give you anemia (see page 33), a sore, red, smooth tongue, diarrhea, and in kids, retarded growth, but it's a most unlikely cause of arthritis. However, if you have all these other symptoms of folic acid deficiency *and* arthritis too, you've got the diagnosis made! (But leave the final decision to your doctor.) If you take 1 milligram of folic acid supplement daily all your symptoms should magically disappear.

Several studies have suggested that 400 IU of *vitamin E* daily will ease the symptoms of arthritis (and at the same time protect against cardiovascular disease). I'm not convinced about the first claim, but am inclined to believe the latter one. Vitamin E is an antioxidant whose time has come.

Vitamin E is one of four vitamins that dissolves only in fat and not in water (the others are A, D, and K). Vitamin E is an essential nutrient, which means that the body must have it and can't make it. This vitamin is a key component of virtually every energy process; it keeps the red blood cells healthy too, and even protects the lungs against pollution. The RDA simply to *prevent deficiency* is only 10 milligrams per day. That may be all you need to keep you going, but I suspect that higher doses may provide additional benefits, as indicated by recent studies of the beneficial effects of vitamin E in persons with heart disease. The richest natural sources of vitamin E are wheat germ and wheat germ oil, and corn, soybean, and sunflower oils—commonly used in salad dressings and margarine. There is not much in peanut, olive, coconut, and fish oils.

Too much vitamin E in your diet isn't likely to make you sick because it's relatively nontoxic. Those of my patients who were enrolled in a trial of vitamin E for the treatment of Parkinson's disease took 3,000 milligrams a day for years without any adverse effects (It turned out not to help). (The RDA of vitamin E is only 8 milligrams for women and 10 milligrams for men!) The problem is that most foods high in vitamin E are also high in fat. That's why so many people prefer the supplements. I recommend no more than 400 to 800 IU per day.

It has been reported that correcting a lack of *selenium* may improve osteoarthritis. The soil is selenium poor in many parts of the world. Recent studies in Sweden have shown that persons with osteoarthritis who live in selenium-deficient areas have fewer symptoms when they take supplements of this mineral. The official RDA for selenium is 55 micrograms for women and 70 micrograms for men. Its richest sources are lobster, Brazil nuts, spices such as garlic and cinnamon, and whole grains. You'll also find some in kidney, liver, meat, and poultry, but fruits and vegetables have very little. How much selenium each of these particular foods contains will depend on the selenium content of the soil in which they were grown (except for lobsters, of course). I do not recommend selenium supplements for arthritis unless you live in an area where the soil is low in selenium and you are unable to meet the RDA in your diet.

Certain diets are said to improve osteoarthritis as, for example, the *"no-nightshade"* diet, which is free of white potatoes, tomatoes, all peppers (except the spices, black and white), tobacco, and eggplant. I have always regarded this claim as nothing more than faddism. But every now and then a patient will insist that this regimen has helped him or her. The majority, however, deny it. There's no harm in trying the no-nightshade diet for three or four weeks and seeing what happens, even though I am not aware of any scientifically controlled studies confirming its benefits.

Then there is the *"Dong"* diet. (Don't jump to conclusions about this one just because of its name.) Dr. Collin Dong was a physician who proposed a diet of fish and vegetables free of all preservatives, and without any fruit, red meat, spices, or milk. I don't know of any scientific studies substantiating the claims made on its behalf, nor can I recommend any diet, including this one, that would have you shun fruit. After all, arthritis is a chronic condition, and no one should go through life without fruit.

The *Airola* diet is one to avoid. It's basically lactovegetarian (a vegetarian diet that includes butter, milk, and milk products), but in addition to avoiding all refined foods, it also calls for periods of fasting and frequent colonic enemas, both of which are undesirable and potentially dangerous.

There are several other foods "guaranteed" to help your arthritis, including extract of the green-lipped mussel, a rare New Zealand mollusk. Forget it. Or you may have heard of chuifong toukuwan, a Chinese herb that does contain some agents that reduce inflammation. I'd stay away from it; some of its ingredients are so toxic they're illegal in this country.

The beneficial action of aspirin and the NSAIDs (nonsteroidal anti-inflammatory drugs) suggests that fish oils might be an effective treatment for rheumatoid arthritis. This subject is currently being studied in many medical research laboratories. Aspirin and NSAIDs counter the effects of prostaglandins, chemicals that promote inflammation. Fish oils have a similar anti-inflammatory effect, and several of my patients with rheumatoid arthritis have told me they have less morning stiffness and joint pain when their diet is rich in fish with a high omega-3 fatty acid content (see the table on page 221 for the most common sources of omega-3). These include sardines, tuna, halibut, mackerel, and salmon. You may possibly improve the symptoms of rheumatoid arthritis if you regularly eat these fatty, cold-water fish. If you cannot afford them or don't like their taste, you may take 6 grams of the supplement capsules every day, bearing in mind the precautions listed on page 201. However, I recommend natural sources of omega-3 if possible.

Every now and then a patient tells me that some dietary intervention or other has made a dramatic difference in his or her arthritis. I can often explain such a result by the inadvertent, serendipitous elimination of a food to which they are allergic. Since some 20 percent of cases of arthritis are associated with food allergy, I suggest to my patients with severe arthritis that they stop eating, one by one, the following foods: soy, coffee, eggs, milk, corn, wheat, potatoes, apples, lettuce, shellfish—especially shrimp—oranges, alcohol, beef, pork, and vegetable oils. The last contain omega-6 polyunsaturated fatty acids, which, unlike the omega-3 found in fish oils, can worsen or provoke arthritis. If the systematic elimination and reintroduction of these foods does not appear to have any effect on your arthritis, then it's back to my physiatrist's original prescription of weight loss, exercise, and physiotherapy.

The entire focus of this chapter has been on the role of diet in the treatment of the *symptoms* of osteo- or rheumatoid arthritis. But I cannot emphasize strongly enough the fact that good nutrition is extremely important in the overall management of these conditions—for a variety of reasons. Being overweight further damages painful joints in people with osteoarthritis, and losing those extra pounds helps them considerably. But it's hard to lose weight if you don't exercise, which many people with severe arthritis can't do. If you lead a sedentary life, you'll need to watch your calories very carefully, while making sure you get enough essential nutrients.

Rheumatoid arthritis presents an even greater nutritional challenge. Because this disease affects the body as a whole, your appetite is often severely impaired. People with rheumatoid arthritis tend to be thin and undernourished and need nutritional supplementation. The many painkillers and other medications you take further reduce your appetite and may irritate your stomach. If you are disabled and living alone, you may not be able to do your shopping often enough to buy fresh fruits and vegetables; the arthritis can affect your jaw or the temporomandibular joint (just below the ear on each side), making chewing difficult and painful. You may need liquid nutritional supplements until the acute stage of the disease is controlled.

In summary, osteoarthritis and rheumatoid arthritis are the two most common joint disorders affecting adults. You can manage them with medication to control pain, weight loss when necessary, and the proper balance of rest, exercise, and physiotherapy. In severe cases, surgery may be required to correct deformities or even to replace damaged and painful joints. However, a large body of anecdotal "evidence" suggests that some foods may aggravate or improve symptoms. The omega-3 fatty acids found in certain deep-sea, cold-water fish appear to have the most credibility. I have discussed some of the other popular remedies, including avoidance of the nightshade group of vegetables, which you may wish to try for a short time—but don't hold your breath waiting for relief.

ASTHMA

EAT RIGHT AND WHEEZE LESS

The characteristic high-pitched, musical wheeze of asthma occurs when the airways (bronchial tubes) to the lungs are narrowed—by mucus, swelling of their lining, or spasm. An acute attack may result from an allergic reaction to something you've inhaled or eaten; a wide variety of noxious odors, including strong perfume and tobacco smoke; infection (usually of the sinuses, bronchial tubes, or lungs); exercise; extremes in temperature or humidity; or emotional stress. Asthma affects 5 to 8 percent of us at every age. Its incidence is increasing; the number of cases in the United States rose by 28 percent between 1990 and 1992.

The many medications that can effectively prevent or control an attack of asthma fall into four categories: sympathomimetics such as albuterol, which dilate the bronchial tree; cromolyn and a newer agent called Tilade, which stop an allergic trigger from throwing the airways into spasm; steroid hormones, by inhalation, tablet, or injection, which reduce inflammation and the excess mucus from which asthmatics suffer; and bronchodilator drugs, whose active ingredients are theophylline and its derivatives, which widen the constricted air passages. These agents *do* work, and asthmatics should always carry the appropriate ones with them. However, there are specific dietary measures that help too. Happily, they do not include camel and crocodile dung, asthma treatments that were popular in ancient Egypt.

If your asthma is caused by *food allergy,* particularly to milk, eggs, seafood, or shellfish (only one in twenty is), the best way to determine which foods to avoid is to keep an accurate food diary and to record *everything* you've eaten. Foods consumed hours or even minutes (but not days) before your asthma attacks may have caused them.

Aspirin, especially in people with nasal polyps, can induce asthma. *Sulfites* (preservatives added to food to keep it looking fresh and to give it a longer shelf life) can also cause asthma in a small number of sensitive individuals. However, in 1986 the FDA banned their use in fresh and raw fruits and vegetables. (I always wondered why the lettuce in salad bars always looked so crisp and fresh even after sitting in the buffet for hours, while ours at home was always wilted.) But you will still find sulfites in wine, beer, dried fruits, avocado dip, shrimp, shellfish, bacon and cold cuts, and many packaged foods (unless otherwise labeled). Check the label of all processed foods because, according to law, food manufacturers must list the sulfite content of any product containing more than ten parts per million. You can find sulfites referred to by these terms: sodium sulfite, potassium sulfite, sodium metabisulfite, potassium metabisulfite, sodium bisulfite, potassium bisulfite, sulfur dioxide, and MSG (monosodium glutamate). The FDA has a GRAS ("generally recognized as safe") list that can give you further information on sulfites. One of the paradoxes in medicine is the presence of sulfites in drugs—including those used to treat asthmatic patients! Occasionally, an asthma patient has been made much worse in an emergency room when he or she was given medication containing sulfites. *Tartrazine* is a dye found in many yellow and yellow/orange packaged foods and beverages. It brightens the appearance of prepared foods, drinks, medications, and mouth-care products, but can on occasion also induce asthmatic attacks in a small number of people *who are also allergic to aspirin.* So don't waste your time checking what you eat and drink for the presence of tartrazine unless aspirin makes you sick too.

Some of my patients swear by royal jelly. They say it keeps them feeling and looking younger. Books on herbal remedies claim that this bee by-product is a tonic with antiaging properties, great for the memory, and especially good if you're the nervous type. Frankly, I am not aware of any scientifically documented benefit from royal jelly. As far as I'm concerned, it's simply an expensive way to get some extra B vitamins and amino acids. Its popularity probably stems from the extrapolation of its dramatic effect on the bees themselves. This milky-white material is secreted by glands in the throats of worker bees and fed to all bee larvae (the immature, wingless feeding stage of the insect). But after two days, those destined to become worker bees are fed honey, while queen bees–to–be are given royal jelly. Presumably because of her different nutrition, the queen bee is twice the size of the others, lays two thousand eggs a day, and lives five to eight years (forty times longer than the workers). Royal jelly comes in capsules, ointments, and creams. If you are happy with royal jelly and can afford it, I'm all for it—*except if you're asthmatic!* There have been reports from Australia that several people with asthma experienced serious reactions—even death—minutes after ingesting royal jelly. There have also been reports of asthma induced by other bee products such as beeswax and bee pollen. If you have asthma, regardless of whether you're allergic to bee venom (the attacks mentioned above occurred in people who were not allergic), royal jelly is not your fountain of youth.

If you know from experience that a particular food will provoke an asthmatic attack, avoid it no matter what skin allergy tests show. You are a better judge of what makes you sick than any test yet devised. In fact, I do not usually perform skin tests for food allergy on my patients because too many "allergic" persons react positively to practically everything except the food most likely to induce an attack!

Although it's important to avoid foods that provoke asthma, you should also know what to eat to help *prevent* attacks. For years, natives in Mexico and South America have been eating *chili peppers* to improve sexual performance, decrease lung congestion, and relieve pain. Really hot chilis consumed regularly (a raw pepper contains 110 milligrams of vitamin C and only 18 calories) will reduce the frequency and severity of your asthmatic attacks; so will drinking a glass of water containing ten to twenty drops of Tabasco sauce, a chili concentrate. (The same "drink" also eases the symptoms of chronic bronchitis and the common cold.) Chili peppers are even more effective if you also eat generous portions of fresh garlic and onions. Contrary to popular belief, chili will *not* usually give you an ulcer or irritate your stomach. If the peppers make your mouth burn, have some milk or chocolate whose casein content (casein is the principal protein in cow's milk) will "cool" it.

None of these centuries-old observations about the use of chili peppers by "primitive" peoples was taken seriously until scientists found that chilis' active ingredient, capsaicin, is an effective topical anesthetic agent. (Capsaicin, marketed commercially as Zostrix cream, is used *topically* for relieving itch and easing the pain of shingles, alleviating the severe discomfort experienced by some diabetics whose nerves have been affected by their disease, and soothing the soreness of arthritic joints.)

Adult asthmatics who drink real coffee regularly (not the decaffeinated form or tea) have 30 percent fewer attacks than do non–coffee drinkers. Indeed, before the era of modern antiasthmatic medications, coffee was the treatment of choice for asthma. Its active ingredient, methylxanthine, dilates the bronchial tree by relaxing the muscles that go into spasm. So if you've left home without your medications and have an asthma attack, get hold of the drugs you need or seek medical attention. In the meantime, drink two cups of strong, brewed coffee. That will sometimes ease your symptoms within the hour and continue to protect you against recurrence for another six hours.

Asthmatics who regularly consume at least three servings a week of omega-3 fatty acids (present in deep-sea, cold-water fish such as salmon, sardines, haddock, and mackerel, as well as shellfish, notably oysters, mussels, crab, and clams) also may experience fewer attacks. (See page 221 for a list of foods containing omega-3.) This should come as no surprise since asthma is due to a combination of immune system malfunction and inflammatory changes in the air passages. Omega-3 fatty acids affect the production of prostaglandins and leukotrienes (see page 332), both of which are potent mediators of the immune system. If you can't eat enough cold-water fish, or don't like it, take commercially available omega-3 supplements (but not if you're hypertensive or have a bleeding disorder). The usual dosage is 3 grams daily, but diabetics should have no more than 2 grams. It goes without saying that the omega-3-rich foods are not for you if you're allergic to fish! The beneficial effects of fish have also been shown to benefit the lungs in other ways. The incidence of chronic bronchitis and emphysema, to which heavy cigarette smokers are vulnerable, is reduced by about 50 percent if they eat two and a half servings of fish every day.

A final thought. Chicken soup is a subject for humor by many stand-up comics whose mothers and grandmothers, including my own, plied them with it whenever they were sick. Maimonides, the famous physician of the twelfth century, recommended chicken soup to his asthmatic patients! Eight centuries later, researchers reported at a meeting of the American Lung Association that chicken soup stops the migration of white blood cells (which increase the symptoms of inflammation) to the respiratory passages. So don't laugh. If you have asthma—or even just an ordinary cold—try some steaming chicken soup. It's a whole lot tastier than crocodile or camel dung!

Dietary intervention is no substitute for modern medication in the management of asthma, but avoiding foods that predictably provoke it and consuming coffee, chili peppers, and fish oils can help.

WHEN YOU'RE A "POWER" ATHLETE

EATING TO SURVIVE AND

MAYBE EVEN TO WIN

Exercise is "in" these days. People of all ages and in every walk of life are getting the message that regular exercise—the kind you enjoy and in amounts you can tolerate—is good for you. Former couch potatoes like myself are working out one way or another. I now walk on a treadmill for thirty minutes at 3.8 miles an hour every morning before breakfast. But there are many other ways to exercise—bicycling (stationary or mobile), gliding on a cross-country ski machine, walking outdoors when weather permits (or in a mall when it doesn't), jogging, even dancing. Many individuals, however, are "power athletes" who prefer prolonged rigorous and demanding activities—endurance and even ultraendurance exercise such as hours of sustained running in marathons.

If you plan to subject your body to such physical stress, you must be nutritionally prepared. You cannot suddenly decide to eat "properly" two hours before an athletic event, after having paid no attention to your diet for weeks, and expect your body to respond optimally. You must begin a nutrition regimen *during your training period* so as to build up your stamina and provide the necessary energy during the competition itself.

If you are a power athlete, the optimum composition of your

diet—how much of what nutrients to take and when to do so—
depends on your age, sex, and body build, as well as the nature,
duration, and level of exertion you perform. The National Research
Council's Commission on Life Sciences, which is concerned with
various aspects of sport, has recommended that women consume 37
to 51 calories per kilogram of weight per day during their training
period and that men have 41 to 58 calories per kilo. (A kilo is 2.2
pounds; so a female weighing 60 kilos or 132 pounds requires about
2,200 to 3,060 calories a day; a man of the same weight needs between
2,460 and 3,480 calories daily.) The more prolonged and intense the
sport, the more calories you should eat; but that also varies with your
particular body frame, height, weight, and lifestyle. For example,
female athletes are usually more concerned about their weight than are
men and are apt to diet accordingly. When they do so, the foods most
likely to be dropped first are calorie-dense dairy products, and this may
lead to a deficiency of calcium, iron, and zinc—minerals important for
bone metabolism and efficient energy expenditure. The consequences
of such a diet are stress fractures, tendinitis, and the early onset of
osteoporosis. Some athletes of both sexes are quite understandably
hesitant about exercising on a full stomach, so they reduce their caloric
intake during training and competition, forgoing the full quota of
energy they need for their workout. The diet of vegan athletes who
shun all animal products may be too high in fiber and low in calories
for the physical stress in which they are engaged.

I can't tell you how to "eat to win," but I can help you eat to
compete. Here are the basic nutritional guidelines for everyone engaging in endurance and ultraendurance activities for more than two
consecutive hours.

The key nutrient for athletes is *carbohydrate*. It provides lots of
energy quickly, prevents or reduces fatigue, and helps restore a sense
of well-being after the workout. Sixty to 70 percent of your total daily
calories should come from carbohydrate. Throughout this book you
will read my recommendations to replace simple, refined sugars with
high-fiber complex carbohydrates. Here is one situation, however,
where that is not usually the case. Power athletes need rapid replenish-
ment of energy. Complex carbohydrates remain in the stomach for a
longer time and are absorbed more slowly than are simple sugars. That
means less available energy. So *do* eat fruits, which are naturally high

in simple sugar that reaches the liver quickly. The best sources for a quick energy fix are lemonade, graham crackers, a cup of frozen yogurt, or some apple juice. The last time I watched the New York Marathon, I saw several runners breaking off small pieces of "power bars" and eating them as they ran. Always read the label on these bars because some of them contain considerable amounts of fat, which, as I explain below, is not something you want to consume while working out. If you have a taste for these convenience snacks, buy those high in carbohydrates and low in fat.

If you are a regular athlete and work out vigorously several times a week, don't worry about eating more carbohydrate than you need; any excess will be converted to and stored as glycogen in your muscles and liver. Later, should you expend a great deal of energy for a long period of time without having eaten enough carbohydrate, your body will call upon its glycogen stores to provide what's necessary.

Ideally, you should consume 5 to 10 grams of carbohydrate per kilo of body weight (roughly 2 to 5 grams per pound) every day while training or competing. That usually works out to about 500 or 600 grams daily. If you exercise vigorously and limit your carbohydrate intake to, say, 100 to 150 grams a day, the glycogen reserves in your muscles and liver will become depleted. There are several ways to restore those reserves. Since it takes about twenty hours to do so, you can limit your exercise for one day before the big event and eat a high-carbohydrate meal of 500 to 600 grams (some athletes call this "carbo loading"). Or, you can exercise lightly for three or four days prior to your workout and eat the same 500 grams of carbohydrate daily, representing 50 to 60 percent of your total caloric intake. The table on page 68 offers a sample meal plan that provides over 500 grams of carbohydrate. Unless you give mind to your carbohydrate needs when you are about to embark on a vigorous endurance exercise activity, your body protein and fat will be drawn upon to supply the necessary energy. That's something you want to avoid because burning off excessive fat too quickly results in the accumulation of toxic substances, which, in effect, poison the body, while breakdown of protein eventually causes loss of muscle mass.

About 15 percent of the power athlete's diet should consist of *protein,* with fat making up the remaining 10 to 20 percent. If you eat enough protein, your body will not break down muscle tissue when glycogen stores are depleted. Consuming sufficient protein also en-sures the continued buildup and strength of muscles. If you are a vegan, i.e., you eat no animal protein, make sure that the protein in your plant foods is of high quality. As I explained on page 12, the "quality" of protein depends on the particular building blocks or amino acids it contains. Some of these amino acids are "essential," that is, they cannot be synthesized by the body and must come from your food. The other amino acids can be "put together" from various dietary proteins. To be sure that as a vegan you are getting the proper mix and full range of these proteins, you may have to combine several in your diet. Examples of such "complementary" proteins are rice and peas; cornmeal and beans; and wheat products and legumes.

Fat provides a concentrated source of energy (9 calories per gram as compared with 4 calories per gram from carbohydrate or protein); it also helps your body absorb four key vitamins—A, D, E, and K. Most of your fat intake, which should be limited to 10 to 20 percent of your total calories, should be monounsaturated (olive, peanut, and canola oils) and polyunsaturated (from various vegetables such as corn and soy). Whatever animal fat you require is present in your protein. Athletes should avoid all fat for three to four hours before and after rigorous exercise because it slows emptying of the stomach. This delays the arrival of nutrients to the tissues that need them. The best time to consume fat is in the evening or after your final workout.

Do athletes need mineral and vitamin supplements? That's an aca-demic question because 60 percent of them take them (the same percentage as in the country at large). But there is no proof that a well-nourished athlete (with the exception of vegans or those who have been dieting) needs vitamin supplements simply because he or she exercises, or that vitamin supplements enhance performance in any way. Avoid megadoses of any vitamin, not only because of their potential toxicity, but because the gut can absorb only a limited amount at any one sitting, and an excess of one vitamin may result in others not being absorbed. Supplements of vitamins A, D, K, and B_6 can cause adverse effects in amounts only ten times greater than the recommended daily allowance. Remember, too, that niacin, particu-larly the long-acting preparations, can damage the liver. All vitamins should be taken *with* meals because that's when they're best absorbed.

It's extremely important for you to replace fluid during vigorous exercise—as much as three or more quarts of sweat are lost in just one hour of strenuous exercise. It's not always possible to drink that amount during exercise, so make sure to have enough fluid on board *before* you get going and replenish it immediately when you have finished. Thirst is not a reliable indicator of your fluid requirements. Most athletes only feel thirsty *after* they have lost about 2 percent of their body water—and that's a lot! So don't hold off drinking until you're thirsty. You need enough body fluid when exercising in order to deal with the heat produced by muscle activity and to maintain a stable core body temperature. Dehydration is also a threat to your vascular system, which needs fluid to function normally.

If you have been exercising continuously for more than two hours, especially in hot weather, it's vital to replenish the sodium and potassium lost in sweat. You need sodium for muscle contraction; it also helps retain the water you drink and contributes to the thirst signal that leads you to drink more. Most healthy individuals have enough sodium stores to cope with what they lose during mild to moderate exercise. I believe we overemphasize the need for extra salt in those circumstances. However, salt replacement is necessary for the mega-workout, especially in hot weather. Potassium loss is a more serious matter. Its lack can cause muscle weakness and potentially fatal cardiac rhythms, so anyone performing vigorous exercise should have extra potassium. You can get it from skim milk and fruit juice and by eating lots of fruit, particularly raisins, bananas, mangoes, tomatoes, figs, prunes, and other dried fruits. The table on page 252 lists the potassium content of foods and their caloric content per serving.

Are specialized *sports drinks* really necessary or any better than plain water? If you work out for less than an hour at a time, all you need is water and/or fruit juice. But if you're really into it and exercising steadily and strenuously for two or more hours, you do require the additional carbohydrates, sodium, and potassium present in such products as Gatorade, All Sport Lite, Power Ade, Hydro-Fuel, First Ade, and others. Despite all the advertising hype, however, I think these products are pretty much all alike, so pick the one with the taste you prefer. If you are diabetic, pay attention to the sugar in these drinks; some people with high blood pressure need to watch their salt intake too, and these drinks have plenty. In both cases, check with your doctor about how much is safe for you to drink and when.

About three to four hours before takeoff, eat about 500 calories' worth of complex carbohydrates—for example, 3 cups of pasta or a large bagel (see the table on page 69). Then, just before you start competing, *drink* 400 to 500 calories' worth of fruit juice, which is low in protein, fat, and fiber. Replace lost fluids *before* you feel thirsty, and continue to do so even after your thirst is quenched. As I mentioned earlier, thirst is not a reliable indicator of the body's fluid needs. On the run, I recommend an 8-ounce glass of a commercial solution every twenty minutes—and drink it cold. It's better absorbed that way. It goes without saying that you should avoid iced tea, coffee, or anything with caffeine that will increase your heart rate. Do not drink carbonated beverages either, because they fill you up quickly and cause bloating.

We tend to focus on what the athlete should consume before and during vigorous exercise. However, what you eat when the event is over is also very important. That's because high-intensity exercise raises your metabolic rate, and you continue to burn extra calories after you've finished exercising, a phenomenon called "afterburn." This excess oxygen consumption can continue for several hours after your workout has ended. Remember too that the glycogen stores I referred to earlier are also depleted by a strenuous workout and need to be replenished. You really require those extra carbohydrates, and the best time to eat them, especially if you're concerned about putting on weight, is after you've finished your workout. So when the event is over and while you are waiting to receive your medal, trophy, or certificate, start eating between 1 and 2 grams of carbohydrates per pound of body weight every two hours for six hours. If you weigh 145 pounds, that means anywhere from 150 to 300 grams every two hours. Avoid high-fiber foods such as whole-grain bread, pasta, and fruit at this time because they slow the emptying of the stomach.

Athletes are suckers for muscle-building aids. Anabolic steroids such as testosterone that do increase muscle mass are universally forbidden—not to mention dangerous and illegal—and many a champion has been disqualified after analyses of blood and urine have exposed their use. Are there any effective, safe, and legal substitutes for these steroids? Chromium picolinate is alleged by some to increase body muscle mass. I am not aware of any proof for that claim, and more than 200 to 250 micrograms of chromium a day can cause anemia. There is no proof either that gamma-orycanol, derived from rice bran oil, builds muscles. L-carnitine, a combination of two amino acids, is widely used by athletes because it allegedly spares glycogen, so it's not depleted as quickly. This purported effect needs more research and I cannot recommend it at this time. I have not been able to find any convincing evidence that Imocine, derived from plants, is an effective anabolic steroid substitute either. Finally, branched-chain amino acids (leucine, valine, and isoleucine) are said to strengthen athletes' muscles. Proteins consist of amino acids, and the branched chains are the smaller molecules among them. The theory behind their use is that they are more easily absorbed than the more complex proteins because of their smaller size. Also, unlike other amino acids, the branched chains act entirely within the muscles. There is active research in this particular area, and it may turn out to be promising, but on the basis of the present evidence, I do not believe that normal people require these branched-chain amino acids. However, if you have an absorption problem because you've had part of your stomach removed, or you have some disease of the intestine causing impaired absorption of nutrients, you may find them helpful.

Exercise, in the right amount, at the right time, and tailored for *you,* is not only good, but necessary. Certain disorders and disabilities require special attention, so work with your doctor to develop your exercise prescription. For example, if you are diabetic, the best time to exercise is one or two hours after you've eaten, because that's when your blood sugar is highest. Since exercise lowers blood sugar for as long as eight hours after you've finished, exertion can result in a low blood sugar level unless you have been calorie fortified. If you must exercise in the morning or three to four hours after you have eaten, check your blood sugar level before you start. (Most diabetics have small, easy-to-use portable devices to measure their blood sugar.) If your sugar level is less than 100 milligrams, eat 30 grams of carbohydrate before you set out (two slices of bread will do it). *And remember always to carry sugar cubes or packets with you to abort the early symptoms of hypoglycemia.* While you're running, leaping, jumping, swimming, or whatever it is you're doing, you'll need carbohydrates to prevent your blood sugar from dropping too low. The amount necessary will vary with the intensity of the exertion—as much as 50 grams per hour for a really tough and prolonged athletic event.

The key to adequate nutrition for power athletes is eating and storing food rich in energy and available quickly. Carbohydrates fit that bill, along with a "touch" of protein and fat, and adequate fluid replacement. The benefit from vitamin supplements and anabolic steroid substitutes is largely wishful thinking.

SAMPLE MENU FOR POWER ATHLETES
(ABOUT 500 GRAMS CARBOHYDRATE)

FOOD	PORTION	CARBOHYDRATE (gm)	CALORIES
Breakfast			
Special K cereal	2⅔ cups	42.6	220
Skim milk	1 cup	12	90
Banana	1 medium	30	228
Snack			
Bagel	1 large (6 ounce)	120	480
Jelly	1 tablespoon	15	60
Lunch			
Pasta, cooked	3 cups	120	480
Tomatoes, stewed	½ cup	8.3	34
Zucchini, steamed	1 cup	10	50
Snack			
Yogurt, nonfat with fruit	8 ounces	31	150
Dinner			
Grilled chicken breast, skinless	6 ounces	0	300
Olive oil, for brushing chicken	1 tablespoon	0	125
White rice, cooked	2 cups	86.6	398
Carrots, steamed	1 cup	10	50
Snack			
Fruit juice	3 cups	90	360
Fruit cup:			
banana	½ small	15	60
nectarine	1 small	15	60
blueberries	¾ cup	15	60
		620.5	3,205

GOOD SOURCES OF COMPLEX CARBOHYDRATES

FOOD	PORTION	CARBOHYDRATE (gm)	CALORIES
Bagel	1 large (6 ounces)	120	480
Bread, white or whole wheat	1 slice	15	80
Chickpeas	1 cup	90	538
Corn	1 cup	41.2	178
Macaroni, cooked	1 cup	39.7	197
Pasta, uncooked	2 ounces	41.8	210
Peas	1 cup	21.4	118
Potato, baked with skin	1 medium	51	220
Rice			
brown, cooked	1 cup	44.8	216
white	1 cup	43.3	199

CANCER

A TALE OF FAT, FIBER,
VITAMINS, AND HEREDITY

The other day one of my patients, several of whose relatives had died of cancer, asked me what she, her family, and her children could do to minimize their own vulnerability. After I reviewed with her the list of known risk factors for malignancy, she was discouraged. "The bottom line, as I see it," she said, "is that just being alive causes cancer. Anything I wear, drink, eat, breathe, and do can apparently give it to me!" She was wrong! While it is true that your genetic makeup; the pollution of air, water, and food; excessive alcohol and tobacco use; solar radiation; a host of chemicals; and certain infections all increase your risk of cancer, there is a lot you *can* do to prevent it.

About 30 percent of all cancers in America are associated with tobacco use; 4 percent are related to exposure to industrial carcinogens (a carcinogen is a substance with cancer-producing potential) such as asbestos, radon, and aromatic amines; compounds used in the manufacture of dyes; benzopyrines; irradiation; and chemicals needed in the rubber and leather industries, in paint manufacturing, printing, metalworking, and hairdressing. Three percent of cancers are the consequence of excessive intake of alcohol (cancer of the mouth, tongue, and esophagus, especially when combined with tobacco, as well as cancer of the liver); 2 percent are associated with pollution. Medications, among them various hormones such as estrogen and testosterone, as well as immunosuppressants and X rays, may contribute to the development of some cancers too.

There is considerable evidence to suggest that at least one third of all malignancies are related to what you eat. If we were to increase our intake of fiber and complex carbohydrates, and drastically reduce the amount of fat we consume, the incidence of cancer in this country would surely decline substantially. It's never too late to change your eating habits, even *after* you have cancer. Although diet at this late stage will not cure you, it may help prevent a second malignancy.

The advice of the American Cancer Society (ACS) remains the last word in the dietary approach to the prevention of cancer as we understand it today. In a twelve-year study by the ACS, being more than 40 percent overweight is associated with a significantly increased incidence of cancer of the uterus, gallbladder, kidney, stomach, colon, and breast. Their general recommendations, on which I elaborate below, stress a diet low in fat and high in fiber, with emphasis on an increased intake of fruits and vegetables, a reduction in the consumption of salt-cured, smoked, and nitrite-cured foods, and moderation in alcohol consumption.

According to the ACS, about 15 percent of your daily calories should come from protein, 20 to 25 percent from fat, and the remaining 60 percent from carbohydrate. Your diet should contain no more than 200 milligrams of cholesterol daily, and anywhere between 35 and 50 grams of fiber. Such a diet is nutritious and satisfying, helps control your weight, is varied, and you can easily follow it for a lifetime.

In devising a diet based on these guidelines, you must first determine *your* caloric needs. Here's a simple way to do it. Allow 10 calories per pound of your ideal weight as your basic requirement. Now refine it further in terms of your particular level of physical activity. If you're a couch potato and lead a sedentary life, add an extra 3 calories per pound; if you're moderately active, increase it by another 5 calories per pound; if you really are the strenuous, physical type, allow 10 more calories per pound. According to these guidelines, someone who weighs 175 pounds and is moderately active should consume the basic 10 calories plus an additional 5, making a total of 15 calories per pound or 2,625 calories per day. To calculate 25 percent of calories from fat, you should know that every gram of fat, when utilized, yields 9 calories, while protein and carbohydrate each have only 4 calories per gram. So if your total daily intake is 1,800 calories, 25 percent is 450 calories. Dividing by 9, the number of calories per gram of fat, yields 50 grams—your daily fat allowance. Calculating the same way will tell you that 20 percent protein amounts to 90 grams, and 55 percent carbohydrate requires an intake of 248 grams.

Now that you have determined the number of grams you're allowed in each food group, you need to know how many grams different foods contain, as well as their portion sizes. This allows you to play the game of food substitution, at which diabetics in particular must be proficient. This information is available from The American Diabetes Association by writing to them at 1660 Duke St., Alexandria, VA 22314, or by phoning (800) ADA-DISC. Their pamphlet will tell you, for example, that 1 teaspoon of olive or canola oil, or mayonnaise, contains 5 grams of fat, as do ten small olives or five large ones; that 1 ounce of *lean* protein such as skinned chicken or turkey, or fish canned in water, contains 3 grams of fat and 7 grams of protein. You can also write to the U.S. Department of Agriculture for Handbook #8, which contains extensive information on the composition of foods. Their address is Department of Agriculture, Agriculture Research Service, Human Nutrition Information Staff, 6505 Belcrest Road, Room 315, Hyattsville, MD 20782.

Doctors used to think that only saturated (animal) fat was bad for you. Indeed, not so many years ago, heart specialists were recommending that we eat large amounts of polyunsaturated fat, derived from vegetables, to prevent heart disease. We now know that such a diet appears to be linked with an increased incidence of cancer. Excessive intake of *any* fat raises the risk of colon and prostate cancer. The exception to that statement may be omega-3, the kind of fat present in fish, which has recently been found to have antitumor properties. (See page 221 for food sources of omega-3.)

To reduce your fat intake, you should avoid fatty meats; substitute skim (nonfat) or low-fat milk for whole milk; and omit butter, whole milk, cheese, and other whole-milk dairy products, cooking fats, and oils from your diet. Dairy products are rich in calcium, but you can get all you need by using nonfat milk products or by taking calcium supplements. (In fact, skim milk contains even more calcium than whole milk.) In the last few years, there has been an explosion of low-fat and nonfat dairy products, including yogurt, sour cream, cheese, and butter substitutes, as well as cakes, cookies, salad dressings, mayonnaise, and frozen entrees. It's all out there—by Kraft, Entenmann, Pritikin, Pfeiffer, Hellmann's, Nabisco, and many, many others. All you have to do is visit your supermarket and read the labels.

Perhaps the most important ACS recommendation is to eat more *high-fiber* foods (see page 116)—at least six servings a day of whole grains, which are present in whole-wheat bread or pita, macaroni, and brown rice, as well as in cereals such as corn and bran flakes. Substitute whole-grain bread for white, and use whole-grain flour in your baking recipes. You can add to the variety of your fiber intake with foods such as air-popped popcorn, baked potato with its skin included, and chickpeas (which, incidentally, make a wonderful salad). Have a high-fiber cereal at breakfast. There are many available, but if you really want a whopping amount of fiber in one sitting, 13 grams per ounce, try Fiber One. A serving of ½ cup contains only 60 calories. The key to tolerating all the fiber you need is to increase the amount you eat gradually. Unless you do, the gas will float you away like a helium balloon! The cramps won't be fun, either. And unless you drink at least eight glasses of water, you may find yourself constipated despite all the fiber!

You should have at least five servings of fruit and vegetables every day. For example, eat a salad or two daily, with different fat-free dressings. Or have some dried fruit as a snack or for dessert—ten dates contain almost 5 grams of fiber; five figs have 9; and five prunes will net you 3. Gradually increase the number of these servings every two weeks until you're getting enough. The fruit and vegetables should be fresh, thoroughly washed, and with their skin intact. It's best to eat them raw. Cooking should be minimal—lightly steamed, braised in water, nonfat broth, or wine (not sautéed in oil), or microwaved. Focus on green and deep yellow fruits and vegetables rich in beta-carotene and vitamin C (e.g., carrots, tomatoes, spinach, yams, winter squash, broccoli, apricots, peaches, and cantaloupe). Beta-carotene, an antioxidant in food that is converted to vitamin A in the body, may, in its natural form, reduce the incidence of cancer of the larynx, esophagus, and lungs. In a recent Harvard study, a daily intake of 25,000 IU of beta-carotene lowered the rate of heart disease as well.

(The table on page 89 contains a list of beta-carotene-rich foods.) Try to get all your vitamins from food whenever possible, and don't take extra vitamin A in supplement form for this purpose because of its potential toxicity. A diet high in vitamin E may reduce the incidence of stomach and esophageal cancer by inhibiting the formation of a potent carcinogen, nitrosamine, in the stomach.

Cruciferous vegetables are plants that have flowers with four petals. The best-known examples are cabbage, broccoli, brussels sprouts, and cauliflower. There is a new hybrid variety called brocci-flower, which is a paler green than broccoli—it looks almost like cauliflower—and has a very pleasant taste. (I wonder whether former President Bush has tried it.) Cruciferous vegetables contain several natural cancer inhibitors that lower the risk of gastrointestinal and respiratory tract malignancies. In some experiments, animals fed a diet rich in these vegetables and then given cancer-producing chemicals did not develop malignancies.

Too much *alcohol* can lead to cirrhosis (scarring) of the liver, which occasionally progresses to liver cancer. Concomitant heavy drinking and smoking pose a special risk of cancer of the oral cavity, larynx, and esophagus as well. Alcoholics are also prone to malnutrition, which can increase vulnerability to malignant disease. Alcohol is a source of hidden calories, with every gram yielding 7 calories, almost as much as the 9 calories per gram in fat, and contains no nutrients.

Avoid eating *salt-cured, smoked, or nitrite-cured foods* on a regular basis because of their documented link to stomach cancer. The meat industry and the U.S. Department of Agriculture have already reduced the permissible amounts of nitrites in prepared meats. In this country, liquid smoke, which is less hazardous than traditional methods of smoking because it absorbs fewer cancer-causing tars, is already widely used in the preparation of ham, smoked fish, and sausages. In countries where large amounts of salt-cured or pickled foods are eaten (Japan is a good example), the incidence of cancer of the stomach and esophagus is much higher. A high-fiber diet, especially one rich in vitamin C (see page 105), may offer some protection against the carcinogenic nitrosamines in these foods.

These dietary recommendations may help decrease your risk of cancer. You should also know that researchers at the Roswell Park

Cancer Institute in Rochester, New York, found that people who drink at least 1 cup of low-fat milk (but not whole milk) every day have less cancer of the lung, cervix, mouth, rectum, and stomach. Following are more specific considerations related to particular malignancies.

LUNG CANCER: TOBACCO'S REVENGE

In 1984, cancer of the lung surpassed colorectal cancer as the leading malignancy in the United States (excluding skin cancers) and remains in the lead. One-third of all cancer deaths in men are due to lung malignancy. Cigarette smokers are at ten times the risk of developing lung cancer than nonsmokers; among those who use two or more packs a day, that risk increases fiftyfold! Your risk also depends on how long you have been smoking and how deeply you inhale. Filters have very little, if any, impact on reducing the risk of lung cancer; neither does lowering tar and/or nicotine. Cancer of the lung has replaced breast cancer as the number-one cancer killer among women in America today because, while virtually every other segment of our society has drastically curtailed the use of tobacco, teenage girls are starting and continuing to smoke in alarming numbers. If all of us were to stop smoking right now, the number of new lung cancer cases in this country, presently 140,000 a year, would probably drop to 35,000 or less—a reduction of 75 percent! If the present trend continues, cancer may one day surpass heart disease as the leading cause of death in the United States, and women may lose their advantage over men in life expectancy.

Tobacco crops are treated with fertilizer rich in phosphates, which are derived from apatite rock containing substantial amounts of radioactive polonium. The latter adheres to the tobacco leaf throughout the entire manufacturing process and gets right into the cigarette. When the smoke is inhaled, these particles enter the lungs and remain there for about six months. Smokers get most of it, but so do others who happen to be nearby, inhaling what the others exhale. Nonsmokers subjected to passive (secondhand) smoke have more lung cancer than persons not so exposed. Radiation from polonium is of the alpha type, which penetrates the cells of the lungs, disrupts the DNA in the nuclei, and is more carcinogenic than the gamma and beta radiation in the environment. In two years, a thirty-cigarette-per-day smoker is exposed to an amount of radiation equivalent to 300 chest X rays!

Unfortunately, some people simply cannot or will not stop smoking, something a reformed smoker finds difficult to understand. I advise such persons (as well as anyone constantly exposed to secondhand smoke or who lives in an industrial environment with hazardous pollutants) to eat a diet rich in fruits and vegetables. Something in these foods helps keep the cells lining the respiratory passages (where many lung cancers originate) growing in an orderly way. It may also neutralize the carcinogenic effect of cigarette smoke itself, as well as the cancer-causing substances in charcoal-broiled meats and industrial wastes. Another reason for smokers to focus on fruits and vegetables is that there is less vitamin A present in the tissues of smokers than in nonsmokers. Beta-carotene, an antioxidant, maintains normal levels of vitamin A in experimental animals and may also do so in humans. If you're at high risk for lung cancer for whatever reason—because you smoke or were exposed to airborne asbestos, or work in milling, mining, textiles, insulation, or cement manufacturing, or if you had too much radiation from your dentist or doctor before its harmful effects were fully appreciated—get enough beta-carotene in your diet in the form of food, not supplements. A recent study conducted in Finland on some twenty-nine thousand smokers not only failed to show any protection from lung cancers by taking 50 milligrams of beta-carotene *supplements,* there was an 18 percent higher incidence of this malignancy. These data will need further evaluation because they are contrary to many earlier epidemiological studies. At this time, I do not advise taking beta-carotene supplements. Nor should you use vitamin A supplements or exceed the RDA of 800 micrograms RE for women and 1,000 for men. Vitamin A toxicity, with its skin, intestinal, and neurological complications, can be very disabling, but unless you're an Eskimo with a passion for polar bear liver, you'll develop it only from taking too many supplements.

CANCER OF THE COLON AND RECTUM:
WHERE DIET REALLY WORKS

I am convinced that a diet high in fiber and low in saturated fat reduces the risk of cancer of the large bowel. This malignancy is the second biggest cancer killer in men (after lung cancer), and the third in women. Some 155,000 new cases are reported each year, and 51,000 die annually from this cancer and its complications. There have been many studies, both prospective and retrospective, establishing a link between diet and colon cancer. (A "prospective" study is one in which subjects are enrolled in a research project and then monitored for a period of time. Their habits and other characteristics are recorded carefully, and at the conclusion of the study, one sees how many have died from whatever disease is being evaluated. A "retrospective" study is one in which we look back at the habits and characteristics of a group that suffers from whatever is being investigated and compare them with the same parameters in nonaffected individuals.) Virtually every study of colon cancer has shown that individuals who regularly eat fruit, vegetables, and grains, and who adhere to a diet low in saturated fat, have significantly less colon cancer. They also develop fewer polyps (benign growths that can turn malignant).

According to more recent research, taking an aspirin every second day may further reduce that risk. This protective effect may also be conferred by other aspirinlike drugs, such as the nonsteroidal anti-inflammatory agents, e.g., ibuprofen.

Calcium may also have an anticancer effect on the bowel by rendering the cells lining the colon less susceptible to malignant change. In several studies, including a fifteen-year dietary survey in Japan, persons with colorectal cancer were found to have diminished body calcium content when compared with persons without cancer. (But they also ate more sugar, carbohydrate, and fat.)

The incidence of colorectal cancer is ten times greater in industrialized countries, including the United States, than it is in third world nations, and this difference is believed to be due to diet.

What is it about fat, any fat, that predisposes you to colon cancer, and how does a high-fiber diet help prevent it? Fat may be harmful because it triggers the release of bile acids from the gallbladder and liver that promote the action of cancer-causing agents, and change the nature of the bacteria that normally reside in the gastrointestinal tract. As for fiber, there may be a protective anticancer enzyme in the various "seed" foods such as maize, beans, and rice. One such enzyme, protease inhibitor, has been isolated and is currently being studied to see if and how it protects against cancer. Many other constituents of fresh fruit such as indole-3-carbinol (I3C) and sulforaphane in vegetables and whole grains may also inhibit the formation of cancer-producing substances. Cruciferous vegetables such as cabbage, broccoli, brussels sprouts, and cauliflower are also protective, probably because of their high beta-carotene and vitamin C content, other micronutrients, and fiber content. In my opinion, antioxidants may protect against cancer too, perhaps because they prevent the cell membranes from being attacked and broken down. Finally, fiber in the diet causes the stool to be larger and bulkier and more quickly passed so that any cancer-causing substance that is present has less contact with the bowel.

Will a high-fiber diet protect you against cancer if you go on eating lots of fat too? It apparently does to some extent, if the Finns and the Danes are any example. Both consume a great deal of fat, much of which is of animal origin (at least 40 or 45 percent of total calories), but the Finns consume much more fiber—and have a significantly lower incidence of colon cancer than the Danes. But why not have the best of both worlds with low fat *and* high fiber?

Selenium is a trace mineral that has been the subject of considerable recent research. There is a higher incidence of cancer, particularly of the intestinal tract and prostate, wherever the selenium level of the soil is low. Malignancies are more common in persons who have a reduced selenium level in the blood, especially if their diet is also lacking in vitamins A and C. Laboratory animals exposed to carcinogenic substances after having been fed selenium develop fewer cancers. Dietary proteins, predominantly of animal origin, are the richest sources of selenium, but how much they actually contain will depend on the amount of selenium present in the soil and water of the environment from which they were obtained.

In summary, you should follow these specific rules, especially if colon cancer runs in your family: Reduce your intake of red meat and other foods containing animal fat; eat lots of fruits and vegetables, legumes, and fiber; make sure you're getting 1,000 milligrams or more of calcium daily; and, unless there's a reason not to do so, take an aspirin every other day. The baby size (81 milligrams), preferably enteric-coated, is enough. But remember, even if you meticulously adhere to this regimen, there is no guarantee that you will not develop colon cancer. You must continue to pay attention to the warning symptoms that can lead to its early diagnosis—blood in the stool, change of bowel habits, recent onset of constipation and diarrhea, unexplained weight loss or abdominal pain—and see your physician for regular screening examinations.

CANCER OF THE UTERUS

I don't know why there is more uterine cancer in the United States than anywhere else in the world. Women between the ages of fifty and sixty-seven are most vulnerable. I suspect that many of the risk factors responsible for other "endocrine" cancers, such as those involving the breast, prostate, and ovaries, act on the uterus too, including its neck (the cervix). For example, women who are at special risk for breast cancer also have a greater chance of developing endometrial cancer, especially if they are overweight. (The endometrium is the lining of the interior of the uterus.) Diabetics are at high risk for uterine malignancies, also probably because they are too heavy. So it would seem that your best chance of avoiding uterine cancer is to control your weight, and that's most effectively accomplished by a low-fat, high-fiber diet.

CANCER OF THE CERVIX

Endometrial (lining of the uterus) and cervical (the neck of the uterus) cancers together rank sixth in incidence in the United States. There are many risk factors for cervical cancer (which is detected by the Pap test) that have nothing to do with diet. For example, regular intercourse begun in the pre- and early teens predisposes you to it, and a virus may be the responsible agent. That is probably why genital herpes increases the likelihood of cervical cancer eightfold. What's more, components of the herpesvirus have been found in the cervical tumors themselves. The papillomavirus, which causes genital and urinary warts, and the chlamydia organism may both predispose you to cervical cancer.

Cigarette smoking is an important environmental risk factor for cervical cancer. Admittedly on theoretical grounds, I recommend a diet rich in fruits and raw vegetables to reduce the chances of that malignancy (just as I do for lung cancer), along with 500 milligrams of vitamin C daily, but that's not nearly as effective as quitting tobacco.

BREAST CANCER: HOW *MUCH* YOU EAT MAY BE MORE IMPORTANT THAN WHAT YOU EAT

The overall likelihood of an American-born woman developing breast cancer is about 10 percent. Your chances of having it increase as you get older. In addition to age, other strong risk factors are a family history of breast cancer, entering puberty earlier than, say, age thirteen, not becoming menopausal until after the fifties, and either never having a child or not until after thirty-five years of age. This malignancy is one of the most intensely studied with respect to the importance of the various risk factors mentioned above, as well as the use of estrogen-replacement therapy, fibrocystic breasts, the importance of early detection, and the role of overweight and diet.

Until quite recently, fat and fiber were believed to be as important in the development of breast cancer as they are in colorectal malignancies. However, a study at Harvard suggests otherwise. In some ninety thousand female nurses, ages thirty-four to fifty-nine, who were first evaluated in 1980 and followed up for eight years, there was no apparent relationship between fat intake and breast cancer. Nor was any protection by fiber demonstrated. I am troubled by this study and am not yet prepared to accept its conclusions. I continue to believe that a low-fat diet protects against breast cancer, although perhaps not as much as originally thought. The problem with the Harvard study is that the subjects were mostly white and belonged to a fairly uniform socioeconomic group. Those on so-called low-fat diets nevertheless obtained 27 percent of their calories from fat. That's not very low. I believe that additional studies with greater restriction of dietary fat are needed to clarify this vital question. In the meantime, I urge all women to continue eating a low-fat, high-fiber diet even if only to protect themselves against colon cancer!

Here's what you can do to minimize your risk for breast cancer. Eat plenty of fruit and vegetables. Lose weight if you need to because overweight increases your risk. If you gain ten pounds at age thirty, your chances of developing breast cancer go up by 23 percent; an extra fifteen pounds raises that figure to 37 percent; and a twenty-pound weight gain is associated with a 52 percent increased risk. If you've already had cancer in one breast, and were overweight at the time it was detected, the recurrence rate ten years later is greater than if your weight was normal. So whether you are at risk for cancer or have already developed it, it's wise to maintain your ideal weight. Tall, postmenopausal women who are heavy have more breast cancer. You can't reduce your height, but you can lose weight!

Despite earlier detection and better treatment, the number of breast cancer deaths remains essentially unchanged. It's such a bad and common malignancy that I grasp at any straw that may conceivably protect my patients. Because geographic areas where the soil is selenium poor have a high breast cancer rate, I recommend that women who are at special risk because their mothers, sisters, aunts, or daughters had breast cancer take a daily multivitamin containing selenium.

There is no evidence to implicate *methylxanthines* found in caffeine (present in coffee, tea, some cola drinks, and chocolates, as well as certain antacids, painkillers, and cold remedies), in the causation of any form of cancer. But I still advise limiting coffee intake to three cups a day and no more than one or two drinks of alcohol daily. Some researchers believe that alcohol increases the risk of cancer somewhat, probably by raising the estrogen level in the body. That's something to bear in mind, especially if you are genetically vulnerable to this malignancy. I also recommend dietary antioxidants from natural sources across the board—beta-carotene, vitamin C, and vitamin E—to anyone vulnerable to *any* kind of cancer, including breast cancer, despite the absence of proof that they are protective.

PROSTATE CANCER: BACK TO THE CULPRITS (FAT AND MEAT)

There are some eighty thousand cases of prostate cancer diagnosed every year, making it the fourth most common malignancy overall. It's a disease of older men, and the incidence increases with age. Blacks are more likely to have it than whites, and it beats me why, but married men are more vulnerable than bachelors. If your father had prostate cancer, you're at twice the risk of developing it yourself. If a brother also had this tumor, your risk is now three times greater than normal. The closer the blood relatives in your immediate family (brothers, uncles, grandfathers) with prostate cancer, the higher your own vulnerability.

The routine use of the prostate specific antigen (PSA) test, together with regular digital rectal examinations, has skyrocketed the number of prostate cancers detected in their early stages. I believe that both these tests should be done every year on every man over the age of fifty, even though some of my "cost-conscious" colleagues say it's "overkill." Failure to do so, in my experience, is "underkill"! I've also noticed that some patients prefer not to have a digital rectal exam. "Just the PSA, please," is what I now frequently hear. The other day my finger detected the second early prostate cancer in as many months even though the PSA was normal! The PSA can be inaccurate when the cancer is very small. So if you're going to do it, do it right—with both the rectal exam *and* the PSA. But don't panic if the PSA is a little high. Benign enlargement of the prostate without any cancer can cause an elevated reading.

Can what you eat or not eat help prevent prostate cancer? A link has definitely been established between a high-fat diet, increased protein intake, and prostate cancer. Fat, especially in whole milk and whole milk products such as ice cream, may predispose you to this malignancy, possibly by raising the level of the male hormone, testosterone, on which the prostate depends for its growth and development. Blacks, whose testosterone level is generally higher than whites, also have more prostate cancer. It's worth noting too that testosterone levels are raised following vasectomy, which every now and then is speculated to contribute to prostate cancer. Meat eaters have two and a half times the incidence of prostate cancer than do vegetarians. Men with high dietary levels of alphalinoleic acid, a component of polyunsaturated fat, have almost three and a half times more prostate cancer. These fatty acids are present only in meat, dairy products, and some vegetable oils. Finally, in an attempt to understand why the incidence of prostate cancer is so much lower in Japan than in the Western world, researchers have been studying various components of the Japanese diet in great detail. Their findings to date suggest that a substance (genisten) present in soybeans, soy meal, and tofu, all of which are consumed in large amounts in Japan, may protect against this malignancy. Genisten has estrogenlike properties that may inhibit the growth of prostatic cancer early in its development. So skip the ice cream and feast on tofu! The Japanese also eat much less fat than Americans, but in the past ten to twenty years, the fat content of their diet has been increasing—and so has the prevalence of prostate cancer!

BLADDER AND KIDNEY CANCER: TOBACCO AGAIN!

There are about sixty thousand cases of these malignancies reported every year—two thirds are bladder cancers, the rest involve other parts of the urinary tract. Cancer of the bladder is primarily a disease of men; only a third of the cases occur in women. It's two to three times more common in smokers than nonsmokers, so that 40 percent of cases in males and 30 percent in females are clearly due to cigarettes. I suspect that nicotine and its by-products, one or more of which are carcinogenic, reach the bladder (and cervix, too—since there is a higher incidence of cervical cancer among women who smoke).

Is there a dietary link to bladder cancer? Remember the fuss when artificial sweeteners in high doses were shown to cause bladder cancer in laboratory animals? As a result, cyclamates were removed from the market in the United States in 1969. (They are still available elsewhere in the world.) An attempt was made to withdraw saccharin too, but the FDA bowed to public opinion and allowed it to be sold, albeit with a warning label about its cancer-producing potential. Saccharin is available but cyclamates are not, even though the evidence against saccharin, such as it is, is more convincing, theoretically, than that against cyclamates! (Aspartame has never been implicated in bladder cancer, even remotely.) Because tea and coffee are diuretics and make you "go" more frequently, a possible carcinogenic effect on the urinary bladder has been suggested. I could find no convincing evidence in the literature that this is so.

Cigarettes are the single most important cause of *kidney cancer*! Thirty percent of these malignancies in men and 20 percent in women are directly due to tobacco, and smokers are twice as likely to develop it as are nonsmokers. As with breast cancer, extra weight is also a factor in women (although not a strong one), perhaps because of the high estrogen levels present in fatty tissue. Here too I believe that smokers should follow a low-fat, high-fiber diet rich in fruit and raw vegetables.

CANCER OF THE MOUTH AND THROAT: THE EVIL WEED

Tumors of the mouth and throat are more than twice as common in men as they are in women, and 90 percent of them develop after age forty-five. The chief offender is tobacco—chewed, dipped (as with snuff), and smoked. In India, 75 percent of these oral malignancies occur in people who chew a mixture of betel nuts, betel leaves, tobacco, and lime. Women in the southern United States who put snuff in their cheeks also have a high rate of mouth cancer. If you smoke more than a pack of cigarettes a day, your chances of having throat cancer are six times greater than those of a nonsmoker. Pipes cause more cancer of the lip, perhaps because of the heat they generate and the pressure of the stem, especially one that is curved. (Sherlock Holmes, however, did not die of lip cancer.) Alcohol alone doubles the risk of cancer of the mouth and throat, but if you smoke *and* drink, you are at fifteen times the risk—even if you have only one cocktail a day, but smoke forty or more cigarettes.

Then there is the *mouthwash* phenomenon. Women who neither smoke nor drink, but who use a mouthwash daily, are at some increased risk for cancer of the mouth. I have no idea why this is so or why the observation has not also been made in men.

The amount and type of fat, protein, and carbohydrates you eat also have a relationship to oral and throat cancer, as does vitamin deficiency. If you're not eating as well as you once did for whatever reason—because you're older, poorer, or can't chew well—supplement your diet with multivitamins.

CANCER OF THE PANCREAS: ONE OF THE WORST

Here's yet another relationship between cancer and cigarettes. Smokers (this time it's only cigarettes, not pipes or cigars) have twice the incidence of pancreatic cancer of nonsmokers. This suggests that the carcinogen involved is present in inhaled smoke, since most pipe or cigar smokers either do not inhale or do so less deeply than cigarette smokers. One study has also raised the possibility of a link among pancreatic cancer, heavy meat consumption, and decreased vegetable intake—the now-familiar story of high fat and low fiber—but this has not been proven.

STOMACH CANCER: BARBECUES IN JAPAN!

This serious malignancy has a five-year survival rate of only 16 percent. It occurs in greater numbers among blacks and low-income groups, and is more common in men than in women. Whereas stomach acid aggravates (but does not cause) ulcers, its *deficiency* is implicated in stomach cancer.

What you eat has a great deal to do with whether or not you develop stomach cancer. Its relatively low incidence and continuing decline in this country may reflect the fact that we're eating more fresh fruit and vegetables than ever before. In Japan, stomach cancer causes more deaths than all other malignancies combined and is almost six times more common than it is in the United States, presumably because of all the pickled, salted, barbecued, and smoked foods the Japanese eat. (Note that in its nutritional guidelines, the American Cancer Society advises reduced intake of these particular foods.)

People with stomach cancer share certain characteristics. Most were not in the habit of eating foods rich in vitamins C and A, which, together with other antioxidants, prevent the formation of nitrosamines in the stomach. (Nitrosamines are potent cancer-producing substances that form when nitrates—chemicals present in some water supplies, cheese, and cured meats—combine with normal bacteria in the intestinal tract.) People with stomach cancer also tend to be poor, so their diet is usually high in refined, processed starch and low in fresh fruits and vegetables. The best way, then, to beat stomach cancer is to cut down on smoked, barbecued, pickled, salted, and cured meats and fish, and eat lots of foods rich in vitamins C and A.

MALIGNANT MELANOMA: THE TANNED CORPSE

Most skin cancers, no matter how late they're found and removed, are not a threat to life. Malignant melanomas, which rank thirteenth in cancer incidence, are the exception. Their worldwide attack rate continues to rise because of our obsession with the sun. (The highest incidence is in Australia, which is near the equator where the strong solar rays are stronger.) If you have a fair complexion or are of Irish descent with red hair, the sun is your mortal enemy!

Malignant melanoma is a cancer that, unless detected early and removed completely, spreads like wildfire—and is fatal. The key to its prevention is avoiding excessive exposure to the sun; the key to its cure is early detection and surgery.

Beta-carotene may reduce the risk of malignant melanoma. So if you suffered serious sunburns as a child, or remain a sun worshiper even though you know better, eat plenty of fruit and raw vegetables— to be on the safe side.

CANCER OF THE LIVER: A STORY OF RACE, ALCOHOL, AND VIRUSES

There are in this country about fourteen thousand new cases each year of cancer that originates in the liver—mostly in elderly black males. Cancer of the liver is the leading cause of death in other areas of the world, especially some parts of Africa. Sixty to 90 percent of cases occur in persons with alcoholic cirrhosis or other late complications of either hepatitis B or alcoholism. Hepatitis B can be prevented by a vaccine, but cirrhosis and its subsequent cancer can be eliminated only by abstinence from alcohol. If you're an alcoholic on the road to cirrhosis, your best bet is to get on the wagon—fast!

In the absence of chronic blood loss, adults should rarely, if ever, take iron supplements because excessive iron deposition in the liver may be a forerunner of malignancy of that organ.

CANCER OF THE ESOPHAGUS: TOBACCO AND BOOZE

Esophageal cancer is a dreadful malignancy that strikes ten thousand victims every year. It affects mostly black males over the age of fifty-five, and urban rather than rural dwellers. It is a cancer in which lifestyle and diet are important, predisposing factors. The major risk is, as usual, tobacco, but this time not only cigarettes, but cigars and pipes as well, especially when combined with even "moderate" alcohol use (one or two drinks every day). Cancer of the esophagus affects mostly poor people whose nutrition is deficient in such vitamins as riboflavin (B_2), and vitamins A and C, as well as in iron and zinc. The best protective dietary regimen I can give you is to avoid alcohol if you're a smoker (and vice versa), eat all the beta-carotene you can in leafy green vegetables, and have lots of vitamin C—a minimum of 60 milligrams a day (the RDA), preferably from fruit or vegetables rather than from supplements.

There are, of course, many cancers to which I have not specifically referred—lymphomas, leukemias, testicular cancer, thyroid cancer, and others. But seven malignancies—lung, colon, breast, uterine, prostate, oral, and skin—account for most cancers and for more than half the deaths. These "major" players are most successfully prevented largely by changing your diet and lifestyle. Much of the confirming data are very strong; others are weak, but I have never seen any evidence that eating lots of fruits and vegetables or following a low-fat diet ever harmed a healthy, well-nourished adult. So while awaiting absolute confirmation of the dietary link to cancer, you're well advised to eat plenty of fruit, vegetables, whole-grain cereals, and dried peas and beans every day. Your dairy products should be of the nonfat variety; you should consume alcohol in moderation because of its association with cancer of the mouth, throat, esophagus, and liver. Remember that booze is high in calories but devoid of vitamins and minerals. Stop using tobacco in any form! Garlic protects laboratory animals against cancer and may do so in humans too. The same kind of bioflavonoids present in anticancer foods such as brussels sprouts and cauliflower are among the many ingredients of garlic thus far identified.

How much dietary fiber should you eat? I suggest at least 35 grams a day, but check it out with your own doctor first, especially if you have any problems with your intestinal tract. Don't be carried away when you embark on a high-fiber diet. Increase your intake gradually. Most people who eat a lot of fiber regularly pass gas liberally, but a sudden, excessive intake will also give you cramping and diarrhea. These gradually subside as you adjust to the diet. You'll know you're eating enough fiber when your stools are soft and regular, and move easily. At that point, don't increase the amount, but continue to drink six to eight glasses of water or other liquids every day. (Coffee and tea don't count because they act as diuretics, promoting loss of fluid from the body.) Whole grains such as wheat, corn, rye, oats, and bran are important sources of fiber that you can find in a variety of cereals, breads, and pasta. The refined flour used to make white bread has very little fiber. Sprinkle miller's bran over your regular cereal or put it in tomato or orange juice, starting with 2 teaspoons a day and working up to 3 tablespoons daily over a two- to three-week period. Psyllium, a soluble fiber marketed as Metamucil, Fiber-All, and several other brands, is also a convenient source of fiber. Four slices of whole wheat bread daily at 5 grams a slice will give you more than twice the daily average intake of fiber in this country. Frozen vegetables are as satisfactory as fresh ones, and if you eat apples, peaches, and potatoes with their skins, you'll get even more fiber.

A high-fiber diet is not entirely risk free. Because high-fiber foods pass through your bowels rapidly, certain vitamins, minerals, and other nutrients like zinc, iron, magnesium, and calcium may be lost in the stool. So if you're consuming very large amounts of fiber and your nutrition is poor to begin with, you may experience important deficiencies. That's what happens in rural Africa and among the elderly poor in this country. Anyone eating a very-high-fiber diet should consider taking supplemental multivitamins and minerals.

Meat eaters should have no more than 6 ounces daily of the leanest cuts of beef and pork, and should trim away all visible fat. Eat your poultry skinless. There should be lots of fish in your diet too, fresh where possible and, if frozen, without sauce. Choose canned fish packed in water, not in oil. You want lots of foods rich in vitamins, and that means the dark green, leafy variety and cruciferous vegetables—broccoli, cauliflower, brussels sprouts, and cabbage. However, other greens are good for you too. Red, yellow, and orange vegetables and fruits also reduce cancer risk because they are rich in fiber, vitamins, and minerals. (My wife makes a wonderful dish of bok choi with mustard greens, rutabagas, and turnips.)

In summary, don't be nihilistic about cancer. As with heart disease, there *are* risk factors that you can avoid. Although doing so does not guarantee protection, it will, without question, reduce your risk. The factors to reduce or eliminate are tobacco use, especially in combination with alcohol, alcohol alone in excess, exposure to the rays of the sun and radiation generally, and fat in the diet. Reduce intake across the board to no more than 20 or 25 percent of your total caloric intake, especially if you are predisposed to colon and prostate cancer (and probably breast malignancy as well). Eating a high-fiber diet adds an additional measure of protection. However, no matter how carefully you orchestrate your lifestyle, early detection and treatment are still your best bet for beating the cancer odds. And remember that giving up smoking remains the most important preventive measure you can take.

FOODS RICH IN BETA-CAROTENE*

FOOD	PORTION	BETA-CAROTENE (mg)
Apricots		
dried	15 halves	8.8
fresh	3 medium	3.5
Broccoli		
cooked	⅔ cup	1.2
uncooked	1¼ cups	0.7
Cantaloupe	⅛ medium	3.0
Carrots		
cooked	⅔ cup	9.8
uncooked	1 medium	7.9
Chanterelle mushrooms, uncooked	3.5 ounces	1.3
Dill, fresh	¾ cup	2.3
Grapefruit, pink	½ medium	1.3
Leafy greens		
beet greens, cooked	⅔ cup	2.5
chicory leaf, uncooked	⅔ cup	3.4
collards, cooked	⅔ cup	5.4
endive, uncooked	⅔ cup	1.3
kale, cooked	⅔ cup	4.7
lettuce		
leaf lettuce	2 cups	1.2
romaine	2 cups	1.9
mustard greens	⅔ cup	2.7
spinach		
cooked, fresh or frozen	½ cup	5.5
uncooked	1¾ cups	4.1
Swiss chard, uncooked	½ cup	3.6
Mango	½ small	1.3
Parsley, fresh	¾ cup	2.7

FOODS RICH IN BETA-CAROTENE* *(Continued)*

FOOD	PORTION	BETA-CAROTENE (mg)
Peaches, dried	7 to 8 halves	9.2
Pumpkin	3.5 ounces	3.1
Red bell pepper	1 medium	2.2
Sweet potato, cooked	½ cup	8.8
Tomato juice, canned	3.5 ounces	0.9
Tomato paste, canned	½ cup	1.7
Tomato sauce, canned	3.5 ounces	1.0
Winter squash, cooked	½ cup	2.4

*Note: To calculate how many milligrams (mg) of beta-carotene you need to reach your RDA of vitamin A (in IU), multiply the amount of vitamin A (say, 5,000 IU) by .6. This will give you the number of micrograms (mcg) of beta-carotene. Then divide that number by 1,000 (because 1,000 mcg = 1 mg). For example,

5,000 IU vitamin A × .6 = 3,000 mcg beta-carotene

3,000 ÷ 1,000 = 3 mg beta-carotene.

So, you would need to consume 3 milligrams of beta-carotene to get 5,000 IU of vitamin A.

CARPAL TUNNEL SYNDROME

VITAMINS

FOR A PAINFUL WRIST

When you have carpal tunnel syndrome (CTS), your median nerve, one of three that supplies the hand, is "pinched." As a result, the thumb and middle three fingers tingle, feel numb, and hurt. Your wrist and forearm may also be painful. The most common cause of CTS is a mechanical one—the result of chronic, repetitive motion and overuse of the hands or wrists—so you're a candidate if you are a typist, computer operator, butcher, carpenter, or store cashier. Tissues surrounding the median nerve become irritated and swollen, and impinge upon it. Carpal tunnel syndrome was much less common among typists when the manual typewriter was still being used. The keys on modern computers and word processors are so much easier to depress that your fingers move much faster, and you don't have even the momentary relief of returning the carriage at the end of each line.

The median nerve can also be affected by several *nonmechanical* conditions. For example, when the immune system is not functioning properly, as occurs in people with rheumatoid arthritis, tendons and ligaments surrounding the nerve swell and compress it; low thyroid function causes retention of fluid, engorging the structures that surround the median nerve; the nerve itself may become irritated in diabetics (diabetic neuropathy), and in people undergoing kidney

dialysis. Finally, carpal tunnel syndrome may come on suddenly during pregnancy, and will often disappear soon after the baby is born.

Treatment of CTS depends on its cause. If it's due to mechanical irritation from repetitive movement, you've got to stop or change that movement, at least until the symptoms subside. You may be given a temporary splint (I have never thought they help much), or have your painful wrist injected with steroids to reduce inflammation and swelling. If the ligaments entrapping the nerve are thick and swollen, the nerve may have to be surgically released. This can now be done by new endoscopic techniques that are much simpler than the more extensive "open" operation.

If your carpal tunnel syndrome is due to an underactive thyroid gland, replacing the missing thyroid hormone will clear the symptoms. Most other nonmechanical causes respond to dietary measures. Taking 150 milligrams of supplemental B_6 daily for about four months (the RDA is only 2 milligrams per day for men and 1.6 milligrams for women) will raise your pain threshold and ease your symptoms. It does not, however, affect the underlying process, which usually runs its course during that time. You don't have to be deficient in B_6 to benefit from it. I have seen impressive, subjective response to this therapy in obviously well-nourished individuals. Although the supplemental B_6 doesn't affect the function of the involved median nerve as measured in objective tests, it still makes you feel better—and that's what really counts. Adding 100 micrograms of supplemental B_{12} daily by mouth or injection (its RDA is only 2 micrograms) may help too, but unlike B_6, its effectiveness has not been confirmed. So if you have CTS due to diabetes or other nonmechanical factors, try vitamin therapy before opting for splinting and surgery.

Why supplements and not just lots of B_6 and B_{12} in your diet? Because the amounts of these vitamins present in food is not great enough to control the pain of carpal tunnel syndrome. But if, for some reason, you're averse to taking supplements, the richest natural sources of vitamin B_6 are liver, oatmeal, bananas, rice bran, wheat germ, chicken, fish, and sunflower seeds, and there is some in avocados and meat too. (See page 364.) You can obtain lots of B_{12} in organ meats such as liver as well as fish, shellfish, muscle meats, eggs, and cheese. (See page 389.)

In most cases of carpal tunnel syndrome associated with pregnancy,

symptoms appear in the last trimester and usually clear within two weeks after the baby is born. However, CTS can also set in after the delivery, especially in women who are having their first baby in their thirties. Here, symptoms generally appear within three and a half weeks after delivery, continue for about six months, and disappear spontaneously.

In summary, if you wake up one morning with a painful hand and wrist, and the pain continues for days, see your doctor. If he or she diagnoses carpal tunnel syndrome, try 150 milligrams of vitamin B_6 a day, with or without supplemental B_{12}, before submitting to a cast, injections, or surgery of any kind. This is especially important to remember if you are diabetic, or do not use your hands every day in hours of repetitive functions. Anti-inflammatory drugs such as ibuprofen will also provide at least temporary relief. Remember, however, that doses of vitamin B_6 higher than the recommended 150 milligrams per day may have a toxic effect on the nerves (neuropathy), causing generalized body pain. If you're pregnant, check with your doctor before taking these (or any) vitamin supplements in high doses.

CATARACTS

WHY IT'S CLOUDY ALL DAY

As we get older, our senses become less acute; we don't hear as well; food doesn't taste quite the same; our sense of smell is not as sharp as it once was; and we need stronger and stronger eyeglass lenses to see and read. The most common cause of impaired vision in otherwise healthy older persons is cataracts—but what you eat *can* prevent or delay their development.

The lens of your eye functions very much like the one in your camera. You can wipe dirt and dust from the latter, but not from the lens in your eye. You'll know you're "growing" cataracts when cleaning your glasses or changing their prescription doesn't make the newspaper print any sharper, and you still keep rubbing your eyes trying to make what you're looking at less cloudy. (Other eye disorders can cause similar symptoms, so never diagnose a cataract yourself. See an ophthalmologist.) The human lens is made of protein and is normally sparklingly clear. As we age, it first begins to turn yellow (making some colors—especially red and blue—less bright) and eventually opaque, so that detail is lost. At this point, you're on your way to a cataract.

Your lens opacifies as a result of oxidation, a biological process

involving oxygen that is accelerated by certain of its end-products called *free radicals*. These free radicals are neutralized by a class of vitamins known as antioxidants, among which the best known are beta-carotene (a plant pigment converted to vitamin A in the body), vitamin E, and vitamin C. That being the case, it seems logical to assume that eating ample amounts of antioxidants throughout life should make you less vulnerable to cataract formation. To test this hypothesis, the diets of some fifty thousand female nurses, ages thirty-four to fifty-nine, were evaluated over a period of ten years. Those who had taken between 250 and 500 milligrams of supplemental vitamin C daily for at least ten years had a 45 percent lower incidence of cataracts.

The best way for you to act on this information is to have plenty of vitamin C in your diet throughout life. Its richest sources are acerola cherries, citrus fruits, vitamin C–fortified juice (raw, frozen, or canned), and leafy green vegetables. Over 90 percent of the vitamin C in our diet comes from citrus fruits and vegetables. (When is the last time you ate acerola cherries?) The "average" American (whoever that may be) is said to consume about 120 milligrams of vitamin C per day. To prevent cataracts, or slow down the progress of those that have already begun to form, you'll need to more than double that amount. (The daily RDA for vitamin C is 60 milligrams for adults, 70 milligrams for pregnant women, and just under 100 milligrams for nursing mothers.) That means more orange or grapefruit juice—or supplements. Page 105 lists some common sources of vitamin C and how much they contain per serving.

Vitamin A was also found to be protective against cataracts in the Nurses' Study. The richest food sources of "preformed" vitamin A are liver, milk, eggs, and liver oils from cod and halibut. But vitamin A has some five hundred different natural constituents called carotenoids, and it's not clear which among them best prevents cataracts. We used to think it was beta-carotene, but carrots, which are among the richest sources of beta-carotene, are not as effective against cataracts as is spinach, which has more of the other carotenoids, but less beta-carotene. But from a practical point of view, I suggest you go the beta-carotene route. You'll find the best sources to be yellow, orange, or red fruits and vegetables, as well as green leafy vegetables. (The latter are green despite their beta-carotene content because of the chlorophyll they contain.) Page 89 contains a list of beta-carotene–rich foods.

Do not conclude from any of the above that you should take vitamin A supplements, too much of which can hurt you. You'll know you're in trouble when you develop headaches, a dry and itchy skin, diarrhea, nausea, blurred vision, emotional swings, yellowing of your palms and soles (but not your eyes), and when you start losing your hair. All these symptoms clear when you stop the excessive intake of vitamin A. (The RDA of vitamin A for adults used to be expressed in International Units, IUs, and was 4,000 to 5,000 such units. In 1989, however, the system was changed to retinol equivalents [RE].) Although the RDA is now officially expressed as 800 RE for women and 1,000 RE for men daily, nearly all supplemental bottle labels still use the old RDAs. To find out how milligrams of beta-carotene translate into IUs of vitamin A, see the beta-carotene table, page 89.

Beta-carotene is not toxic like vitamin A, and what's more, fruits and vegetables high in beta-carotene are also abundant in vitamin C, other vitamins, and fiber. They're also low in fat and calories. By contrast, foods rich in preformed vitamin A, such as liver and other animal organs, eggs, milk, and fish-liver oils, generally contain fat and cholesterol, and are highly caloric. Try to consume 25,000 IU of beta-carotene per day from natural food sources.

Although vitamin E, also an antioxidant, does not play a major role in the dietary prevention of cataracts, it helps keep cell membranes in the lens intact and may reduce the risk. Most people have enough vitamin E in their normal diet, and supplements are not warranted at this time for cataract prevention.

Finally, here is yet another area in which tobacco rears its ugly head. Cigarette smoking speeds up the formation of cataracts in both men and women, perhaps because it generates lots of free radicals that can damage the lens. So if you haven't quit yet, this is another good reason to do so.

In summary, the relationship between antioxidants and cataracts is still somewhat controversial. Some trials are currently under way and will hopefully clarify the issue. In the meantime, the best way to reduce your chance of developing cataracts is to make sure you consume between 250 and 500 milligrams of vitamin C per day. That's easily done by eating at least five servings of fruits and vegetables every day to include two servings of sweet potatoes, winter squash, or spinach, which are rich in vitamin A and its many carotenoid constituents. I also recommend 25,000 IU of beta-carotene daily, preferably from food. And finally, stop smoking.

CHRONIC FATIGUE SYNDROME

IT'S *NOT* ALL IN YOUR HEAD!

Is there really such an entity as Chronic Fatigue Syndrome (CFS)? If so, what causes it? Is there any treatment? These fundamental questions about a common and troublesome group of symptoms remain unanswered and are the source of an ongoing, often acrimonious controversy among patients and doctors alike.

If you have the constellation of complaints characterized as CFS, chances are that you're under forty years of age and previously enjoyed good health. Then, you got the "flu" or a bad cold that you weren't able to shake, that continued for weeks or months on end. You remain exhausted even after a good night's sleep; you often lack the energy or drive to get out of bed in the morning; you have trouble concentrating; the slightest task is too much for you; you may run a low-grade fever from time to time, usually under 100 degrees F; your throat is occasionally sore and the glands in your neck are tender; you don't have much of an appetite; and you're depressed. You tell your doctor how bad you feel; he or she examines you from head to toe and comes up with nothing. Even at the height of your symptoms, the physical exam and all the routine blood tests are completely normal! The next thing you know, you are being asked seemingly irrelevant questions about your love life, or how things are going at work and at home.

You have the feeling that your doctor thinks this is all in your head, and that maybe you should see a shrink. You're right. That's how most physicians react to such patients!

Until quite recently, I wasn't at all sure that CFS was a "real" disease. Given the normal workup, I concluded that most of these people were probably stressed, depressed, and anxious, and that their physical symptoms were of psychological origin. Other physicians, groping for clues, have implicated the Epstein-Barr virus (EBV) because its antibodies are often present in the blood of these individuals. Since EBV causes infectious mononucleosis, these doctors conclude that CFS is caused by the reactivation of that viral infection.

The EBV theory and the measures taken to "treat" it by fad therapists (expensive intravenous megavitamin therapy) have little or no support among most "establishment" physicians. EBV antibodies are only a *marker* of previous mononucleosis infection and are present in the blood of more than 90 percent of all Americans! In my opinion, there is no way to justify giving megavitamins by vein at exorbitant cost to these people.

Although I do not believe that the Epstein-Barr virus is responsible for CFS, I am convinced that some as-yet-unidentified virus is. That would explain why so many people with these complaints have some subtle abnormalities in their MRIs, nuclear scans, and PET scans of the brain.

It's challenging for a doctor to treat someone with symptoms the cause of which are unknown. Here's what I do in my own practice. First, I perform a complete physical exam, followed by comprehensive blood analyses, a chest X ray, and any other tests that are appropriate. If *all* the results are normal, and I have no other explanation, I accept the diagnosis of CFS. Now here's the hard part. No physician should ever tell a patient that there is nothing to be done, and that he or she should simply go home and "wait it out"! No one who is sick—and these people are, even though we don't know why—will accept such advice anyway. Most, in their desperation, will go "doctor shopping" and end up in the "care" of some quack who rips them off (in this case, with costly intravenous megavitamins).

I reassure my patients with CFS that their symptoms are probably due to a viral infection and that the best and safest treatment is sound, *oral* nutrition. I prescribe a generous intake of protein—approximately

one half gram for every pound of body weight, provided that they
have normal kidney function. (One does not want to burden a sick
kidney with an extra protein load that it cannot handle.) That adds up
to about 80 grams a day for a 180-pound man, which you can consume by eating 10 to 12 ounces of lean, skinless chicken, turkey, or
fish. (A woman who weighs 135 pounds should have 60 grams or 8
ounces of lean protein.) Egg whites are an excellent source of high-
quality protein without fat, and they make tasty yolk-free omelets.
Your diet should also contain three or four servings of fresh fruit daily
and four or five servings of fresh vegetables (steamed or in salads) as
well as 2 or 3 cups of skim milk or nonfat yogurt. Your remaining
calories should come from such complex carbohydrates as pasta,
potatoes, and whole-grain breads. Limit your intake of oil and fat,
most of which should be monounsaturated (olive or canola oil). On
theoretical grounds, I recommend multivitamin supplements because
of their vitamin B complex content, as well as the trace metals and
minerals, such as magnesium and zinc that they contain. The supplement should meet 100 percent of the RDA (virtually all of them do),
and contain no added sugar, salt, or chemical additives. Check the
label to make sure of that. If you're taking vitamins, always do so
during or immediately after a meal to enhance their absorption. Also,
although I am not aware of any proof of their efficacy in people with
CFS, I prescribe 1,000 milligrams of vitamin C and 400 IU of vitamin
E—in the hope of strengthening the immune system and enhancing
resistance. Yes, it's the same shotgun vitamin therapy as the intravenous route that I decry, but unlike the latter, it won't put you in the
poorhouse or subject you to the risk of a vitamin overdose.

Other doctors recommend 1 gram of omega-3 fatty acid supplements a day because fish oil reduces inflammation and may, at least
theoretically, have some beneficial effect. If that concept appeals to
you, I suggest that you get your omega-3 from natural fish sources—
mackerel, salmon, tuna, whitefish, bluefish, anchovies, and herring.
(See the table on page 221.)

There has been a great deal written by practitioners of alternative
medicine about the "yeast connection" to CFS. In their view, *Candida*
is the culprit, and they prescribe a diet low in yeast and drugs to
eliminate this organism. I am not convinced by any evidence that this
is so, but frankly, I have no better explanation.

Chronic Fatigue Syndrome is real; don't let anyone convince you otherwise. Unfortunately, the only "treatment" that makes any sense, given how little we know about it, is a nutritious diet and oral vitamin supplements. Time and nature will eventually heal you. Don't waste your time and money on exotic and useless intravenous megavitamins.

THE COMMON COLD

WHAT, IF NOT VITAMIN C?

During the winter months, someone—my wife, children, friends, or patients—asks me almost every day what to do about a nagging cold. I tell him or her not to take antihistamines. They're good for allergies, but can make your nose even more stuffy and aggravate your cough if you have a cold. You're better off taking a cough suppressant if you need one (most over-the-counter preparations are effective), and an oral decongestant such as pseudoephedrine or phenylephrine. Nose drops or sprays are helpful too, but if you take them for more than three or four consecutive days, their "rebound" effect can leave your nose stuffier than ever. For relief of aches and pains, I prefer a non-steroidal anti-inflammatory drug such as ibuprofen (Motrin) over acetaminophen (Tylenol) or aspirin, the latter two of which may spread a cold by promoting shedding of the virus that causes it. Like most doctors, I used to advise steam or cold mist inhalations to relieve nasal congestion, but was chagrined to read the other day that they are of no use whatsoever for that purpose. Still, if you think they help you, there's no harm in using them, provided the water inside the humidifier is clean.

Colds are the most common infections of man, but no medical text I've ever read tells you what (or what not) to eat or drink when you have one—whether to feed a cold or to starve it. Your doctor's advice is likely to be based on his or her personal experience (and bias) rather than on scientific reports. Here are some of my own personal preferences and observations.

Diet, other than what you feel like eating, has very little effect on the symptoms, severity, or duration of your cold. However, chili peppers may relieve nasal stuffiness. Large quantities of fluid, especially fruit juice (assuming you have no other illness such as diabetes, kidney trouble, or heart failure that might preclude your doing so), helps liquefy the secretions in your nose and respiratory passages.

The argument about whether vitamin C is a useful treatment for the common cold continues to rage, notwithstanding the volumes of testimony and "evidence," pro and con. The world is full of experts on this question. They range from anyone who has ever had a sniffle, to the late Dr. Linus Pauling, multiple winner of the Nobel Prize in medicine. Despite the public controversy, several of my colleagues and patients do take extra vitamin C themselves, either overtly or secretly, when they have a cold or feel one coming on. That's either because Linus Pauling was its chief proponent, or because large doses of vitamin C are rarely, if ever, seriously toxic, although megadoses can cause diarrhea.

I have reviewed the major research reports concerning the effect of vitamin C on the common cold published during the last twenty years. There are a few that claim it can shorten the duration and severity of symptoms, but for every such positive report, there are twenty that conclude it is ineffective. So I compromise by telling my patients to get extra vitamin C—from food. The table on page 105 lists the most common sources of vitamin C and its content per portion. Acerola cherries have far and away the most—1,600 milligrams per cup—but yellow peppers and papaya also have an abundance, and are much less expensive. If you have a cold, drink lots of citrus fruit juice (orange or grapefruit), which naturally contains about 15 milligrams of vitamin C per ounce, but is often fortified with extra amounts. Remember that vitamin C is easily destroyed by cooking and leaches out into cooking water, so you're better off eating your fruit and vegetables raw. If you add sodium bicarbonate while cooking vegetables to preserve their color, you will significantly reduce their vitamin C content.

The Pauling "lobby" claims that researchers who did not find vitamin C effective were simply not giving their subjects enough of it. They recommend 4,000 milligrams daily to *prevent* a cold, and several times that amount if you've actually got one! Other C enthusiasts go even further, asserting there is no upper limit, and that you should take all you can until you develop diarrhea, then back off! Most physicians, even those who take some vitamin C themselves, do not go nearly that far, and recommend a limit of 2,000 milligrams daily. If you are persuaded that vitamin C will help your cold, take whatever amount you've decided on in *divided* doses during the day to minimize the likelihood of stomach irritation. Fortunately, vitamin C is water soluble and not retained by the body even when consumed in huge quantities. Whatever your body can't use is excreted in the urine. Maybe that's the reason so many of my patients have told me that taking high doses of vitamin C makes them void frequently, and keeps them from sleeping well at night.

I am not impressed by the claims made for zinc lozenges in the treatment of the common cold.

Many patients, some ear, nose, and throat specialists, and just about every parent I've ever met believe that milk stimulates mucus formation and should be avoided when you have a cold. The most recent test of this theory debunks it. Swallowing milk may leave your throat *feeling* like you have more mucus, but you really do not.

There are some natural remedies that may ease the symptoms of a cold. If you add a few drops of eucalyptus oil to a vaporizer, your stuffy nose may open up a little; patients have told me that lungwort tea improves hoarseness, that herb tea with ephedra is an effective decongestant, and that elm bark tea suppresses a cough. I suppose I'm old-fashioned, but I worry about taking any product, natural or man made, whose ingredients have not been tested as thoroughly as any other medication. It's not that I think herbs are ineffective. On the contrary, I fear some of their undocumented, potential side effects. Several major pharmaceutical houses have entered into negotiations with shamans and witch doctors throughout the world in a plan to analyze the potions and herbs they believe help their "patients," and I expect that some good will come of this joint venture. However, until those data are forthcoming, I remain cautious about the use of most herbs.

As far back as the twelfth century, Maimonides, one of the fathers of modern medicine, recommended chicken soup for upper respiratory infections. (The Chinese use it too, but they add ginseng to it.) Since then, mothers everywhere, Jewish and non-Jewish alike, have been following his advice! Researchers in Miami reported in the prestigious *New England Journal of Medicine* that chicken soup is an effective decongestant. It's probably the safest (and most delicious) cold remedy you can take!

In summary, use vitamin C when you have a cold if you're persuaded that it helps, but do so in divided doses and limit yourself to 2,000 milligrams a day. Have some hot chicken soup, but make sure it's not too salty if you have heart or blood pressure problems. Best of all, wash your hands frequently after exposure to someone with a cold, including your own child, because cold viruses spread by physical contact. It may be safer to kiss someone with a cold than to shake his or her hand!

VITAMIN C CONTENT OF FOODS

FOOD	PORTION	VITAMIN C (mg)
Acerola cherries, uncooked	1 cup	1,644
Broccoli, uncooked	½ cup	41
Elderberries, uncooked	1 cup	52
Gooseberries, uncooked	1 cup	42
Grapefruit		
pink or red	1 medium	94
white	1 medium	78
Grapefruit juice		
bottled or canned	8 ounces	72
fresh	8 ounces	94
frozen, from concentrate	8 ounces	83
Kale, boiled	½ cup	27
Kiwi	1 medium	75
Lemon	1 medium	31
Lime	1 medium	20
Mango	1 medium	57
Orange	1 medium	80
Orange juice		
bottled or canned	8 ounces	86
fresh	8 ounces	124
frozen, from concentrate	8 ounces	97

VITAMIN C CONTENT OF FOODS *(Continued)*

FOOD	PORTION	VITAMIN C (mg)
Papaya	1 medium	188
Pepper		
hot chili, uncooked	1 medium	109
green	½ cup	45
red	½ cup	95
yellow	1 large	341
Persimmon		
Fuyu (Japanese)	1 medium	13
Hachiya (Californian)	1 medium	17
Potato, baked with skin	1 medium	24
Strawberries	1 cup	85
Tomato	1 small	24
Tomato juice	6 ounces	33

CONGESTIVE HEART FAILURE

WHEN THE SPIRIT IS WILLING,

BUT THE PUMP IS WEAK

Several different diseases or disorders can injure the heart, leaving it unable to pump blood effectively to the rest of the body. When that happens, you are in "congestive heart failure." The most common causes of such damage are one or more heart attacks; long-standing, untreated high blood pressure; infection by a virus that infiltrates and destroys the heart's fibers; a leaky or narrowed valve that creates extra work for the cardiac muscle; and the direct toxic effect of excessive alcohol. In some cases, the heart muscle fibers are weakened without any cause that we can diagnose. How long it takes for any of these "insults" to make the heart "fail" depends on how severe they are and how long they have been present.

Your heart is one tough muscle. In order to continue its normal pumping action in the face of adversity, it can temporarily compensate for or overcome the forces that are weakening it. Initially, it does so by getting progressively bigger and thicker just as other muscles in your body do when overworked. As long as that process can continue, you will not experience any symptoms of failure. But there is a limit to how large and thick the heart can become. After it has exhausted its reserves, it dilates and weakens. When that happens, it can no longer expel the normal amount of blood with each contraction. As the heart continues to stretch and thin out, it becomes weaker and weaker. The tired heart begins to beat faster in an attempt to get more of its blood out. Eventually, even this increased effort is not enough, and blood backs up into the lungs where it replaces some of the air. You now begin to experience the major symptom of heart failure— shortness of breath—at first only when you exert yourself, but eventually even at rest. Because lying down increases the amount of blood returning to the lungs from the lower part of the body, you'll prefer to sleep elevated, or even to sit in a chair during the night.

In addition to causing congestion in the lungs, heart failure deprives vital organs of the blood they require to function normally. The beleaguered kidney, for example, now excretes less salt in the urine. Excess amounts of salt then accumulate in your body, causing it to retain fluid. Your legs begin to swell first, then your abdomen.

Heart failure is also accompanied by generalized weakness (your muscles do not get their fair share of blood, either), loss of appetite, and poor nutrition. You may gain weight, but the scales are deceiving. The extra pounds are due to fluid and mask the loss of muscle that occurs when the heart is weak.

The best way to treat heart failure is to correct the underlying problem. That may mean having a faulty valve replaced, controlling your high blood pressure, abstaining from alcohol if it is having a toxic effect on your heart muscle, or undergoing a coronary bypass operation to improve blood flow to the deprived cardiac muscle. In very severe cases, where large amounts of cardiac muscle have been irreparably destroyed, nothing short of a heart transplant will do.

There are several different kinds of medications that can help the weakened muscle to cope, sometimes for a long while. They range from powerful diuretics (water pills) that get rid of the retained fluid, to agents that improve the strength of the heart's contractions (digitalis) or ACE inhibitors. The latter, angiotension-converting enzyme inhibitors, are drugs that prevent the formation of angiotension II, a very powerful, natural blood pressure–raising substance. The prototype of these agents is captopril (Capoten), which dilates the arteries and lowers blood pressure, thus reducing the workload of the heart. Many of these "miracle" drugs are relatively new. Before they became available, the only effective way to treat heart failure was to severely restrict intake of sodium (salt) and fluid. Patients were limited to 1 gram of sodium or less a day. That was truly draconian! It meant eliminating *all* salt from cooking, removing the shaker from the table, forbidding many commonly used foods, and even making patients hunt for salt-free bread, milk, and other basic foodstuffs. Fluid deprivation was also most unpleasant. I can think of nothing worse than unquenched thirst. This regimen was unappetizing and extremely difficult to adhere to, took the joy out of life, and in the long run left patients even weaker than ever because of malnutrition. The treatment was worse than the disease!

Fortunately, modern cardiac drugs, such as the ACE inhibitors and diuretics have made rigid salt and fluid restriction obsolete. Because today's powerful diuretics are able to remove so much of the retained sodium, most people with heart failure may now eat enough of it to make their diet palatable. Severe sodium restriction is not only unnecessary, it's also undesirable. And even though doctors discourage "pushing" fluids in these people, no one with heart failure should suffer from thirst.

We consume an average of 4 to 5 grams of salt (sodium) daily, but need no more than 2. That's what I recommend for everyone, with and without heart failure. The table on page 249 is an example of a daily menu that contains about 2 grams of sodium. You will not exceed that amount if you remove the salt shaker from the table and avoid obviously salt-filled foods such as delicatessen products, most packaged luncheon meats, lox, potato chips, bacon, hot dogs, sausage, olives, dill pickles, soy sauce, and the like. The table on page 248 lists a number of salt-rich foods to avoid, and the table on page 247 charts the sodium of a number of popular beverages. I allow my patients to add ¼ teaspoon of salt per day to their cooking to make their food palatable (a full teaspoon contains 2,300 milligrams of salt). If your food needs still more oomph, try the many tasty sodium-free herbs and salt substitutes now available (see page 243). I'm certain you'll find one you like. But check their labels. Some of them contain potassium, which is occasionally retained by the kidneys in people with heart failure, and which can hurt you in these circumstances. You must also be aware of the hidden sources of salt such as milk shakes, fried potatoes, and canned soups.

Just because you have heart failure is no reason to be physically inactive. I'm not suggesting that you run a marathon, but neither should you become a couch potato. Walk as much as you comfortably can—every day (but wait for an hour or so after eating). However, rest is also important. You should relax *in bed* for an hour or two every day, depending on how bad your heart failure is. This will return more blood from the legs and abdomen to the heart, which can usually handle a brief extra load such as this. The resulting increase of blood pumped to the kidneys helps improve their function so they excrete more salt. While you're in bed, do some passive leg exercises to keep the blood moving and prevent blood clots from forming.

The process of digestion makes energy demands on the heart too. Every time you eat, the stomach calls for more blood. So have smaller meals, more frequently. *What* you eat will also depend on the medications you're taking. For example, diuretics may cause the loss of potassium and magnesium, which you may have to replace in your diet or by taking supplements.

If your cardiac muscle is weak you should continue to follow the low-fat low-cholesterol, high-fiber diet on page 119. See also page 116 for a list of the fiber content of various foods.

CONSTIPATION

A DIET FOR HARD TIMES

Which one of the following words beginning with "C" does not belong with the others—*cancer, high cholesterol, condoms, constipation*? If you picked *condoms*, you're wrong! The right answer is *constipation*, because it's the only one of the four with which *everyone* has had some experience at one time or another!

Most Americans are almost obsessed with their bowels. Perfect strangers glare at you from your TV screen demanding to know whether or not you're "regular"! Little Johnny's farewell from Mom on his way to school in the morning may well be "And did you move them after breakfast, dear?" I have seen men and women in the throes of a heart attack, wired to a multitude of monitors, receiving oxygen, occasionally even sick enough to have been given the last rites, worried less about death than with their failure to "eliminate" that morning! I have patients who, sitting across my desk while I'm having a sandwich at the office, think it's appropriate and important to describe not only their evacuation schedule but the appearance of their stool as well. I can understand such preoccupation with sex, a good meal, great theater, spellbinding music, even stamp collecting—but constipation?

I have never known anyone to become sick because he or she didn't have a bowel movement for a day or two. People worry about constipation, but most don't even know what it is. Would you believe that among fifteen thousand men and women in England who were asked whether they suffered from constipation, fully 10 percent of those who had a *regular movement every single day* said yes, they did? One third of those who "enjoyed" as many as *six* movements a week were of the same opinion. Americans obviously have a similar misconception; otherwise, why would we spend more than $200 million every year on over-the-counter laxatives?

There is no law of nature that demands you have a bowel movement every single day. How often you "go" depends on your diet, your level of physical activity, your daily fluid intake, what medications you're using, whether you have any other health problems that may slow down your intestinal tract (as, for example, a sluggish thyroid gland), and the interaction in your own body among the various complex muscular, neurological, and anatomic factors. It's very much like sex; some of us enjoy it as often as twice a day, while others are satisfied with a session every few weeks.

Given the wide variation in "normal" bowel function, you shouldn't use the term *constipation* loosely (no pun intended). Save it to describe *hard and dry* stools that you pass much less frequently than usual *for you*. So defined, it is estimated that there are almost 5 million "constipees" (don't look for this word in the dictionary; I made it up) in the United States alone—more blacks than whites, more men than women, and more persons over age sixty than under. They are apt to have less money and leisure time, and are usually not as well educated; they consume fewer calories, eat fewer high-fiber foods such as fresh fruit and vegetables, whole grains and beans, and are apt to drink more tea and coffee, but less water.

Chronic constipation is much more common in the Western world than in most "underdeveloped" countries because of how we've changed our diet over the last hundred years. Much of the food we now eat is "refined"—more digestible, tasty, caloric, fattier, and with much less fiber. A century ago our forebears ate 40 grams of fiber a day; our current average consumption is about 10 grams daily. No wonder the incidence of constipation has doubled.

If you are chronically constipated for whatever reason, you probably have a lazy bowel. Unless you ply yourself with larger and larger doses of laxatives, you'll be straining whenever you do "go." This is not the kind of exercise people should have; its most immediate reward is hemorrhoids, and if you have coronary artery disease, all the pushing and forcing on the toilet can induce heart pain (angina). Further down the road, chronic constipation also contributes to diverticulosis, little outpouchings in the wall of the bowel, that can become inflamed, infected, and even rupture (see diverticulitis, page 155), requiring emergency abdominal surgery; and can even result in hiatal hernia, colon cancer, and gallstones.

Can you turn the clock back once you've become a confirmed constipee? Can you ever again become regular? Only if you restore the fiber eliminated from your diet. Lots of water helps too, but won't do the job without the fiber.

There are two kinds of dietary fiber—*soluble* and *insoluble*. *Insoluble fiber* is composed largely of cellulose and lignin that is present in whole grains such as wheat germ, wild rice, wheat bran, buckwheat, cornmeal, millet, rice bran, and whole wheat. *Soluble fiber* is found primarily in oats, oat cereal, oat bran, barley, legumes such as lentils and soybeans, vegetables including artichokes, beans, broccoli, brussels sprouts, cabbage, carrots, cauliflower, onions, and squash, and fresh fruit such as apples, apricots, bananas, berries, dates, peaches, pears, and prunes. The richest sources of soluble fiber are oat bran and psyllium (commercially available as Metamucil, Fiber-All, and other brands).

If you eat 35 to 40 grams or more daily of total fiber, at least four or five of which should be of the "crude" or insoluble variety, your bowel movements will be regular and soft. Your constipation will be but a memory! There are many different ways you can combine the various fiber sources in your diet so that you get enough and enjoy it. However, to satisfy your insoluble fiber quota, I recommend you include ½ cup of any "superfiber" cereal, which contains 12 or 13 grams of fiber, ½ cup of 100 percent bran, which contains about 8½ grams of fiber, or ¾ cup of bran flakes with 5 grams, or 2 tablespoons of raw miller's bran, which provide 5 grams. (Miller's bran is a coarse, high-fiber supplement that is very effective in small doses. You are more likely to find it in health food stores than in supermarkets.) I suggest that if you are a fiber novice, you start with 1 tablespoon of miller's bran and increase the amount gradually to a total of 4 tablespoons daily. In resistant cases of constipation, you may need two or three times that amount. You can put miller's bran in yogurt or sprinkle it over your breakfast cereal. Look at the fiber sources on page 116 for the fiber and caloric content of foods per serving. Select a variety to make your meals more interesting and tastier, and to provide additional nutrients. For example, sprinkle a couple of teaspoons of wheat germ on your high-fiber cereal; eat brown, not white, rice (the extra cost at the Chinese restaurant is well worth it); use whole wheat, not white, bread; add buckwheat to your ravioli (the Russians call it *varenekes*). Remember too that fiber is filling; the best way to lose weight and to keep it off is to follow a high-fiber, low-fat diet forever.

Don't get carried away in your enthusiasm to eat a fiber-rich diet by starting with 35 or 40 grams right off the bat. Fiber is potent stuff. As with exercise, you should start with small amounts and work your way toward your target, increasing the fiber in your diet no more often than every two weeks. If you take too much fiber too fast, you are going to have lots of embarrassing and foul-smelling gas and end up (no pun intended) with an itchy rear end. This is especially true if you eat coarse bran, which can irritate the anal canal.

Your dietary fiber should consist of a mix of the soluble and insoluble forms. Four pieces of fresh fruit and one salad every day is a good way to start. One cup of berries contains 2.5 grams; the average pear provides over 4 grams; 3.5 ounces of dehydrated cabbage will give you 10 grams! (But who eats dehydrated cabbage?) And there are so many other delicious high-fiber foods to feast on—dates, apples, peaches, cauliflower, and a variety of nuts, to name but a few. Here is an ideal, fiber-rich sample menu, but you can devise an equally good one yourself: for breakfast, a glass of orange juice, ¾ cup of bran flakes (containing 5 grams of crude fiber), and two slices of whole wheat toast (almost 4 grams of crude fiber). At lunch, in addition to the main course, have two more slices of whole wheat bread, a green salad, and four or five dates, prunes, or dried figs. You can enhance the fiber content of dinner with an appetizer portion of a cold cabbage salad as well as a hot, steamed, high-fiber vegetable such as cauliflower or broccoli. You'll find still another example of a high-fiber menu—and a low-fiber one for comparison—at the end of this chapter.

Don't forget legumes. They provide the same number of calories as cereals, but contain almost four times as much protein. The most popular legumes in this country are beans of every variety (lentils, peas, and one of my favorites, chickpeas). They all give you gas, but you can degas them somewhat by soaking them overnight in water and discarding the soaking water, in which event you needn't cook them as long either. (My wife does not soak legumes overnight. She just heats the water to a boil, leaves the beans in it for two or three minutes, then soaks them in "new" water for about an hour.)

If you're eating all the fiber I recommend, you *must* drink a minimum of eight glasses of fluid (water, fruit juices, and sodas, but not tea or coffee because of their diuretic effect) during the day—two glasses with every meal and two or three in between (except if there is some reason for you not to do so, e.g., if you have severe heart failure or certain kinds of kidney trouble). Unless you do, your stool will become hard and impacted (dry), despite the fiber.

In addition to getting plenty of fiber and fluids, being physically active will also help prevent constipation. Thirty minutes of brisk walking every day is all you need to help keep your bowels in working order.

Each of us has his or her own bowel habit. Most people "move" either before or after breakfast. If you habitually ignore the urge, you will lose that "rhythm," your movements will become haphazard, and you will become constipated. Respond as quickly as possible to every evacuation notice! Nature does not like to be ignored.

If you've been chronically constipated, don't expect results from fiber overnight. It generally takes at least one to three weeks to work, but work it does! (The most tangible evidence is seen in hospital patients who have been confined to complete bed rest. Their constipation is much less troublesome if they eat two slices of whole wheat bread every morning.) In the meantime, an enema, suppository, or laxative will give you quick results. Casual, occasional constipation does not usually require a visit to your doctor, but if it persists for several days or more, be sure to tell him or her about it. Don't get into the habit of relying on laxatives. They can be habit forming. By contrast, a high-fiber, low-fat diet has many health benefits beyond curing your constipation—and has no side effects.

Now and then constipation is more than just a consequence of your diet and lifestyle. It may be due to countless drugs, e.g., diuretics—water pills—that dry you up; the codeine in cough mixtures or some medication you have been taking to lower your blood pressure; antidepressants and other mood-altering drugs; or calcium channel blockers such as verapamil for the treatment of various cardiovascular disorders. Other causes of constipation are hypothyroidism, when all the body processes ranging from libido to bowel movements slow down; a polyp; or even a cancer obstructing the exit of the stool from the body. So despite its usually benign connotations, sudden, continuing, or recurring constipation should always be looked into (no pun intended) by your doctor.

We usually think of constipation as a problem plaguing adults, not children. However, youngsters may also suffer from constipation—usually because of what they do or do not eat, as well as parental overconcern with bowel habits. Children these days are into junk food—fatty, refined, and sweet. It's a wise parent who helps his or her child develop a taste for, or at least become accustomed to, a high-fiber diet—the earlier, the better. It's much easier when consuming such foods comes naturally than enforcing their consumption after constipation has set in. For a child with constipation, daily servings of raw bran (which can be nicely mashed with a banana for younger children), as well as lots of fruits and vegetables, will usually unplug them. Cut down on their milk intake too, at least temporarily until the problem is solved, because milk can be constipating.

In summary, constipation is common and preventable. My prescription? Fiber, water, exercise, and "moving" when your body tells you to.

FIBER CONTENT OF FOODS

FOOD	PORTION	FIBER (gm)	CALORIES
Beans/legumes			
black, cooked	1 cup	7.2	227
broad beans, cooked	1 cup	8.7	186
chickpeas, cooked	1 cup	5.7	269
green peas, cooked	½ cup	2.2	67
kidney, cooked	1 cup	6.4	225
lentils, cooked	1 cup	7.9	231
navy, cooked	1 cup	6.6	259
pinto, cooked	1 cup	6.8	235

FIBER CONTENT OF FOODS (Continued)

FOOD	PORTION	FIBER (gm)	CALORIES
soybeans, immature seeds, cooked	3½ ounces	1.4	118
soybeans, mature seeds, cooked	3½ ounces	1.6	71
Bread/grains			
barley, pearled, light	½ cup	15.6	352
bread, whole wheat	1 slice	2.0	80
brown rice, cooked	½ cup	1.6	108
buckwheat	3½ ounces	9.9	335
bulgar, uncooked	3½ ounces	1.7	359
flour, whole wheat	½ cup	5.3	200
macaroni, whole wheat, uncooked	2 ounces	5.6	210
Oatbran Pita Bread (Sahara)	1 small	3.6	132
popcorn, air-popped	3 cups	3	75
whole grain cracker (Ry-Krisp)	½ ounce	2.5	40
Cereals			
All-Bran (Kellogg's)	⅓ cup	10	70
All-Bran with Extra Fiber (Kellogg's)	½ cup	14	50
Branflakes (Kellogg's)	¾ cup	5	90
Cornbran (Quaker)	⅔ cup	5.4	109
Corn Flakes (Kellogg's)	1 cup	1.0	100
Fiber One (General Mills)	½ cup	13	60
miller's bran	2 tablespoons	5.0	16
oat bran, uncooked	⅓ cup	4.9	76
100% bran	½ cup	8.4	76
rice bran	1 ounce	6.1	88
wheat germ, toasted (Kretschmer)	¼ cup	3.3	103
Dried fruits			
dates	10	4.2	228
figs	5	8.7	238
prunes	5	3	100
raisins, seedless	⅓ cup	2.6	150

FIBER CONTENT OF FOODS *(Continued)*

FOOD	PORTION	FIBER (gm)	CALORIES
Fruits			
apple, fresh	1 medium	3	81
apricots, fresh	3 medium	1.4	51
banana	1 medium	1.8	105
blackberries, fresh	½ cup	3.3	37
blueberries, fresh	1 cup	3.3	82
cantaloupe, fresh	1 cup	1.5	42
kiwi, fresh	1 medium	2.6	46
orange	1 medium	2.9	59
peach, fresh	1 medium	3	37
pear, fresh	1 medium	4.3	98
raspberries	1 cup	5.8	61
strawberries	1 cup	3.9	45
tomato, uncooked	1 small	1.6	26
Vegetables			
artichoke, cooked	3½ ounces	2.8	24
asparagus	½ cup	1.2	19
bamboo shoots	½ cup	2.0	21
broccoli, uncooked	1 cup	2.4	24
brussels sprouts	½ cup	3.4	30
cabbage, red, uncooked	½ cup	0.7	10
carrot, uncooked	1 medium	2.3	31
cauliflower, uncooked	½ cup	1.2	12
corn, cooked	½ cup	3	89
cucumber	1 medium	3	42
eggplant	½ cup	0.6	11
endive, curly, or escarole, uncooked	3½ ounces	0.9	20
lettuce, butterhead, Bibb, or Boston	2 leaves	0.2	2
lettuce, iceberg	1 leaf	0.2	3
lettuce, romaine	½ cup shredded	0.5	4
onion, uncooked	½ cup	1.3	30
peppers, sweet, uncooked	½ cup	0.8	13
potato, baked with skin	1 small	4	160
snow peas	3 ounces	2.0	35
spinach, uncooked	½ cup chopped	2.0	21

FIBER CONTENT OF FOODS *(Continued)*

FOOD	PORTION	FIBER (gm)	CALORIES
summer squash, all varieties, cooked	½ cup	1.3	18
squash, winter, all varieties, cooked	½ cup	2.9	39
tomato, uncooked	1 small	1.6	26
zucchini, uncooked	½ cup	0.3	9

SAMPLE HIGH-FIBER MENU

	SERVING	FIBER (gm)	CALORIES
Breakfast			
General Mills Fiber One	½ cup	13	60
Skim milk	½ cup	0	43
Fresh peach, sliced	1 medium	3	37
Coffee or tea, black	1 cup	0	5
Snack			
Nonfat vanilla yogurt	6 ounces	0	150
Fresh berries	½ cup	1.5	22.5
Lunch			
Black bean soup	½ cup	4.9	103
Sandwich:			
white meat turkey	3.5 ounces	0	147
whole-grain bread	2 slices	4	160
yellow mustard	1 teaspoon	0	4
lettuce	½ cup	0.5	4
tomato, sliced	½ small	0.8	13
Apple	1 medium	3	81
Diet cola	12 ounces	0	0
Snack			
Popcorn, air-popped	3 cups	3	75
Butter substitute (Molly McButter)	½ teaspoon	0	4
Dinner			
Red snapper, grilled	6 ounces	0	218
Brown rice	½ cup	1.6	108
Steamed carrots with herbs	½ cup	1.5	35

SAMPLE HIGH-FIBER MENU *(Continued)*

Salad:	SERVING	FIBER (gm)	CALORIES
lettuce	1 cup	1	8
tomato, sliced	½ small	0.8	13
cucumber, sliced	½ cup	0.5	7
green pepper rings	2	0.8	6.5
fat-free dressing	2 tablespoons	0	20
Regular noncola soda	12 ounces	0	144
Snack			
Crunchy sundae:			
vanilla ice milk	6 ounces	0	138
wheat germ	1 tablespoon	1.5	52.5
raisins	2 tablespoons	1.3	75
		42.7	1,733.5

SAMPLE LOW-FIBER MENU—WHAT *NOT* TO EAT!*

	SERVING	FIBER (gm)	CALORIES
Breakfast			
Corn flakes	1 cup	1	100
Skim milk	½ cup	0	43
Orange juice	½ cup	0	60
Coffee or tea, black	1 cup	0	5
Snack			
Glazed doughnut	1 small	0	230
Lunch			
Sandwich:			
white meat turkey	3.5 ounces	0	147
white bread	2 slices	2	160
yellow mustard	1 teaspoon	0	4
lettuce	½ cup	0.5	4
tomato, sliced	½ small	0.8	13
Apple juice	8 ounces	0	116
Snack			
Potato chips	1 ounce	1.5	150
Regular 7UP	12 ounces	0	144

SAMPLE LOW-FIBER MENU *(Continued)*

	SERVING	FIBER (gm)	CALORIES
Dinner			
Grilled red snapper	6 ounces	0	218
Mashed potato (made with whole milk and margarine)	½ cup	0	111
Steamed broccoli	½ cup	2	22
Snack			
Apple pie	⅙ pie	<u>1.6</u>	<u>231</u>
		9.4	1,758

*At first glance, this low-fiber menu looks pretty close to its high-fiber cousin. Now look more closely at the subtle changes. By having fresh fruit instead of fruit juice, brown rice instead of mashed potatoes, substituting whole-wheat bread for white, and making a few other small changes, you can add over 30 grams of fiber to your diet—painlessly!

CYSTIC FIBROSIS

WHEN THE "WORST" FOODS

ARE THE BEST!

I recently attended a fund-raising dinner to benefit the Cystic Fibrosis Foundation. I asked a woman sitting next to me whether she was there because she had a special interest in cystic fibrosis. No, she told me, she was simply someone's guest. She went on to say that all she knew about cystic fibrosis was that it is a disease of the lungs caused by heavy smoking, and that the best way to treat it is to kick the habit. Among the speakers that evening was a researcher in cystic fibrosis who described the exciting advances in gene therapy that we hope will soon prevent, control, and even eradicate this disease. After his talk was over, a woman seated on my other side leaned over and whispered, "Isn't it too bad that there aren't such breakthroughs in the really important diseases, not just in rare ones like cystic fibrosis?"

Both these women were misinformed about this illness. Cystic fibrosis (CF) is the most deadly and *common* genetic disease of white Americans, affecting one infant in every twenty-four hundred live births. It is much less prevalent in blacks (one in seventeen thousand live births) and in Asians (one in ninety thousand).

Cystic fibrosis is a hereditary disorder; it can be passed from generation to generation and it is *not* caused by smoking. Persons who have only one CF gene are "carriers." They do not have the symptoms of the disease, but can transmit it to their children. (Five percent of Americans are "carriers.") A child who inherits two CF genes from a mother and father who are carriers, is born with cystic fibrosis. Cystic fibrosis has never, to the best of my knowledge, ever been passed on by someone with the disease, because males with CF are, as a rule, infertile. That's because the various ducts through which the sperm must pass are affected by the disease in the same way as are other ducts throughout the body (see below).

My dinner partner who thought that cystic fibrosis is a disease of the lungs was only partially correct. It also affects the intestinal tract, pancreas, and sweat glands. The lungs of children with CF appear to be healthy at birth, but pulmonary symptoms of the illness develop within weeks or months. Glands in the respiratory passages (bronchi) normally produce thin mucus designed to keep the airways moist. In people with CF, the mucus becomes very thick and plugs the ducts that carry it. These secretions back up into the glands and ultimately damage or destroy them. So the first symptoms of cystic fibrosis are those of bronchitis (cough, sputum, and recurrent upper respiratory infections), which become progressively worse. These chronic infections cause recurrent attacks of low-grade fever and difficulty breathing. Eventually the disease process involves the entire respiratory tree, including the lungs themselves. When the infection overwhelms the lungs, death occurs from respiratory failure, and many people with CF do not survive beyond their twenties or thirties. Newer and more powerful antibiotics help control pulmonary infections, and there are medications to thin the mucus, but these are basically stopgap measures. The only hope for an absolute cure lies in altering the faulty genetic structure.

Cystic fibrosis makes enormous energy demands on the body that must be met virtually from birth by substantial additional calories. Nature helps by endowing these infants and children with ravenous appetites. When a youngster with recurrent respiratory problems just can't get enough to eat early in life and has recurrent respiratory problems, you should suspect cystic fibrosis. But this craving and need for so much food have their problems. The abnormal amount of thick mucus causes gagging and vomiting. Food is not well absorbed because there is a lack of the enzymes necessary to digest it—which leads us to consider the pancreas, the other major organ affected by this disease.

The pancreas makes several digestive enzymes in addition to insulin. While the latter diffuses or seeps into the bloodstream, the digestive enzymes are carried to the intestine in a series of ducts. The bile that is needed to digest fat in the intestine reaches its destination through ducts from the liver, where it is made, and from the gallbladder, where it is stored. In people with cystic fibrosis, all these ducts become obstructed by thick mucus, just as they do in the lungs. Since their digestive enzymes never get out of the pancreas and into the intestine (duodenum), what they eat just sits in the gut, undigested and unabsorbed, accounting for many symptoms of the disease. For example, the enzyme *lipase* normally breaks up large fat globules into smaller ones that can be absorbed. But when it can't reach the duodenum, as happens in 90 percent of people with cystic fibrosis, the fat you eat is excreted undigested. The fat-filled stools of people with CF are voluminous, loose, foamy, and foul smelling. In addition to malodorous diarrhea, kids with cystic fibrosis are also malnourished because the fat they excrete takes with it the four fat-soluble vitamins: vitamin A, necessary for the healthy lining of various organs and for night vision; vitamin D, needed for bone growth; vitamin E, for which there seems to be a new benefit reported almost daily stemming from its antioxidant role in neutralizing harmful free radicals; and vitamin K, required for normal blood clotting and whose deficiency causes hemorrhages. (Sometimes a child with cystic fibrosis will bleed vigorously from a simple cut.) Vitamin B_{12}, though not a fat-soluble vitamin, is also often poorly absorbed in people with cystic fibrosis, resulting in the same blood and neurological complications that occur in pernicious anemia, a disease of B_{12} deficiency.

The pancreatic enzymes *trypsin* and *chymotrypsin* split dietary *protein* in food into its more digestible amino acid components. People with CF lack these enzymes too, so the protein in their diet goes the way of fat—undigested and unabsorbed. Without enough fat or protein, they become malnourished and anemic; growth is retarded and virtually every organ in the body is underdeveloped.

The pancreatic enzyme *amylase* helps digest *carbohydrate,* but its role is not as crucial as that of the fat- and protein-digesting enzymes because other processes are also involved in carbohydrate digestion. So when amylase fails to make it to the intestine, some carbohydrate in the diet is digested nevertheless. That's why carbohydrate, not fat or protein, is the staple of the cystic fibrosis diet.

CF wreaks even more havoc within the pancreas itself. As more and more pancreatic ducts become blocked, the resulting buildup of pressure in the organ progressively destroys it. With the loss of many of the insulin-producing cells, less insulin is produced. Thirty percent of people with cystic fibrosis who reach adult life (the median survival is twenty-eight years) become diabetic for this reason. Once that happens, they lose even more calories because, in addition to not absorbing much of what they eat, they now excrete sugar in their urine.

The *sweat glands* and the *parotid glands* (the ones below the ears that make children who have mumps look like bunny rabbits) of people with CF pour out abnormal amounts of salt in their perspiration, saliva, and tears—the only condition in which this happens. In fact, the disease can be diagnosed by analyzing the salt content of sweat. So a person with CF needs extra salt in the diet and even more in hot weather and when exercising.

Once you appreciate what cystic fibrosis is all about, you can see why diet plays such a critical role in its management, and why someone with CF needs lots of calories, fat, carbohydrate, protein, salt, and even water (the latter because of the vomiting and diarrhea that are so common in this disease). Until quite recently, doctors were between a rock and a hard place in helping their patients fulfill those needs. Replacing salt and water is relatively easy, but it was a challenge to ensure enough fat and protein; if simply added to the diet, they were excreted intact because the enzymes necessary to digest them were not available. Fortunately, there is now a way to deliver these enzymes in adequate amounts.

The new formulation that makes this possible consists of *enteric-coated microspheres* containing pancreatic enzymes extracted from pigs; *enteric* means that the pill's coating won't dissolve and release its enzymes until they're ready to be absorbed by the intestine. (Before this technology was developed, enormous amounts of the enzymes were necessary to have even a minimal effect, and their toxicity made them intolerable.) People with CF take one to three of the enteric-coated capsules with meals and one between meals. The exact dosage depends on how much functioning pancreatic tissue you have left as well as what kind and how much food you've eaten. The enzyme capsules should never be opened, crushed, or chewed because doing so destroys their enteric coating. Those who find them hard to swallow can add them to puréed or other semisoft food (but not dairy products such as milk custard, which also destroy the coating). While these enzyme supplements do not result in completely normal digestion, they do enable most people with cystic fibrosis to absorb more fat and protein without as much diarrhea.

The question of nutrition in cystic fibrosis used to be academic because so many persons with this disease died young. Newer antibiotics, chemicals that liquefy the mucus, and pills with more efficient delivery of digestive enzymes have resulted in a much longer life expectancy. The new genetic therapy on the horizon is grounds for even more optimism. Proper diet is now an essential part of living with CF. The right diet should provide enough protein (20 percent of the total calories) to ensure optimal growth and development and extra calories for energy—anywhere from 50 to 120 percent more than the RDA needed by healthy persons of comparable age, sex, and weight. Do not rely on charts. Children who are small for their age, thin, and chronically tired are either not eating enough of the right food or are not absorbing it. You cannot overfeed these children! At the same time, avoid nutritionally empty foods. Every morsel someone with CF eats should be calorie dense—which means that 35 to 40 percent of daily calories should be in the form of fat. Don't fill up on a large bowl of popcorn when what you really need are the calories in the one small pat of butter you put on it. Don't worry about the extra fat and cholesterol; getting the calories you need now is much more important to your health than the risk of heart disease later.

The best way to get the required calories is to gradually increase portion sizes, with plenty of calorie-dense snacks throughout the day. Offer a child with CF food that he or she really enjoys. If meals cause breathing problems, softer or liquid foods will reduce the work of chewing. The diet should be very high in complex and simple carbohydrates (65 percent or more of total calories) because, the new enteric-coated microspheres notwithstanding, that's what people with cystic fibrosis digest best. Avoid sugar if you're diabetic or prediabetic, but if diabetes is not a problem, eat plenty of simple sugars such as sweets because they are more easily absorbed than the complex carbohydrates. That's a reversal on most of the recommendations made about carbohydrates throughout this book. If you are lactose intolerant (as many people with CF are because of deficiency of the enzyme lactase), avoid milk and its derivative foods (see table on page 299). Eat plenty of fish, especially the deep-sea fatty variety. They are a good source of protein and fat and also contain many essential fatty acids (see page 221). Eat as many eggs and as much butter and soy and corn oil as you can tolerate, and be sure to take high-potency vitamin and mineral supplements. Most nutritionists recommend twice the RDA of each constituent. I agree that that's sufficient for vitamin A, but I recommend the others in even higher doses. For example, I advise 400 IU of *water-soluble* vitamin E (the fat-soluble preparations will not be absorbed), 400 IU of vitamin D, and 1,000 micrograms of vitamin B_{12} daily. To determine your need for additional vitamin K, your doctor will need to test your blood clotting. If a potential for abnormal bleeding is found, you need additional vitamin K: 2.5 to 5 milligrams once a week for infants under one year of age and twice a week for older children and adults. Your multivitamin preparation should also contain trace metals and minerals such as zinc, copper, selenium, and iron. If your caloric intake is too low, as gauged by your weight, energy, growth, and development, you may need to drink commercial, prepared liquid products such as Ensure or Sustacal. There are many such brands on the market; sample a few to see which one you like best. Fourteen percent of the calories in Ensure are from protein, 31 percent are from fat, and 55 are derived from carbohydrate. An 8-ounce glass of Ensure provides 240 calories. Ensure Plus High contains 360 calories per 8-ounce glass. Sustacal has the same caloric content as Ensure, but 24 percent of its calories are derived from protein, 21 percent from fat, and 55 percent from carbohydrates.

You should have lots of salty food to compensate for what is lost from the sweat glands, as discussed earlier. All processed foods in the typical American diet provide enough salt for most people with CF. For a list of high-sodium foods, see the table on page 248. Infants who are breast-fed may need an extra 1/8 to 1/4 teaspoon of salt per day because of the low sodium content of breast milk. (This translates into approximately 288 to 575 milligrams of sodium, since 1 teaspoon contains 2,300 milligrams.) If your baby is on formula, add salt to the formula to stimulate a taste for it since it is so necessary in this disease. When the weather is hot, or when engaging in strenuous exercise, people with CF need even more.

In summary, cystic fibrosis is probably the only disease in which you can disregard just about every usual, conventional dietary recommendation doctors give. Eat all you can and forget your weight. Add lots of salt to your food; the adult diet should contain at least 4 to 6 grams from food or the salt shaker. Eat plenty of simple, refined sugars and as much fat as you can. When gene therapy becomes a reality, your plugged ducts will open up, your pancreas will function normally, you will breathe easily with lungs free from infection, and you'll have to watch your fat and cholesterol like everybody else!

DIABETES:

HOW SWEET YOU ARE,

AND MAYBE EVEN FAT!

There are about 10 million diabetics in this country—0.2 percent of all children, 1 percent of young adults, 6 percent of middle-aged persons, and 8 to 10 percent of the elderly. Half of them don't know they have the disease because, like high blood pressure, diabetes may remain "silent" for years without causing any symptoms whatsoever. It's detectable only by a blood sugar test. Diabetes is serious. It almost triples your risk of heart disease, is responsible for half of all amputations and a quarter of the cases of kidney failure, and is the leading cause of blindness in the United States.

You don't become diabetic because you're a sugar freak. True, there's too much in your blood, but the root problem lies with insulin, the hormone that converts sugar into usable energy. In some diabetics, the cells of the pancreas do not produce enough insulin; in others the insulin is plentiful, but doesn't work properly.

Diabetes was known to the ancients in various civilizations—in Greece, Rome, India, Egypt, and other countries. (The Greeks called it diabetes mellitus, *mellitus* being the Greek term for "honeyed." They were clearly aware that diabetic urine is high in sugar.) Over the centuries, and as recently as the early 1900s, this disease was managed in one of two ways. Some doctors felt that the sugar lost in the urine should be replaced, and prescribed *high*-carbohydrate diets; others speculated that a *low*-carbohydrate intake would be more effective. But all treatment of diabetes was essentially guesswork until 1921, when Banting and Best discovered insulin.

Diabetes is not a single disease, even though all diabetics have high blood sugar. The type that begins in childhood or adolescence almost always requires insulin (and so is called insulin-dependent diabetes mellitus—IDDM) and is frequently life threatening. By contrast, diabetes that develops in adult life can usually be controlled by diet and weight loss, without the need for insulin (and is designated non–insulin-dependent diabetes mellitus—NIDDM). Death and disability rates in this latter group, though higher than normal, are much less than in the childhood form.

The underlying causes of these two types of diabetes differ fundamentally. The immune system, which can normally distinguish between what is good and bad for the body, goes berserk in juvenile diabetics, attacking and killing many of the insulin-producing cells in the pancreas. No one knows how or why this happens in some children and not in others. According to the most widely accepted theory, a viral infection early in life sends the wrong signals to the body's defense mechanisms. Whatever the trigger, the result is a deficiency of insulin. The sugar these youngsters eat enters the bloodstream after being absorbed from the stomach and is delivered on schedule to every tissue in the body. But that's as far as matters go. The sugar—a concentrated source of energy—just sits there, unable to penetrate many of the tissues and to fuel them, because that requires insulin—of which there is not enough available. So, with nowhere to go and nothing to do, the sugar circulates in the blood until it reaches the kidney and is passed in the urine. The tissues, deprived of carbohydrate, turn to protein and fat to carry out their life-sustaining biological processes. Burning protein, however, causes wasting of muscles; metabolizing fat instead of sugar leads to the accumulation of toxic by-products that can result in coma and death. Replacing the missing insulin spares fat and protein, avoids the complications of their metabolism, and is lifesaving.

There is no shortage of insulin in diabetics whose condition starts in midlife, usually after age forty. The pancreas continues to produce it in normal amounts, but the cells on which it is supposed to act are resistant to its effects. Many of these diabetics are overweight, and when they lose enough pounds, the cells become more responsive, allowing the insulin to metabolize blood sugar. When that happens, their blood sugar drops without the need for additional insulin.

There is another subtype of diabetes, virtually limited to young blacks. In its early stages, there is a temporary lack of insulin, but as the disorder evolves, insulin is no longer needed.

The classic symptoms of all three types of diabetes—thirst, frequent urination, weight loss despite an increased appetite, and itching, leading to coma and premature death—are all the result of too much sugar that is underutilized by the body, and of the substitution of fat and protein as the first-line providers of energy.

Although the diagnosis of diabetes is obvious if you have these telltale symptoms, your sugar may be elevated for years before they appear. That's why routine screening to measure the sugar level in the blood is so important for everyone, especially if you have a family history of the disease. Actual numbers will vary somewhat with the technique used, but, generally speaking, a *fasting* plasma glucose level should normally fall between 70 and 115 milligrams. Values between 115 and 140 milligrams constitute a gray area. A reading greater than 140 milligrams is diagnostic of diabetes. (However, certain medications, such as steroid hormones and diuretics, may bring out a latent tendency to diabetes, and the increased levels return to normal when the drug is stopped. So remember to tell your doctor if you're taking these medications if you're being tested for diabetes.)

Diabetes can lead to a variety of complications, especially when blood sugar levels have not been assiduously treated. Nerves can become diseased ("diabetic neuropathy"), causing numbness in the feet or shooting pains throughout the body; arteries everywhere can become narrowed—resulting in a stroke when the brain is involved; a heart attack when the coronary arteries are hit; blindness when the blood vessels in the eye are affected; pain in the legs when the arteries supplying the leg muscles are diseased; and kidney failure when the circulation of that organ is compromised. It is no small wonder that the life expectancy of diabetics at any age is only two thirds that of the general population and that diabetes is a major cause of death in this country. Insulin and oral hypoglycemic agents do not cure diabetes, but they do control sugar levels and reduce the frequency and severity of its symptoms and complications.

In treating any diabetic, child or adult, the goal is to keep the blood sugar as close to normal as can be safely and comfortably achieved. Until quite recently, many doctors were too permissive in this regard. But a landmark study in 1993 laid to rest any question about the importance of tight control. *The best way to minimize the crippling and killing complications of diabetes is to keep blood sugar levels as close as possible to normal.* This is especially important in children, in whom the key to successful treatment is the proper balance of diet and insulin. Since growth and development are so critical for them, young diabetics should be prescribed a diet that will allow them to mature normally, however many calories that takes. What they eat can be counterbalanced with appropriate amounts of insulin. But there are guidelines to follow. Youngsters' diets should consist of the following: up to 20 percent of calories from protein, 25 to 35 percent from fat, and 50 to 60 percent from carbohydrate. (This is very similar to the diet recommended for diabetic adults, except that it provides all the calories and protein needed for children's rapid growth.) To avoid hypoglycemia, kids should have three meals a day, along with a snack at mid-morning, mid-afternoon, and bed-time. Every diabetic should have available, understand, and make use of diabetic food-exchange lists that explain the relationship among various foods, their portion size, the number of calories they contain, and their composition of fat, protein, and carbohydrate. These lists are available from the American Diabetic Association (ADA) or your own doctor. However, the measure of success in managing diabetes in a young person is not how little insulin he or she can get away with, but whether he or she is able to grow normally and has a near-normal range of blood sugar.

If you're an adult diabetic, and your blood sugar remains unacceptably high even though you've been following your diet faithfully and have lost weight, you may need oral sugar-lowering drugs. The right combination of insulin, drugs, and diet should eliminate the nadirs and spikes in your blood sugar levels. In my opinion, it's better to have your sugar a little higher than optimal than too low, because low levels can impair brain function and, if severe and prolonged enough, can lead to loss of consciousness. It is especially dangerous in the elderly in whom it can result in neurological or cardiac crises.

There has been a major change recently in the dietary advice doctors and the American Diabetic Association are giving their diabetic patients. Time was when fat and protein were "in" and all carbohydrates were taboo. That approach was subsequently modified and fat was virtually forbidden in order to slow down the process of arteriosclerosis, to which the arteries of diabetics are especially vulnerable. At the same time, the restriction on complex carbohydrates (but not simple sugars) was relaxed, so that more pasta, bread, beans, and vegetables were permitted. The rationale behind the distinction among the different sugar sources was based on the "glycemic factor" concept, according to which sugar enters the bloodstream at significantly different rates depending on the source. So complex carbohydrates were believed to be better than candy because their sugar was released much more slowly and therefore did not raise blood sugar levels abruptly. Fructose, the sugar in fruit, was thought to elevate blood sugar less than dextrose and glucose. It therefore did not stimulate the same need for insulin and as a result was preferable as a sweetener.

Here's what has changed. The ADA now says that it's okay to have moderate amounts of fat as long as it's of the monounsaturated variety. Unlike saturated and polyunsaturated fat, monounsaturates such as olive, canola, and most sunflower and safflower oils do not accelerate the process of arteriosclerosis. But when using monounsaturates, you must still take into account their caloric content. The ban on simple sugar has also been relaxed because the validity of the glycemic factor concept has been questioned. Although there is some variation in the speed with which different carbohydrates enter the bloodstream as sugar, it's not nearly as much as we once thought. It's the *total* carbohydrate content of the diet and not the type of carbohydrate that counts. Sugars are apparently *not* digested significantly more rapidly than starches. But although sucrose produces the same glycemic response as rice, bread, and potatoes, that doesn't mean you can have sucrose *and* other carbohydrates. It's one or the other, the critical

factor being the total carbohydrate makeup of your diet. With regard
to the use of fructose as a sweetener, even though it does produce less
of a rise in the blood sugar than do sucrose and other carbohydrates,
it also raises the level of "bad" LDL cholesterol. So diabetics whose
cholesterol level is high to begin with may continue to eat fruit, but
should back off from fructose sweeteners. Another drastic change of
opinion relates to sugar substitutes such as sorbitol, mannitol, and
xylitol, which are the components of most sweets touted for diabetic
patients. The ADA does not believe they are any better for you than
sucrose, and the same is true for fruit juice concentrates, molasses,
honey, corn syrups, dextrose, and maltose. A carbohydrate is a carbohydrate is a carbohydrate.

There are three main sugar substitutes, all of which are noncaloric
and will not raise your sugar. Saccharine and aspartame are available
in the United States, but cyclamate is not. Some diabetes specialists
believe that a 200-microgram tablet of chromium picolinate, which
can be bought without a prescription, helps control blood sugar levels.
(The beneficial effect of broccoli on diabetes is probably due in part
to its high content of chromium and the fact that it is rich in complex
carbohydrates. This is not a food that can be forced. Just eat as much
as you like! There is no upper limit!)

The American Diabetic Association can provide you and your
doctor with a specific diet plan based on caloric requirements tailored
to your height, weight, and age. Following are the principles on which
these diets are based. Carbohydrates, mainly beans (the best for diabetics), pastas, and vegetables high in fiber, should constitute 50 to 60
percent of your total caloric intake. Onions are especially good because they contain sugar-lowering chemicals similar to the oral sul-
fonylureas (antidiabetic drugs).

Fat should make up 30 to 40 percent of your total daily calories with
15 to 25 percent coming from monounsaturated sources. Remember
that there are three kinds of fat—*polyunsaturated* fat (present in vegetable oils), *monounsaturated* fats such as olive oil and canola oil (avocados
and prepared mustards are also good sources), and *saturated* fat, present
in animal and dairy products. Saturated fat is the least desirable because
it promotes hardening of the arteries, especially in diabetics. I suggest
you limit its intake to 7 percent of total calories consumed, but you

may have up to 10 percent of calories from polyunsaturated sources. Also, your diet should contain less than 200 milligrams of cholesterol per day—approximately the amount in one egg.

With 50 to 60 percent of your calories coming from carbohydrate, and as much as 30 or 45 percent from fat, you have approximately 10 to 20 percent left for protein—basically meat, poultry, and fish. Emphasize the fish and poultry, and go easy on the red meat.

Limit your intake of *alcohol* to 4 ounces of wine a day (but avoid the sweet ones such as sauternes or Rieslings), 12 ounces of beer, or 1½ ounces of spirits—but less is preferable. Avoid all mixers containing sugar. (Gin-and-tonic lovers will be happy to learn that there is a sugar-free tonic water virtually indistinguishable from the real thing.) Remember, however, that alcohol contains 7 calories per gram, is metabolized like fat, and should be counted as a fat exchange. One drink equals two fat exchanges. Also remember that booze on an empty stomach can cause hypoglycemia. If you're having a hard time getting your sugar under control, you're better off omitting all alcohol until your condition stabilizes.

If you're diabetic, there are several important considerations that you should always keep in mind: (1) the total number of calories you consume; (2) the proportion of fat, protein, and carbohydrate in those calories; (3) the kind of fat you eat; (4) the intervals between when you eat, when you take your insulin or oral hypoglycemic agent, and when you are physically active; (5) the need to increase your caloric intake when you exercise or have fever; and (6) the necessity of never missing a meal no matter how busy you are.

As I mentioned above, it's critical to provide a diabetic child with enough calories to ensure normal growth and development. You can "cover" whatever extra amounts are necessary with enough insulin to keep the blood sugar as close to normal as possible. This can be a tricky business, and often requires the ongoing involvement of an expert in nutrition who can monitor the child's food intake and correlate it with his or her growth response. Frequently, you'll need to adjust your child's diet in response to infections and other problems. It's therefore important to have accurate diet charts—all of which should be recorded and kept by a professional such as a registered dietician, preferably one who specializes in diabetes. On the other hand, if you're overweight, middle-aged, and diabetic, you must cut back your calories enough to *lose* weight. A sedentary individual needs no more than 1,500 to 2,000 calories a day. If you're more physically active, you may need 2,000 to 2,500 a day. I strongly disapprove of liquid diets and powdered food substitutes to lose weight. It is better, safer, and more effective in the long run to develop and enjoy a natural diet to which you can adhere for more than just a few weeks.

Exercise is beneficial and important for diabetics, but remember that it lowers blood sugar so don't work out while the insulin activity in your system is at its peak. The curve of insulin action depends on the kind you're taking (regular, Lente, or Ultralente). Discuss this carefully with your doctor. If you exercise regularly, try to do so the same time each day. Don't engage in vigorous, sweat-inducing physical activities if your sugar is not under good control. If you are taking insulin and plan to exercise strenuously for more than one hour, have 15 grams of carbohydrate or one bread exchange before you begin. Take some food along in case you develop symptoms of hypoglycemia.

Diabetics, even those who don't engage in heavy physical activity, should always carry some form of sugar in their purse or pocket to correct low blood sugar. If you sense an attack of hypoglycemia coming on (you feel faint, nervous, or sweaty, are trembling, can't think straight, are hungry, or have palpitations, headache, or double vision), drink a full glass of orange juice and eat some regular candy (not a diabetic brand) immediately. Having more insulin on board than your body needs at the time (because you've eaten less than the amount called for by the insulin dose you normally take, have missed a meal, or have been exercising too much) can leave you hypoglycemic. Remember that if your brain has been temporarily deprived of sugar, it takes a while for normal function to return after sugar levels have been restored. So if you've just been through a hypoglycemic attack, wait for at least an hour after taking sugar before you drive your car or do anything else that requires skill and concentration.

Diabetics taking insulin should eat their three meals at fixed intervals determined by the type and dosage of their insulin and when its peak sugar-lowering effect occurs. Timing is very important, especially with respect to the distribution of your carbohydrate intake. Eat 15 percent of your daily carbohydrates at breakfast, 5 percent at your mid-morning snack, 25 to 30 percent at lunch, and 30 percent at dinner. Hold the balance in reserve for afternoon and bedtime snacks. What these meals and snacks consist of will depend on your total calorie intake. Eat fruit with your meals as dessert rather than as snacks. You should know the caloric content of everything you eat.

Diabetes can come on during pregnancy, usually in the third trimester. So every pregnant woman should be tested for diabetes, especially if she is obese or has a family history of diabetes. This is done by obtaining a blood sugar, generally at the twenty-sixth week. If the reading is high, insulin may be necessary. Gestational diabetes usually disappears after delivery, but you should have a glucose tolerance test four to sixteen weeks after giving birth because there is a 20 percent chance that you will develop adult, non–insulin-dependent diabetes within ten years. This possibility is very important for you to discuss with your doctor and is virtually certain if your glucose tolerance test remains abnormal several months after your baby is born. If you have diabetes, regardless of whether or not you need insulin, and are planning to have a baby, it's very important that you get your blood sugar under good control—both before and during your pregnancy. Poorly managed diabetes greatly increases the risk of birth defects in your infant. Their incidence can run as high as 20 percent when the mother's blood sugars are constantly too high. So keep your sugar as close to normal as you can, below 105 milligrams if possible, and preferably by diet, but with insulin or the oral antidiabetes pills, if necessary. These medications have not been shown to harm the fetus.

Being diabetic these days is much less complicated and debilitating than it used to be. Delicious sugar substitutes, low-fat foods, and monounsaturates that do not speed the onset of arteriosclerosis, a better understanding of the role of carbohydrates, and newer, more effective forms of insulin have all made life easier. Still, you do have to follow certain rules to maintain the balance between the energy you consume and what you expend. Perhaps the most important advance, however, is the appreciation that keeping your blood sugar levels as close to normal as possible is the key to preventing the long-term complications and premature death associated with this disease.

DIARRHEA

TOO DRY FOR TEARS

Most of us experienced *noninfectious diarrhea* at some time or another when we were very young. Just ask your parents. This illness, which may or may not be accompanied by vomiting or any other *apparent* evidence of infection, is very common in infants and children. (Its adult counterpart is called *acute gastroenteritis*.) Noninfectious diarrhea is actually a misnomer because it *is* usually caused by infection by a virus or bacterium—and it *is* contagious. Bear that in mind if there are other children at home.

The absence of fever in an adult with diarrhea is reassuring, but don't let it lull you into a false sense of security when it occurs in a child. For in only a day or two, an infant with the "runs" can become seriously dehydrated—and that's a virtual emergency. You can recognize dangerous dehydration when the child urinates less than usual (dry diapers are a tip-off; the body is holding on to every drop of water it contains); when he or she is extremely thirsty, very tired, or irritable; when the eyes or the "soft spot" on the top of the head are sunken; when crying produces no tears; or if the child's usual drooling has stopped. Don't wait for any of these danger signals to appear before you act; by that time the dehydration is at a dangerous stage.

The key to treating ongoing diarrhea in anyone is to replace the lost fluids as quickly as possible, but the *kind* of fluid one gives children is critical. Many of the commercial colas, fruit juices, and "sport" drinks such as Gatorade are loaded with sugar and *should not be given to infants and children with diarrhea*. If you have an infant at home, always keep on hand one or two bottles of oral rehydration solution, which you can buy at most supermarkets. (Some of the trade names to look for are Rehydralyte, Ricelyte, and Pedialyte.) They contain not only the needed water but the specific minerals that are being lost as a result of the diarrhea. The most recent addition to the antidiarrheal infant formulas—my old Latin teacher would have preferred my saying "formulae"—is Isomil-DF. It differs from the others in that it contains soy fiber, which apparently stops the diarrhea sooner than the standard soy formulas without the added fiber. Getting kids who are sick with diarrhea to take *any* rehydration solution is not easy, so use tiny amounts. For example, until their diarrhea stops, continue to give infants under two years of age at least ½ cup every hour, even if they have been vomiting. They may prefer to sip from a teaspoon or medicine dropper every minute or so. Give children older than two years a full cup every hour. These rehydration measures, which are in addition to and not in place of the child's usual diet, will usually stop the diarrhea. So carry on with formula-feeding your infant (breast milk contains lactose, which should be avoided). If your child eats solids, emphasize such binding foods as bananas, noodles, hot cereals, cooked rice, and rice water.

Whenever your child or infant develops diarrhea, alert his or her pediatrician, especially if it's just before the weekend. If your child's diarrhea persists for longer than twenty-four hours, see the pediatrician immediately.

In treating *adults* with diarrhea, the goal is to replace the lost fluid and to replenish salt, potassium, and other minerals excreted in the diarrhea, or, as doctors put it, to restore "electrolyte balance." Although this is very important in adults, it is even more critical in terms of time in infants and young children. Electrolyte balance can be achieved by drinking lots of clear bouillon and fruit juices. Pectin, which is present in applesauce, apple slices (skinless), and apple juice (which should be drunk at room temperature because cold juice aggravates the diarrhea), can help control symptoms. After the stools are a little more firm, you should begin to add, gradually and in small amounts, low-fiber foods such as refined starches (pasta, rice, mashed potatoes) and some protein (I recommend boiled chicken). Avoid dairy products for a few days because the enzyme lactase necessary to digest them may have been depleted by the diarrhea. Increase the fiber in your diet until you reach the amounts you were eating before you got sick.

There have been several diarrhea epidemics in the northeastern United States due to bacterial infection of eggs. So don't eat any that are cracked, and always cook your eggs for at least three minutes. If an outbreak has been reported in your area, you should forgo Caesar salad for the duration, or prepare it without the raw egg. If the meat you're planning to serve is frozen, allow it to defrost in the refrigerator a day or two before cooking—but no longer than that. Leaving it out all day at room temperature permits the growth of bacteria that cause diarrhea. After thawing meat in the refrigerator for approximately twenty-four hours, it should be cooked. It's safe to keep any cooked, leftover meat in the refrigerator for about three days. Beyond that, the meat loses nutrients and spoilage can occur.

The specific organism causing noninfectious diarrhea is not always apparent. Replacing the fluid and nutrients lost in the diarrhea can be critical to an affected child's survival. Gastroenteritis in adults, as a rule, usually clears up spontaneously, but fluid and nutrient replacement is also important. A word of caution, however. Although it is wise and appropriate to focus on the hazards of diarrhea in the very young, you should be aware that the elderly are also especially vulnerable—for several reasons. Their bodies do not correct the chemical imbalances resulting from diarrhea as efficiently as do younger adults', and their thirst mechanism may also be impaired, so that they may be more dehydrated than they realize.

DIET AND INFERTILITY

WHEN WHAT YOU EAT

IS INCONCEIVABLE

If a woman is having trouble becoming pregnant, what she and her spouse eat can sometimes make a difference. Moreover, modifying the diet is a lot easier—and a whole lot cheaper—than getting involved with artificial insemination, in vivo fertilization, and surrogate motherhood. So I contacted several specialists in the field to ask what nutritional advice they were giving their infertile patients. Not a single one of them does. They are all knee-deep in hormonal manipulation and in the newer exotic techniques of ovum implantation. Now, mind you, I'm not knocking any of those approaches. They often work when all else fails, but if you've been trying to have a baby and can't, check out these simple nutritional guidelines first.

Thin is beautiful in our society, but *too* thin may not be compatible with motherhood. Fat is where some of the precursors of estrogen—crucial for fertility—are transformed into this key female hormone. So you need a little padding to enhance that process. If, for example, you're five and a half feet tall and have lost about twenty pounds by diet and exercise, you may have the figure of a model, but chances are your periods have become irregular or sparse, or you've stopped menstruating altogether! That's because your estrogen level has dropped. Putting some of that weight back on may be all you need to become pregnant. Being excessively thin or dieting too stringently is simply not conducive to conception. Constant strenuous exercise can also render you infertile. Your periods may be irregular or absent because of loss of fat and estrogen even though you haven't lost any weight.

You know that you can harm your baby by smoking and drinking once you're pregnant, but are you aware that caffeine can reduce your chances of conception? In one recent study, the equivalent of three cups of coffee a day decreased the incidence of fertility by 27 percent. Smaller amounts of caffeine, whether in cola, tea, or coffee, also had an adverse effect, albeit a smaller one. So if you're trying to have a baby and have not met with success, eliminate caffeine and see what happens. That means staying away from caffeinated coffee, tea, and colas; chocolate and cocoa; and certain over-the-counter sinus and cold medicines (check the label). For the caffeine content of foods, see the table on page 45.

If you have nontropical sprue and an intolerance to gluten (a protein present in wheat, rye, oats, and barley), you may not be able to conceive until you follow a gluten-free diet (see page 311 for a list of foods to avoid).

Infertility used to be blamed solely on women. History is full of accounts of monarchs who abandoned their wives because they failed to "produce" a son. It never occurred to them or our forebears that the fault might conceivably (no pun intended) be the male's. We now know that that is so in at least 50 percent of cases. What might a man be doing that would render his sperm unequal to the task? Subsisting on junk food, smoking, and topping it off with booze for energy is not likely to make your sperm vivacious enough to seek, find, penetrate, and fertilize an egg. Researchers have studied sperm that didn't have "what it takes" and found them to be borderline in their vitamin C content. Supplements of 1,000 milligrams a day restored some of their vitality. I've found no evidence that vitamin C supplements can cure infertility, but it certainly makes sense to recognize the importance of adequate nutrition. Since your body can't store vitamin C, you need to consume foods rich in that vitamin daily. See page 105 for a list of vitamin C–rich foods.

Zinc is another matter. As described in the chapter on diet and sex, correcting true zinc deficiency can improve sexual performance and libido in men. That's the rationale for the oyster legend (see page 147). There is ample evidence in animal and human studies that zinc deficiency can lower the sperm count, and that replacing the missing zinc will increase the number of sperm and permit conception in previously infertile couples. The ovum (female egg) also requires zinc, so women too need to get enough in their diet. You require at least 15 milligrams every day, 20 milligrams a day while pregnant, and 25 milligrams daily while breast-feeding. Also, unless you're getting enough zinc, you will absorb more lead from the environment, and that too reduces fertility. Although there is no evidence that supplemental zinc in the absence of deficiency is of any benefit, it's not unreasonable to supplement your diet with 25 milligrams of zinc daily if you've had no luck in the conception arena. Remember, however, that too much—50 milligrams or more per day—can leave you copper deficient. The table on page 151 lists zinc-rich foods.

The failure to conceive is a complex problem with many possible causes. A thorough infertility workup of both partners will often determine the reasons, and the problem can frequently be corrected. But proper diet and the recognition and correction of nutritional deficiencies are the base on which all other treatment should be built. Severe dieting, weight loss, and habitual strenuous athletics all decrease a woman's fat stores and the amount of available estrogen, interfering with fertility. Excessive alcohol, tobacco, and a diet low in vitamin C and zinc may render a man infertile.

DIET AND SEX

WHY "SPANISH FLY" HAS NOTHING

TO DO WITH AVIATION

The other day my wife went to visit our son in Boston. I was planning to have a quiet dinner alone when a friend invited me out for some seafood. After I ordered fresh Malpeque oysters, my host looked askance, amused—and suspicious. "Camilla won't be back for a few days, will she?" he asked. "That's right," I replied. "So why the oysters?" You know very well what he was implying, but the truth is I asked for the oysters because I love them and not for their alleged aphrodisiac effect!

Throughout the ages, many foods have been said to stimulate desire and improve sexual performance, but scientists are still looking for one that really does (as are the rest of us). Countless myths have fallen by the wayside, but many persist, at least in the mind if nowhere else. These include the belief that ginseng, artichokes, asparagus, various shellfish, and celery, to name but a few, confer enhanced sexual power. Everyone has his or her own list. It takes only one or two apparent "hits" with a given food to convince most people that it is a sexual stimulant.

Before you get all hot and bothered in anticipation of what you will read in these next few pages, let me remind you that loss of desire or libido, the need for a boost of some kind, as well as the inability of a man to "perform," may be either psychological or physical. Before you experiment with any medication or food, ask your doctor for a good going-over. All the ginseng, or even oysters, will not have the slightest impact if the blood supply to your penis is diminished because of arteriosclerosis of the arteries that feed it, or if the nerves that control erection have been damaged by some toxic agent or by diabetes. Your ardor will not be enhanced by anything you eat, drink, or inhale if your thyroid gland is underfunctioning and every organ system in your body is on "hold." Also, there are many medications that impair performance and desire. These include agents to lower high blood pressure, notably the beta blockers such as Inderal and Tenormin, diuretics, and several "psychotropic" drugs prescribed to improve your mood or lessen your depression.

If there are no apparent physical causes for your problem (and there are many more than those mentioned above), consider consulting a sex therapist to determine whether you have a psychological hang-up that can be eliminated. These professionals really can help. Stress and fatigue, two common reasons for lack of interest in sex, are eminently treatable. Do not sell psychological factors short; they are more important than you may want to believe.

Some individuals resort to alcohol, cocaine, LSD, mescaline, morphine derivatives, marijuana, or amphetamines to increase sexual prowess. The truth is, if taken often enough, they all have the reverse effect. Remember Spanish fly? It's made from the dried bodies of the Spanish beetle fly, and all it does is irritate the genitourinary tract, a sensation that some people confuse with desire. Yohimbine, on the other hand, a chemical from the bark of a tree in South America, may have some aphrodisiac properties because it acts on the nerve centers in the spine that control erection. It's available by prescription and should only be taken under your doctor's direction because there's a little poison in every medication, and yohimbine is no exception. Some of my patients who have tried it say it helps, most say it doesn't. Clearly, the search must continue.

If you have a special interest in the history of aphrodisiac foods and potions, read *Medicine Through Antiquity* by B. L. Gordon, published some fifty years ago, and *Aphrodisiacs: The Science and the Myth* by Peter Taberner. Both contain some fascinating accounts of how and why our forebears came to view certain foods as sex potentiators. For example, according to a theory called the Doctrine of Signatures, propounded millennia ago, we humans are a microcosm of the world in which we live, and every one of our organs has a corresponding entity in nature that, when consumed, can enhance its function. Since oysters are shaped like the male testes, they were assumed to be endowed with sex-enhancing qualities. For hundreds of years, men have been eating them with that hope in mind. Casanova really went at it with a vengeance, allegedly consuming fifty every night at dinner! (I'm surprised he didn't develop hepatitis A, whose virus is found in raw oysters taken from contaminated waters, or some other infection. I doubt he knew that adding a splash of hot sauce such as Tabasco kills the germs in oysters within a minute—at least in the test tube. As an oyster lover, I would not alter their taste in this way. I prefer a little lemon juice, and nothing more!)

Casanova notwithstanding, there is a possible rationale for the oyster legend since they are the richest source of zinc. I am not aware of any scientific studies proving that zinc is really a sexual stimulant, but some urologists recommend it anyway because large amounts are found in the male ejaculate. Even a mild deficiency of this essential trace element can reduce the sperm count, lower the level of testosterone, and interfere with normal function of the immune system. (Persons with too little zinc in their diet are unusually susceptible to infection.) Also, some baby boys born with poorly developed sex organs (infantilism) are lacking in zinc. Correcting this deficiency improves their sexual status. Based on these observations, some urologists are recommending zinc to men with impaired libido, especially those who are likely to be deficient in it, as, for example, anyone with alcoholic liver disease, malabsorption problems (see page 307), individuals with rheumatoid arthritis taking penicillamine, persons with chronic kidney disease or sickle-cell anemia, and poorly nourished older people. (One out of every eight men and women in this country above the age of fifty-five eats less zinc than the RDA calls for.) Whether the extra 10 or 15 milligrams, either in supplements or in oysters, will heighten your sexuality is something you should determine for yourself—especially if you like oysters. But regardless of its impact on your love life, extra zinc may enhance your overall nutritional status if you are indeed lacking in it.

The RDA for zinc is 12 milligrams a day for women, and 15

milligrams for men. You sexy oyster eaters won't have any trouble meeting that quota, since six medium raw oysters contain 76 milligrams! Some zinc is also present in lean beef, veal, pork, lamb, chicken, and herring, and to a lesser extent in grains, legumes, nuts, vegetables, and fruit. However, 3 ounces of oysters (that's about six of average size) contain at least ten times more than 3 ounces of beef! Because more people eat beef than oysters, the former is the single most important source of zinc actually consumed in the United States. If oysters are not your cup of tea, you can be virtually certain of getting all you need in 5 to 7 ounces of lean meat, poultry, or fish daily. If you do crave oysters, however, be sure to check their sources. Raw oysters from contaminated waters will give you hepatitis A, a viral infection that won't do much for your sex drive. The table on page 151 contains a comprehensive list of zinc-containing foods, and how many calories they contain per portion. Try to fill all your zinc needs with food, because too much in supplement form can interfere with copper and iron metabolism.

The truth is that the possible relationship between oysters and libido has actually become kind of a joke—like the one my friend made when I ordered them while my wife was out of town. I have never come across anyone who dislikes oysters but eats them anyway just to improve his sex life. *Ginseng,* however, is another matter. Millions take this herb seriously—for whatever ails them. There is a worldwide, multimillion-dollar industry based on ginseng, most of which now comes from the Far East.

Ginseng is a root with a long history. The Chinese have been using it for centuries. Early American colonists, including our own Daniel Boone, were ginseng devotees too. In the past twenty years, there has been a resurgence in interest in this root in this country. Although some form or other is grown throughout the world, the traditional, classic product is the Panax variety of Chinese origin. It is widely used in the United States and elsewhere by athletes, by menopausal women (hoping to help control their hot flashes and other symptoms of estrogen deprivation—see page 316), by both sexes as a tonic, and by men to enhance sexual prowess. The name Panax comes from the Greek *panacea,* and the word *ginseng* itself means "root of man" because the intact root is shaped like the human body. According to the

Doctrine of Signatures, that's why it's supposed to be good for so many different conditions.

Despite all the claims made on its behalf, sexual potency included, I could not find any credible research by Western-trained scientists confirming ginseng's biological activity. Russian doctors claim that it does have substances that act on the glandular (endocrine) system and that it is good for the circulation as well. But the most fervent enthusiasts are the Chinese, who in the last ten years alone have published three hundred scientific articles documenting a wide range of actions by ginseng on the nervous, cardiovascular, endocrine, and immune systems. They believe it not only has strong sex-stimulating powers, but also possesses significant antistress and antiaging properties. In fact, ginseng is officially approved in China for several clinical uses. However, the medical establishment in this country will have nothing to do with it, at least officially. Furthermore, some varieties have been shown to be quite toxic. One of the major problems with ginseng, in my opinion, is that there is virtually no quality control on many of the brands sold in this country.

Another word of warning: Even though the package says it contains a certain amount of ginseng, you may be getting either less than you think or none at all! Researchers in Sweden who recently tested fifty such products sold in eleven different countries, including the United States, found a great variation in their ginseng content, and six of the brands contained none of the plant's root, from which active ginseng is derived. In addition to ginseng, one preparation was found to have ephedrine, a dilator of the bronchial tree, decongestant, and heart stimulant. If you'd happened to be taking some of that before an athletic competition, and your urine or blood was tested for drugs, you'd have flunked!

I have no personal recommendations one way or another with regard to ginseng. I do not use it myself, either when my wife is at home or away, and I do not recommend it to any of my patients. However, there is considerable advertising for it, and some persons will decide to try it. Remember, however, that this herb is not under the jurisdiction of the FDA. If you decide to use it, do not exceed the recommended dose on the box. The usual dose of the Panax herb is one capsule three times a day, or as tea (one cup a day is what most ginseng devotees drink), or 1 or 2 teaspoons in water taken on an empty stomach. Ginseng can make you nervous or jittery, so don't take it at bedtime. Avoid it too if you have high blood pressure or suffer from chronic headaches because ginseng has been known to aggravate both. Be aware that it can also cause vaginal bleeding, especially if you're menopausal. If this occurs, report it to your doctor.

Most foods and potions alleged over the years to enhance sexual powers are harmless, but some can create problems. For example, repeated use of Spanish fly (cantharides) can hurt the genitourinary tract. Folklore about the power of powdered rhinoceros horn taken with wine has helped put that animal on the endangered species list. If you want to experiment, stay with the following exotic substances, which are at worst harmless: Jasmine oil, when inhaled or rubbed into the body, is reputed to increase sexual desire; cardamom, a common ingredient in curry, is said to increase libido when inhaled; the scents of iris, lilac, magnolia, narcissus, orange, sandalwood, vanilla, wood aloe, and many others are all touted to be sexual stimulants too. You won't find any of this documented in medical books, but if you happen to find a scent that stimulates you or the object of your affections, by all means use it.

The latest news in the sex-enhancement arena comes from Dr. Vijay Kakar at the Thrombosis Institute in London. He recently completed an experiment on two hundred people and has concluded that regular cold baths not only increase resistance to viruses but also stimulate the circulation, abolish chronic fatigue, and improve sexual potency. Funny, I always thought cold water had the reverse effect. But according to Dr. Kakar, that's only if you do it occasionally and without prior training. He recommends a three-month period of cold baths during which your body becomes tolerant of the low temperatures. Daily cold baths, he says, stimulate sexual desire by increasing the production of testosterone in men and estrogen in women. At last word, Dr. Kakar wants to validate his findings with five thousand additional subjects. If you're interested, write to him at the Thrombosis Research Institute in London. There may still be an opening for you! That's all for now on this subject. My oysters are waiting.

FOODS HIGH IN ZINC

FOOD	PORTION	ZINC (mg)	CALORIES	CHOLES-TEROL (mg)	FAT (gm)
Beans/legumes					
black beans, cooked	1 cup	1.92	227	0	0.9
chickpeas, cooked	1 cup	2.51	269	0	4.3
lentils, cooked	1 cup	2.5	231	0	0.7
red kidney beans, cooked	1 cup	1.89	225	0	0.9
split peas, cooked	1 cup	1.96	231	0	0.8
vegetarian baked beans (Heinz)	1 cup	3.55	235	0	1.1
Beef					
liver, braised	3.5 ounces	6.07	161	389	4.9
tenderloin, untrimmed, broiled	3.5 ounces	5.3	244	85	14.3
Cashews, dry roasted	1 ounce	1.59	163	0	13.2
Cereals					
All-Bran (Kellogg's)	⅓ cup	3.75	70	0	1.0
bran flakes (Kellogg's)	⅓ cup	3.75	90	0	0
wheat grain (Kretschmer's)	⅓ cup	3.18	57	0	2.3
Product 19	1 cup	15	100	0	0.2
Shredded Wheat	1 ounce	0.93	102	0	0.6
Special K	1⅓ cups	3.75	110	0	0.1
Cheeses					
cheddar	1 ounce	.88	114	30	9.4
cottage, 2% fat	1 cup	.95	203	19	4.4
Gouda	1 ounce	1.11	101	32	7.8
mozzarella	1 ounce	.63	80	22	6.1
ricotta, part skim	½ cup	1.66	171	38	9.8
Swiss	1 ounce	1.11	107	26	7.8
Fish/shellfish					
crab, Alaskan king, cooked	3 ounces	6.48	82	45	1.3

FOODS HIGH IN ZINC *(Continued)*

FOOD	PORTION	ZINC (mg)	CALORIES	CHOLES-TEROL (mg)	FAT (gm)
herring, Atlantic, cooked	3 ounces	1.08	172	65	9.9
herring, Pacific, cooked	3 ounces	0.58	213	84	15.1
lobster, Northern	3 ounces	2.48	83	61	0.5
mussels, blue, cooked	3 ounces	2.27	147	48	3.8
oysters, Eastern, raw	6 medium	76.4	58	46	2.1
oysters, Pacific, raw	3 ounces	14.13	69	55	2.0
Dried fruits					
dates	10	0.24	228	0	0
prunes	10	0.45	201	0	0
raisins, seedless	⅔ cup	0.27	300	0	0
Fresh fruits					
apricots	3 medium	0.28	51	0	0
banana	1 medium	0.19	105	0	0.6
blackberries	½ cup	0.20	37	0	0
blueberries	1 cup	0.16	82	0	0.6
cantaloupe	1 cup	0.25	57	0	0
papaya	1 medium	0.22	117	0	0
peach	1 medium	0.12	37	0	0
pear	1 medium	0.20	98	0	0
persimmon, Japanese	1 medium	0.18	118	0	0
raspberries	1 cup	0.57	61	0	0
strawberries	1 cup	0.19	45	0	0
watermelon	1 cup	0.11	50	0	0.7
Meat/poultry					
chicken, light and dark meat, skinless, roasted	3.5 ounces	2.1	190	89	7.4
lamb, domestic, leg, choice, roasted	3.5 ounces	4.85	204	92	9.2

FOODS HIGH IN ZINC *(Continued)*

FOOD	PORTION	ZINC (mg)	CALORIES	CHOLES-TEROL (mg)	FAT (gm)
lamb, domestic, shoulder, cubed and stewed	3.5 ounces	6.58	223	108	8.8
pork center loin, lean, broiled	3.5 ounces	2.23	231	98	10.5
turkey, ground patty, cooked	3 ounces	2.36	188	57	11.4
veal, ground, broiled	3.5 ounces	3.87	172	103	7.6
veal, top round, braised	3.5 ounces	4.03	203	135	5.1
Milk					
skim	8 ounces	0.98	86	4	0.4
2% fat	8 ounces	0.95	121	18	4.7
Vegetables					
asparagus, cooked	6 spears	0.38	22	0	0.3
beets, boiled	½ cup	0.21	26	0	0
broccoli, uncooked	½ cup	0.18	12	0	0
broccoli, frozen, chopped, and boiled	½ cup	0.28	25	0	0
brussels sprouts, boiled	½ cup	0.25	30	0	0.4
carrot, uncooked	1 medium	0.14	31	0	0
carrot, frozen, boiled	½ cup	0.18	26	0	0
collards, boiled	1 cup	0.14	34	0	0
cucumber, uncooked	⅙ medium	0.12	7	0	0
green beans, boiled	½ cup	0.23	22	0	0
mushrooms, uncooked	½ cup	0.17	9	0	0
onion, uncooked	½ cup	0.15	30	0	0
peas, boiled	½ cup	0.95	67	0	0
radish, uncooked	10	0.13	7	0	0

FOODS HIGH IN ZINC *(Continued)*

FOOD	PORTION	ZINC (mg)	CALORIES	CHOLES-TEROL (mg)	FAT (gm)
spinach, boiled	½ cup	0.69	21	0	0
squash, summer, all varieties, boiled	½ cup	0.35	18	0	0
squash, winter, all varieties, baked	½ cup	0.27	39	0	0.6
tomato	1 medium	0.11	26	0	0
Yogurt, low-fat, with added nonfat dry milk solids	8 ounces	2.02	144	14	3.5

DIVERTICULOSIS
AND DIVERTICULITIS
YOU'RE JUST TOO REFINED!

Diverticulosis is a condition in which tiny, fingerlike projections or outpouchings form in the wall of the large bowel (colon). I don't know who does the counting, or how, but I am told that more than 30 million Americans, most of them over fifty years of age, have this condition. It accounts for some 200,000 hospital admissions every year in the United States alone, at a current cost of about $300 million.

Diverticula (the plural of diverticulum) probably result from long-standing increased pressure within the bowel. What is most likely to cause such elevated pressure over the years? Chronic constipation. Why do people become constipated? *Because, among other reasons, they do not drink enough liquids or eat enough fiber.* Who on earth would eat such an unhealthy diet? Why, you and I and most people living in the Western world! Are we absolutely sure of this relationship between diet and diverticulosis? No, but the circumstantial evidence is very convincing. In most industrialized nations, where a low-fiber diet is the norm, the incidence of diverticulosis is high. By contrast, where the national diet is rich in indigestible fiber, as it is in much of Africa and Asia, this condition is relatively uncommon. When rural inhabitants in these countries move to the cities, abandon their traditional diet in favor of a more "civilized" one, and begin eating refined foods, they too develop diverticular disease of the colon!

In the vast majority of persons, bowel diverticula are silent. But in some, these little outpouchings bleed, or become inflamed and infected. When that happens, you have graduated from the relatively benign diverticulosis to the miserable *diverticulitis,* attacks of which result in abdominal pain (usually in the left lower portion), fever, possibly either constipation or diarrhea, and in about 2 percent of cases, blood in the stool. It's now too late for the preventive diet described below. At this point, treatment of the acute attack consists of antibiotics to control infection, no solid food, only clear liquids, or, if the symptoms are severe enough, intravenous feeding. Should the infected diverticulum develop an abscess or burst, emergency surgery may be required. When diverticulosis is accompanied by repeated bleeding, or when attacks of acute diverticulitis become frequent, surgical removal of the portion of bowel containing the diverticula may be necessary.

The good news is that you can often prevent diverticulosis and its complications with a high-fiber diet. What exactly is fiber, how much are we now consuming, and how much do we need? The answers to these questions offer an example of how we have made an about-face in medicine in recent years. Not so long ago, doctors were actually prescribing *low-fiber* diets in order not to "aggravate" the bowel, especially one with diverticula. We now know that this is precisely the opposite of what they should have been telling their patients!

Fiber is the indigestible constituent in plant foods (grains, fruits, and vegetables). There are two kinds of fiber, soluble and insoluble. The former dissolves in water, the latter does not. The richest sources of *soluble* fiber are oat bran and psyllium (found in Metamucil and its generic equivalents), but it is also present in beans, barley, legumes, and certain fruits and vegetables. Pectin, a soluble fiber, is found in a variety of fruits—apples, oranges and other citrus fruits, strawberries, broccoli, and carrots. One of the extra benefits of soluble fiber is its mild but definite cholesterol-lowering action. *Insoluble* fiber, also called "roughage," is the cellulose and hemicellulose in the skin of fruits and vegetables, and the outer layer (the bran) of corn and wheat kernels. It provides bulk to the stool, makes it soft, and speeds its passage through the bowel. This prevents constipation and all its problems, ranging from diverticulosis to possibly cancer of the bowel and even hiatal hernias and gallstones. We should be eating anywhere from 35 to 50 grams of fiber every day. Instead, the average American consumption falls far short of that, somewhere between 10 and 20 grams per day! See the table on page 116 for a list of the fiber content of various foods. At the end of this section you will find two sample menus—one that gives you plenty of fiber, and one that doesn't. Which comes closer to what you eat?

We should nurture in our children early in life a taste for foods rich in fiber. Serve them plenty of fresh and dried fruits and fresh vegetables daily (focus on those with the highest fiber content—apples, oranges, berries, dates, figs, and pears; as well as brussels sprouts, corn, cucumbers, potatoes, and carrots). Don't even let them know that there is such a thing as white bread; give them whole wheat instead. Your kids should have high-fiber cereal at breakfast. But make sure they also get into the habit of drinking plenty of water, because unless they do, all that fiber may actually cause constipation! Developing such eating habits in childhood reduces the chances of constipation and diverticulosis later in life.

So much for your kids. Is it too late for *you* to start on a high-fiber diet, especially if you already have diverticulosis? It's all the more reason to do so. I believe that eating 35 to 50 grams of fiber a day will sharply reduce the likelihood of diverticulitis and/or bleeding. You can ensure enough fiber in your diet by adding miller's bran (crude unprocessed wheat bran) to your cereal, fruit juice, or soup. Start slowly, with only 1 tablespoon once or twice a day, and increase the amount every two weeks to as much as 4 tablespoons a day. But do not take any more than you are comfortable eating, because too much fiber too quickly can cause distressing amounts of gas, bloating, cramps, and diarrhea. *Psyllium* is another good fiber supplement. Again, start with 1 or 2 teaspoons a day in water, soup, or fruit juice and work your way up. (For more information on high-fiber foods, see Constipation chapter, page 111.) Remember to drink lots of water—at least eight to ten 8-ounce glasses every day to avoid a dry, impacted stool.

There is a potential downside to a high-fiber diet for older people, children, and pregnant women in whom adequate nutrition is especially important. Eating fiber has a greater satiety effect than most other foods—you feel full when you eat enough of it. This may reduce the appetite, and that's not desirable if you're underweight or have greater nutritional needs. Also, when the amount of indigestible fiber in the diet is increased, extra fat and nitrogen may be lost in the stool so that less calcium, vitamins, and other minerals are absorbed from the gut. The amounts are not usually significant in most healthy, well-nourished adults, but they may be in those vulnerable persons mentioned above. The best way to ensure that you're getting the vitamins and minerals you need is to take a multivitamin and mineral supplement that satisfies the recommended dietary allowances.

Doctors used to caution anyone with diverticulosis against eating any foods that contained seeds, on the assumption that one or more might penetrate a little sac, irritate and perhaps infect it, and cause an attack of diverticulitis. Reasonable enough in theory, but wrong in practice. No one knows what actually precipitates an attack of diverticulitis or bleeding, but seeds and nuts do not. Also, they are good sources of fiber, so enjoy them if you want to.

The table on page 119 provides a sample menu for you and your children that will ensure the right kind of diet to prevent diverticulosis, and hopefully reduce the chances of complications if you already have it. If your diet looks more like the menu in the table on page 120, eat more roughage and stop being so refined!

FEEDING YOUR INFANT

EAT MORE AND WEIGH LESS

You've just had a baby! Your own mother probably bottle-fed you because years ago many women in the "developed" countries believed that an "ideal" formula devised by man was better for their infants than anything nature could provide. We now know that there is no commercial product as good for a baby as mother's milk—something even the makers of infant formula concede, right on the label! Human milk contains unique antibodies that protect against infections and allergies, its fat content is better digested than any other, it is bacteria free—and it's guaranteed fresh! What's more, breast-feeding creates an eternal bond between mother and child that no formula, however complete, can duplicate.

Having said all that, I also feel very strongly that how a woman chooses to nourish her infant is a very personal matter. Some mothers cannot breast-feed for physical reasons, but even those who simply prefer not to do so should not be made to feel guilty about it. After all, millions of us were bottle-fed without adverse effects. More important for the baby than the bottle-feeding-versus-breast-feeding issue is its mother's contentment.

If you do decide to breast-feed your baby, your doctor will want to be sure that you don't use any drugs or medications incompatible with nursing, or have any serious ailment such as TB; that your HIV test is negative (the AIDS virus has been found in human milk); and that your nipples are suitable for nursing. Even if you had hepatitis years ago, and your blood is always rejected by the blood bank when you try to donate it, it is safe to breast-feed. However, your doctor will probably immunize your baby with the hepatitis vaccine. Don't worry about your breasts being too small; breast size has nothing to do with successful nursing; big breasts simply contain more fat. It's the number of milk-producing glands within them that counts, and these are usually plentiful even in small breasts.

Once you've decided to breast-feed, start as soon as possible after delivery, and plan to do so for at least three months—preferably for six, even if you are working. Either adjust the feeding schedule so that you nurse morning, noon, and night, or express the milk with a breast pump and make it available on demand when you are away from home. Try not to use artificial nipples, pacifiers, water, or formula during the first few weeks. After all, you want the baby to become accustomed to and feel secure with one kind of oral stimulus. Switching to and from these others only confuses him or her.

All right, you're all set and can't wait to get started. But psychologically you have one important reservation—your weight. After you gave birth you hoped to lose some of the twenty-five pounds or so that you gained. Now you are told that nursing your baby requires an extra 500 to 700 calories per day to make enough high-quality milk and to compensate your body for the loss of all the nutrients flowing out of your nipples. That means 2,500 to 2,700 calories a day for the first six months of breast-feeding as compared to the 1,800 to 2,000 calories you consumed before you became pregnant. And if you continue to nurse for longer than six months, you'll require even more calories because (1) you will have used up all the fat reserves acquired during pregnancy (see below), and (2) as the baby grows, so does his or her appetite, which must be satisfied.

These extra calories do not necessarily mean that you will gain weight. As a matter of fact, you are more than likely to *lose* some despite the increased caloric intake because eight of the twenty-five pounds you put on during those forty weeks was body fat—earmarked by nature to be used later specifically for breast-feeding. They provide as much as 150 calories per day every day you do so. During the first three months, this fat will melt away. Also, because breast-feeding helps you burn calories more efficiently, you'll lose more if you breast-feed than if you don't! Repeated pregnancies *without* breast-feeding may actually leave you fat later on.

To ensure the best-quality milk for your infant, do not cut any nutritional corners. That means no crash dieting. Remember too that although caffeine does not make its way into the milk, too much of it, say more than three or four 5-ounce cups a day, can suppress the amount of milk you produce. Unless you play by all the rules of the nutritional game, both you and the baby will be the losers. However, when push comes to shove, nature prefers to shortchange *you* rather than deprive your infant. Anything the baby needs over and above what you provide in your diet will be taken from *your* body stores. Unless you have plenty of minerals and vitamins in your diet and adequate overall nutrition, your bones may become depleted of calcium, and your body's iron reserves may be reduced as well. Be sure to consume at least 1,200 milligrams of calcium a day while nursing. (Such calcium loss occurs only during lactation, not in pregnancy.) Even with enough vitamin and mineral supplements, you may still lose about 5 percent of your bone density in the first six months of nursing. Imagine how much more that would be without nutritional supplementation. Happily, this bone loss begins to be restored twelve months after delivery. Whether nursing beyond nine months causes any permanent loss of bone density is still being debated, but I do not believe there is enough evidence at the present time to justify your stopping breast-feeding after nine months unless you wish to do so.

You may eat essentially whatever you like when nursing your baby, so long as your daily intake of calcium, iron, zinc, and other minerals and vitamins is adequate. The best way to ensure that is to *continue your prenatal vitamins while nursing*. You also need 15 grams of *extra* protein a day for a total of 65 grams, during the first six months of lactation, and an extra 12 grams per day for the next six months. Two to 3 cups of milk daily will satisfy that need.

There is one important qualification to the "permission" to eat what you like while nursing. Go easy on the sweets and fruits for the first two or three months of nursing. It takes that long for the infant to become accustomed to them, and if you eat them any earlier, they may give the baby diarrhea. Also, if you, members of your family, or your other children have allergies, there are certain measures that can make a difference. You must control the dust mites in your home—by lowering the humidity (on which mold and mites thrive), vacuuming regularly, and cleaning draperies and carpets every three or four months. Also, children raised in a smoke-filled environment have a 25 percent greater chance of developing allergies if even only one parent is allergic, and two of every three will develop them if both parents are allergic. With respect to diet itself, you should not be eating sushi and other raw fish, steak tartare or other uncooked meat, and soft, unpasteurized imported cheeses, all of which leave you vulnerable to listeriosis and other infections (see page 387). Both mother and infant should avoid such common allergens as eggs, fish, nuts, and cow's milk for the first year of life. Nor should you feed the infant any soy products, wheat, or oranges. Fifty-eight breast-feeding mothers and their babies who followed such a regimen for one year, had only one-third the incidence of allergies as compared to those who ate a normal diet. Their children also developed less asthma (4 percent versus 19 percent) and eczema. So it appears that any inherited predisposition to allergy is triggered by environmental factors such as smoke pollution, which, when controlled, can make a difference.

For nine long months you may have had nary a drink—no cocktails, no beer, no wine. Is it safe for you to indulge now—very modestly, once in a while? I believe it probably is, but I suggest that you limit yourself to two or three drinks a week, and no more than 1 or 2 ounces of liquor, 8 ounces of wine, or a bottle of beer per session. The reason for this restriction is that, while alcohol may turn you on, it turns your infant off. It's true that after you take a drink, the baby will suck a little harder for the first minute or so, but the total amount of milk consumed will actually be less. The belief that beer increases the volume of breast milk has persisted for generations. When this hypothesis was actually tested under scientific conditions, it was found to have no basis in fact. And there are better ways to obtain the vitamins in beer. Consuming large quantities of any alcohol while breast-feeding is a complete no-no.

Although you were assured that continuing a vegan diet (a strict vegetarian diet that includes no dairy products) during pregnancy wouldn't harm your baby, you did, in fact, liberalize your diet to some extent—just to be sure. Now you're anxious to go back to the real thing—no animal (including fish) or derivative foods whatsoever. Is it okay to do so if you are breast-feeding? Yes. A vegan diet will fulfill all your nutritional needs and those of your infant *if you take oral supplemental B₁₂.*

You must drink eight to twelve glasses of liquid a day, of which three or four should be low-fat milk—for its protein and calcium content are actually higher than that of whole milk. An 8-ounce glassful every hour or two during the day is a good way to be sure you get all you need.

Just before the very first feeding, when they check their nipples to make sure the milk is flowing, mothers sometimes panic. Is this deep-yellow fluid milk? No, it's not. It's colostrum, and that's what the baby will be drinking for the first few days. It's nature's way of breaking the newborn in, so to speak. Remember that, until now, your infant has taken nothing by mouth. Colostrum is easy to digest; it contains less fat and carbohydrate, but more sodium and potassium than milk, and it's loaded with antibodies that protect against bacteria and viruses. It also has a laxative action that rids the infant's gut of secretions and other waste products accumulated while it was still in the womb. Colostrum prepares your child's intestinal tract to handle your milk later on, with its full complement of fat, protein, carbohydrates, hormones, and growth factors.

Infants have a well-developed sense of taste and smell at birth, so they appreciate your varying your diet while nursing. They can't tell you this, but after a few weeks they actually enjoy a "good meal," which you can provide by eating tasty foods, most of whose odors and aromas find their way into the milk (just as they reach your breath, saliva, stool, urine, and sweat.) When garlic was added to the diet of nursing mothers in a recent experiment, their babies without exception sucked harder and longer than usual, and literally had to be pulled away from the nipples. By contrast, 25 percent of all kids fed the same boring bottle day in, day out, lose their appetite until the formula is changed. Variety, it seems, really is the spice of life. Sometimes, of course, a particular food you're eating may not sit well with your infant. There's no way of predicting what it will be, but onions, tomatoes, even carbonated drinks are among the common offenders. Sometimes, it's not what you eat that upsets the baby, but how much. I remember one mother telling me that bingeing on a bag of peanut butter cookies resulted in the baby having diarrhea the next day. Cramps, diarrhea, irritability, even vomiting are the key symptoms to look out for when you suspect that something new in your diet is not agreeing with the baby.

Although it has not been demonstrated in humans, it is well documented in animals that what the mother eats while nursing influences her child's food preferences later in life. When nursing mammals are given a wide variety of food, their weanlings will accept them all when they're on their own. But when the mothers are restricted to one kind of hay, mash, or fodder, that's what the offspring will stay with once they're weaned.

Breast-feeding is not always simple and easy. Some women get the hang of it without any trouble whatsoever. Others find the engorged breasts uncomfortable or complain that their nipples are constantly sore or leaking. Also, the mechanism that causes the milk to flow is under the control of a nerve-hormone reflex that can be disrupted by stress or anxiety. When that happens, the milk just doesn't come out in quantities that satisfy the infant, and a vicious cycle of maternal/baby irritability ensues. Discuss your nursing techniques, problems, or fears with your doctor or consult the nearest chapter of La Leche League, listed in the phone directory.

I have thus far limited this discussion on infant feeding to the mother who nurses her baby. If you choose to bottle-feed, buy one of the commercial formulas. Do not use whole cow's milk, which contains more protein than the infant can digest or the kidneys can handle in the first year of life. Evaporated milk is not ideal either because, even though it is easier to digest, it lacks some important ingredients. The quality and content of needed vitamins, minerals, and proteins in commercial formulas are regulated by law and are as close as you can get to mother's milk. If your child is lactose intolerant, use a soy-based product. Here is an interesting observation about these soy feedings. Unlike mother's milk, soy has no cholesterol whatsoever. You would think that's good, wouldn't you? Nature, however, doesn't agree! Infants living exclusively on soy formulae produce *more* cholesterol *internally* to make up for what is missing in their diet! It makes one wonder, doesn't it, about how soon to put our children on low-cholesterol diets (see page 215). I have always felt that nature's way should take preference over the recommendations of any scientific or governmental agency, no matter how learned or prestigious!

Here are some key facts for nursing mothers to remember: (1) Breast-feeding makes for healthier babies and fewer problems later in life, but whether or not you choose to do so is a very personal matter. (2) You should continue the high-quality nutrition you enjoyed during pregnancy and continue taking vitamin supplements. (3) A good portion of the weight you gained during pregnancy was earmarked for use during breast-feeding. So the extra calories you have to consume while breast-feeding won't make you gain weight. (4) If you cut corners nutritionally, you'll be harmed much more than the baby. Nature will deplete your body's reserves of essential vitamins and minerals before it deprives the child. (5) Infants respond to different tastes and aromas in mother's milk. Make life interesting for your child by varying your diet while breast-feeding.

FLATULENCE

WHEN IT'S TIME TO RATION GAS

The other day was an event of sorts. It was the first time I had ever encountered the term *fart* in the American medical literature. Why, even when running this section through the spelling checker on the Microsoft program of her computer, my secretary was informed that *fart* is not in its dictionary! This stark, no-nonsense word, written or uttered, is considered to be in bad taste in this country. Yet in England, prestigious medical journals such as *The Lancet, The British Medical Journal, The British Heart Journal,* and *The Journal of the Royal Society of Medicine* all use *fart* as casually as we do *cough*. So hats off to the sixteenth edition of *The Merck Manual* for its courageous stance on *fart*!

Too much gas can be a problem above or below the belt. Most burps and belches (the former are more subtle, elegant, and discreet; a belch is apt to be loud and gross) originate in the stomach and are due to swallowed air, excessive amounts of carbonated beverages drunk too quickly, or baking soda or other liquid "indigestion" medications like Epsom salts. Gas expelled from the rectum—our friend the fart—is usually caused by fermentation of food by bacteria normally present in the intestine, or by certain medications like cholestyramine and colestipol (widely prescribed to lower cholesterol levels).

Swallowing air is a nervous habit aggravated by stress or anxiety. Those who gulp it, even in large quantities, generally do not realize they are doing so. Eating quickly, salivating excessively because of poorly fitting dentures, chewing gum, and smoking all increase the amount of air you swallow. If you have a burping or belching problem, eat smaller meals more slowly rather than fewer larger ones, do not stoop or lie down soon after a meal, keep your belt or girdle loose, don't gulp liquids, and sip, don't quaff, your carbonated drinks. I also advise my patients to put a pencil or soft eraser between their teeth when they feel tense. (Try it yourself, right now, and see whether you can swallow any air with it.)

There is always some gas in the intestine and we all pass it, surreptitiously, when possible. It's not the kind of thing with which you want to go public! I was amused and surprised when reviewing the medical literature on this subject to learn how many studies have been done on virtually every aspect of farting. For example, you wouldn't believe the number of devices there are for measuring and analyzing the gas content of the lowly fart! Some of our most brilliant scientists have worked long and hard to glean the following information that I am certain will be of great interest to you. Normal people like you and me fart an average of thirteen times a day, but someone with a gas-forming problem may do it as often as twenty times an *hour*! No, this is not a typo—twenty times an hour is correct! This is not usually a problem when done in the privacy of one's home, car, or office, but it can be embarrassing at a press conference, in an elevator with just one other person there, or at a board meeting while the chairperson is making his or her report. And imagine the reaction to the music if you're a dentist bending over to fix someone's teeth or a psychiatrist listening to a patient's problems!

In the section on Flatulence in the sixteenth edition of *The Merck Manual,* the following different types of farts are described: the "slider," also known as SBD (silent but deadly)—slow and noiseless, which can be devastating in a crowded elevator (imagine the "Who, me?" expression on everyone's face including that of the perpetrator); the "pooh," noisy but not necessarily aromatic; the "staccato" or "drum beat," quite pleasant when passed in private; the "bark," fine when you're alone but awful at a P.T.A. meeting.

But farting can be fun—and even profitable! It can also make you famous! Le Pétomane was a popular French entertainer at the Moulin Rouge in Paris years ago. His talent lay in his ability to generate unlimited quantities of intestinal gas that he could control with great precision. He delighted his audience by playing, rectally, a number of different tunes, including "La Marseillaise," the French national anthem! But for those of us not interested in making a career of it, excessive abdominal gas is something to be avoided. You can, to a great extent, do so by eating the right food.

Gas in the bowel is produced by normal bacteria in the gut, acting on undigested food. As you might expect, the worst offenders are high-fiber foods, since insoluble fiber is indigestible. Virtually every kind of pea and bean—soy, navy, lima, kidney, or dried—is especially bad that way. Their designation, "the musical fruit" (except that they are legumes, not fruits), is well deserved. But don't let that stop you from eating them. Their benefits far outweigh this inconvenience, and you'll have fewer problems with fiber if you follow these suggestions. Change to a high-fiber diet gradually. For example, begin by substituting whole-grain for white bread, use brown rice instead of white, and have no more than two servings a day for a week or two. As you increase the amount of fiber in your diet, drink more water. Dry fiber can cause constipation. Vary the types you eat; select widely among fresh vegetables and fresh fruit, as well as bran cereals, fresh salads, bean soups, and legumes (see the table on page 116 for a list of foods and their fiber content). You can "de-gas" most legumes to some extent by soaking them for several hours and then discarding the soaking water. Remember, however, that doing so leaches out some of their nutrients. There is also a flavorless over-the-counter product called Beano that, when added to bean dishes, will prevent or significantly reduce any resulting gas. Other potential gas formers are cabbage, peppers, any uncooked starch, broccoli, cauliflower, brussels sprouts, radishes, cucumbers, raisins, garlic, onions, and foods that are eaten extremely hot or cold. No two people react in the same way to the same dish. A particular food will produce "Marseillaise"-tooting amounts in some and barely a bubble in others. Some laxatives, too, produce gas by speeding the transit of food through the bowel and interfering with adequate digestion.

I remember reading about a thirty-year-old man whose quality of life was seriously impaired by too much intestinal gas. He averaged thirty emissions a day, whose characteristics he recorded over a two-year period. He invented a "flatus graph" that enabled him to document the volume and frequency of each "outburst" so that, for example, he was able to distinguish between a "squeaker" and a "blast." He also analyzed the composition of the gas passed and found it contained predominantly hydrogen and carbon dioxide, indicating that it originated in the bowel. (Gas in the stomach due to swallowed air consists mainly of nitrogen.) In order to identify the offending foods, he fasted for two days and then reintroduced 130 different ones in sequence. He found the most "flatulogenic" for him to be milk and its products, onions, beans, celery, carrots, raisins, bananas, apricots, prune juice, pretzels, bagels, wheat germ, and brussels sprouts. By avoiding them, he dramatically reduced his abdominal gas and was able to resume a normal life.

I am not suggesting that you dedicate yourself this way for two years in order to manage your excessive gas. There are, however, certain less-complicated steps you can take. First, make sure that you are not lactose intolerant, meaning you have an inherited deficiency in the enzyme lactase, which digests lactose, a sugar present in milk and its derivatives. Undigested lactose sits around in the bowel, fair game for gas-producing fermentation by bacteria. You can make that diagnosis in your own home. Just record everything you eat for a few days and keep track of your gas situation. Then omit all dairy products for about five days, and see whether or not your farting frequency falls. If it appears that the situation has improved and you suspect that milk or dairy products are the source of your digestive problems, take another two days to check it out further. Have your usual dinner, then nothing more until the following morning. With your breakfast, be sure to drink a full glass of any kind of milk—the fat content does not matter. If you develop gas, bloating, abdominal cramps, or diarrhea in the next six hours, lactose is very probably the root of your problem. There is one more step you should take to clinch the diagnosis. Buy some Lactaid or Dairy Ease tablets (they are available without a prescription) at a drugstore or supermarket. The next morning take three lactase-containing tablets five minutes before eating the same breakfast. (Add them the night before to the milk you're going to be drinking.) If the symptoms you had yesterday do not reappear, you are lactose intolerant because you responded to the missing enzyme.

Using lactase supplements allows most lactase-deficient persons to eat dairy products in moderate amounts without discomfort. (It is especially important for females of all ages to have at least 1,000 milligrams of calcium a day, easily obtained from dairy products, in order to reduce the risk of osteoporosis later in life.) Remember, too, that lactose content varies considerably among dairy products. For example, hard cheese contains relatively little, as compared with milk. Lactose-free milk is now widely available in most supermarkets.

Angina, a heart attack, or a serious abdominal problem are often mistaken for "gas." I always warn my patients to tell me whenever they have chest discomfort or belly pain that they think is due to too much "air." They are often right, but that phone call can save their lives if they are wrong!

Farting is a subject of humor, and I doubt that your insurance carrier will reimburse you for its treatment. But what is funny for one person can be uncomfortable and a source of serious embarrassment for another when there is too much gas in the bowel clamoring to be released. In most cases, the problem is caused by bad eating habits, especially swallowing air.

In summary, eating the right foods at the right pace, not gulping liquids, sipping instead of chugging carbonated beverages, and eating smaller meals more slowly will control most burps and belches. Certain foods, especially those that are rich in fiber, can be fermented by the normal gas-forming bacteria in the bowel. Building up your fiber intake gradually will usually reduce the amount of gas in the bowel. Lactose intolerance results in considerable bloating and gas after eating milk and milk products. Lactase supplements go a long way toward reducing this problem. Even if you do have lots of gas, make sure that your chest discomfort or abdominal pain are not due to heart or bowel trouble. Despite the abundance of over-the-counter antigas remedies, excessive gas in the gut is rarely eliminated by medication.

FLUID RETENTION

WHEN YOU'RE EITHER VERY SICK—

OR SIMPLY MENSTRUATING

Fluid can accumulate in abnormal amounts anywhere—in the brain, in the lungs, under the skin, in the belly, the fingers or feet, or around the eyes. Edema, the medical term for fluid retention, is either limited to one area (a bee sting usually causes localized swelling) or is generalized, so that most of the body is waterlogged. Diseases of the kidney, liver, heart, and thyroid are the usual causes of widespread edema, but it may also be due to oral contraceptives, cyclical hormonal changes, exposure to high altitudes, or a reaction to poisoning. Whatever the reason for the fluid retention, its treatment usually includes restricting salt in your diet (because salt retains water), taking diuretics (medications that cause the body to eliminate water and salt), and, in severe cases, reducing fluid intake.

Many otherwise healthy women complain of chronic fluid retention during or just before their period, when estrogen promotes the accumulation of salt and water. Fluid retention that is constant and not cyclical is called "idiopathic edema." (The word *idiopathic* is not an insult and has nothing to do with your intelligence. It means "of unknown cause.") Women with idiopathic edema are usually on their feet a great deal. Blood pools in their legs, from which fluid leaks into the surrounding tissues. At its peak, this edema may result in a weight gain of as much as ten pounds, generating a vicious circle. Alarmed by their weight gain, these women often go on a crash diet. Their bodies respond by eliminating less salt and retaining more water. They now resort to diuretics that do provide short-term relief, but whose chronic use leads to even more salt retention that persists for days after the diuretic has been stopped.

Take diuretics for short-term relief when the swelling is severe and does not respond to the decreased salt intake, but use only the smallest effective dose. The best time to take a diuretic is before going to bed because most salt retention occurs during the night. Of course, the price you'll pay for such wise timing is frequent excursions to the john. You should also be aware of the potassium- and magnesium-losing properties of most diuretics and make sure to replace both minerals in adequate amounts.

Are there any natural diuretics you can use to eliminate retained water? The major ones are alcohol and caffeine—neither of which is effective in idiopathic edema or premenstrual fluid retention. Beer keeps you "going," both because of its alcohol content and the volume of liquid associated with its consumption. Some of my patients tell me that cranberry and apple juice also have a diuretic effect. I cannot find any reference to this action in the medical literature, but since both are good for you anyway, there is no harm in trying them.

The best way to deal with fluid retention, whether you think it's idiopathic or premenstrual, is first to make sure that it is not due to some other condition. Check with your doctor. Then restrict your salt intake to no more than 2 grams a day. (For details about a low-sodium diet, see sample menu on page 249. See also the table on page 248 for the sodium content of foods, and the table on page 247 for that of beverages.) Identify and then avoid foods loaded with salt, such as pickles, bacon, cold cuts, frankfurters, soy sauce, sauerkraut, tomato and V8 juices, and bouillon. I know people who eat sushi, not only because they like it, but also because it is low in calories. They then dip the sushi in those little bowls containing soy sauce, 1 ounce of which has over 1,500 milligrams of sodium! Fruit and vegetables have no salt to speak of, so you can enjoy them in unlimited quantities. Dairy products, on the other hand, do have significant amounts. Don't worry about salt-free bread. Two grams a day allows you to eat as much "normal" bread as you like, from the sodium point of view. Fats and oils contain no salt, but I don't recommend them for the many negative effects on your health emphasized throughout these pages. Switching from club soda to seltzer water is a good idea too. The former has 75 milligrams per 12-ounce serving, while seltzer water has none! Finally, 1 teaspoon of salt contains 2,300 milligrams of sodium, so don't add any to your cooking and remove the salt shaker from your table. If you use only 1 teaspoon of salt to cook a recipe that serves four, you personally will end up with almost 600 milligrams from that dish! Common hidden sources of salt, of which you should be aware, are soups, processed foods, french fries and the milk shake that goes with them, baking powder, baking soda, MSG, sodium sulfite, and sodium benzoate. Look for them on food labels.

FOOD ALLERGY
FINDING THE CULPRIT

It's easy to tell that you're allergic to a particular food, say, shrimp or lobster, if you break out in hives every time you eat it even before the dessert arrives! But pinpointing the culprit food is not always that obvious, if you've had several different dishes. What's more, the "allergic reaction" you're experiencing (it's not limited to the skin) may not be caused by the actual food in question, but by an additive it contains, such as monosodium glutamate (MSG—remember the Chinese Restaurant Syndrome?), or a coloring agent such as tartrazine, or by sulfites added to foods to prevent them from wilting and browning, or by tenderizers, pesticides, or an impurity in the manufacturing process. The next time you have the very same food, you may get away scot free if that offending ingredient was omitted. Don't confuse food allergy with food *intolerance*. You don't have to be allergic to something for it to make you sick. Food that is spoiled, infected, or contaminated may leave you nauseated or give you stomach cramps, symptoms that mimic and may be mistaken for food allergy. These symptoms may never recur. You can be "intolerant" of virtually any dish if you have a peptic ulcer, a large hiatal hernia, a worm or other parasite in your gut, gallbladder trouble, reflux into your food pipe, or any one of a score of other conditions. If milk or any food that contains it gives you gas and cramps, that's probably not allergy but lactose intolerance due to a congenital deficiency of the enzyme that digests lactose, the sugar present in milk (see page 295). Some people have other enzyme deficiencies that cause symptoms when they eat certain foods (see page 307). But none of this has anything to do with food allergy.

Only 2 percent of adults, and no more than 8 percent of children, are truly allergic to a given food or additive. These numbers change because so many children outgrow their allergies. In such cases, something in the offending food, usually a protein, reacts in a complex way with cells in your stomach that are coated with a special protein. This union results in the release of antibodies that act on different parts of the body—and that's what causes your allergic symptoms. They may range in severity from very mild (hives or an upset stomach) to life threatening, and usually involve the skin, lungs, or intestinal tract. If your skin is the target organ, the wrong food can give you a rash, wheals, itching, swelling of the lips or tongue, and in children, a chronic condition called atopic dermatitis. When the lungs are affected, you may wheeze or cough; when the intestinal tract reacts, you may have a combination of nausea, vomiting, diarrhea, and cramps. You may also develop a migraine headache. Occasionally, a profound reaction to an offending food—*anaphylactic shock*—may result in total collapse and even death unless treated quickly with adrenaline.

Every once in a while an allergic reaction is so bizarre that it defies diagnosis. One of my patients went from doctor to doctor and dentist to dentist for months because of a recurring burning sensation in her tongue and mouth. She underwent a battery of relevant tests—her gums and dentures were carefully examined; her teeth were X-rayed; and her blood was tested for toxic substances. Everything was reported to be normal. After a great deal of meticulous medical detective work, she was found to be allergic to fresh strawberries. As soon as she stopped eating them, the burning in her mouth disappeared. (I have never seen it myself, but I've heard that removing a food to which an autistic person is allergic can result in improvement of his or her condition.)

The severity of an allergic food reaction will vary with your age, how much of the food you've consumed, whether your stomach was full at the time, how the food was prepared, what parts you ate (for example, whether the chicken or apple was skinned), whether the food was fresh or the fruit overripe, and how soon the symptoms occurred after eating. Any food that's going to give you an allergic reaction will usually do so *within an hour*. Don't blame a rash, headache, or diarrhea on something you ate last week!

If you are allergic to one particular food, related products may also give you symptoms because there is considerable cross-reaction. For example, if you develop hives after eating prunes or nectarines, don't be surprised if cherries, apricots, almonds, and peaches cause the same reaction; if eggs make you wheeze, chances are so will chicken, turkey, goose, and game fowl. Such cross-reactivity extends from species to species, so that if you're allergic to cow's milk, you will react similarly to goat's milk and vice versa. Allergy to specific foods also often runs in families.

With all the attention paid to food, we tend to forget the importance of additives in dietary allergic reactions. The best known are sulfites (see page 57), which can result in asthmatic attacks in vulnerable persons. They are present in a variety of foods and beverages, especially wine. So always check the label, since manufacturers must list the sulfite content of any prepared food or drink. Their use in fresh fruits and vegetables in salad bars was banned in 1986 in the United States. Any coloring or dye, including tartrazine, or FDC #5, as well as sodium benzoate, nitrites, and nitrates in processed meats, can induce an allergic reaction too. Always check the label of any prepared food before you eat it.

The best way to identify a food allergy is to keep a diet diary. Write down what you ate and when. Then record the nature of any reactions—wheezing, skin rash, headache, nausea, vomiting, excessive gas, blurred vision, diarrhea, fever, or abdominal cramps—as well as how soon symptoms came on after eating the food in question.

Why bother with a diet diary if you can have a skin test for allergy? In my experience, almost half the patients I've had tested demonstrate a positive—i.e., allergic—reaction to foods that they have no trouble with! A negative test, however, is another matter. If you do not react to something, then you can bet you're not allergic to it.

Food allergy is sometimes so tricky to prove that you may need more than one method to make the diagnosis. The RAST (radioallergosorbent) test is another way to determine food allergy. Antibodies to specific foods are added, one at a time, to a sample of your blood serum (that's what's left after the blood has been spun in a centrifuge and its solid components, the blood cells, have been separated out). A positive reaction indicates the presence of allergy.

Foods most likely to cause an allergic response are cow's milk, shellfish, chocolates, nuts, eggs, wheat, soybeans, and peanuts (which, you may be surprised to know, are a legume and not a nut). As little as one five-thousandth of a teaspoon of the food in question can cause death if you are severely allergic to that food. The cheapest and often most reliable way to identify the culprit is to eliminate suspicious foods from your diet one by one. If your symptoms improve or disappear, reintroduce the suspected food to see whether they return. Do not take any antihistamines or steroids while you are conducting this experiment because they can obscure a positive result. Remember not to eat out, either at a restaurant or a friend's home, while you're trying to identify an offending food because you never know all the ingredients of a dish—especially sauces, soups, and dressings—that you yourself have not prepared. Your doctor can tailor an elimination diet to your needs. Rarely, when all the conventional elimination diets (and there are several) fail to reveal the allergic culprit, you may have to go on to a total elimination diet in which you eat and drink only a commercially prepared allergen-free formula while reintroducing foods one by one.

An important complication of elimination diets continued for any length of time is nutritional deficiency. So limit each to two weeks, and take vitamin and mineral supplements while you're experimenting. As you reintroduce each food, make a note of the symptoms it produces, how soon after eating they appear, and how long they last. Also pay attention to how the food was prepared and whether the skin or any other part of it was removed. If you suspect that a particular food induces a profound allergic reaction, then perform the "challenge" to prove it with a doctor present who can treat you immediately should you become very sick.

Once you've identified the food to which you are truly allergic, you must watch out for it wherever you eat. It's not always obvious—you may have to ask. For example, peanuts can be hidden in chili and you'd never know they're there unless you inquired—or develop a reaction. The same is true for MSG, sulfites, and other additives whose presence in prepared food is documented on the label. But in restaurants or in someone's home, where there are no labels, you have no choice but to review the ingredients with whoever has done the cooking. We usually associate MSG with Chinese food, and whenever I eat in an Asian restaurant, I invariably hear someone asking the waiter whether any dishes contain MSG. You can and should ask for it to be omitted if it doesn't agree with you. But meat tenderizers with MSG are commonly added in many other restaurants, so always ask about them.

There are many palatable substitutes for foods to which you are allergic. If you're allergic to chocolate, you can use carob instead. You'll never know the difference. If you're allergic to eggs and need a substitute with the proper consistency for a recipe, combine 2 tablespoons of flour, ½ teaspoon of oil, and 2 tablespoons of milk. (Commercial egg substitutes contain albumin, which is allergenic.)

Allergy in infants may present special problems. Preemies do not tolerate the protein in cow's milk and should be breast-fed for at least a year. If that's not possible, then they should be fed with soy formula. If an infant who previously thrived on milk develops gastroenteritis for whatever reason, the infection in the lining of the stomach may make the child intolerant to milk, causing diarrhea and cramps. In such cases, stop the milk until the child is feeling better.

If you have previously experienced a severe reaction to any food, you should always carry with you a kit containing adrenaline (it requires a prescription) with which you can inject yourself in an acute crisis. It's especially important to have it handy if you're eating out—anywhere.

GALLSTONES

TOO MUCH FAT, TOO LITTLE FIBER—
AND TOO MUCH FASTING

Fifteen million American women and 5 million men—8 percent of all Americans, including 73 percent of Pima Indian women (a nation living in Arizona)—have gallstones. In half the cases, the stones are "silent," and were discovered serendipitously in tests performed for some unrelated purpose.

Until fairly recently, people with gallstones were advised to have their gallbladders removed, regardless of whether or not the stones were causing any symptoms. (In the typical gallstone attack, there is severe pain under the bottom of the breastbone and in the right upper part of the abdomen, sometimes accompanied by fever and possibly jaundice as well.) The rationale for this aggressive approach was that gallstones are prima facie proof that the gallbladder is diseased and so will eventually have to come out anyway. The sooner done, the better, the reasoning went, while you're in otherwise good condition and able to withstand an operation. What if you just happened to have a flare-up of your gallstones and needed surgery when you might not be as good physical condition? That logic resulted in the 600,000 gallbladder operations performed year after year that sent more surgeons' kids through college than perhaps any other operation. (Hysterectomies and coronary bypasses are now paying for that education!)

Most doctors I know no longer offer this advice to people with "silent" gallstones because, in the great majority of cases, they never need to be removed. Also, there are several modern alternatives to major surgery should intervention become necessary. These include dissolving the stones with medication, shattering them with sound waves in a few very selected cases, or performing laparoscopic surgery without a major incision of the abdominal wall. As a result of all these innovations, the number of "open" gallbladder operations at last count has dropped to 475,000 annually—and is still falling.

What you eat can help prevent the formation of gallstones and reduce the frequency of their attacks. To appreciate why this is so, you must understand how and why gallstones form. The gallbladder is a small, pear-shaped sac on the undersurface of the right side of the liver. It contains a bitter, yellow-green liquid called bile, which is made by the liver and excreted through its ducts into the gut. The function of bile, which is composed of water, cholesterol, other fats, bile salts, and a reddish pigment called bilirubin derived from the red blood cells, is to break up larger globules of fat into smaller, more digestible ones. The liver never stops making bile, even though it is really needed only after you've eaten some fat. Most of it would be wasted if nature, in his or her infinite wisdom, had not given us a gallbladder in which to store what is not being used. Because its capacity is limited to ¼ cup, the gallbladder concentrates the bile in order to accommodate the copious amounts produced. Now, when you eat a fatty meal requiring extra bile, the gallbladder contracts and squirts it into the duodenum (small intestine) through its ducts. To contract efficiently on demand, the gallbladder must be free of disease. When it isn't, possibly because of a low-grade infection within its walls, the bile thickens into sludge in which tiny crystals (most often calcium) form. These are usually coated with cholesterol (in 80 percent of cases) or, in the remaining 20 percent, with the bilirubin pigment—and voilà, you have a stone.

The most dramatic symptoms of a gallstone attack occur when one or more stones in the gallbladder pass into the duct leading to the intestine. Most doctors believe this happens when the gallbladder, responding to a call for more bile after a fatty meal, contracts to squirt bile into its ducts. In so doing, it also extrudes a stone or two! The duct contracts vigorously and in paroxysms (spasms) in an attempt to pass the stones. These contractions are what cause the characteristic severe, colicky pain of a gallbladder attack. If the duct becomes obstructed by the stones, bile backs up into the liver and then into the bloodstream, leaving the person jaundiced (meaning the skin and whites of the eyes turn yellow, the urine dark, and the stool light) until the stone is passed and the blockage is relieved.

Why do some people develop gallstones and others not? Who is vulnerable? Is it genetics, as in the Pima Indian women? Twice as many women as men have gallstones, presumably because of their hormonal makeup. The walls of the gallbladder normally make little wavelike movements that stir the bile so that sludge does not form as easily. Estrogen diminishes these protective contractions. So if you have a family history of gallstones, you may want to consider a contraceptive other than The Pill (it contains estrogen), especially if you are under thirty years of age. Pregnancy also raises estrogen levels, which is why women who have had babies are more likely to develop gallstones later on.

There are other risk factors. For example, even if you are only 10 percent overweight, you are twice as likely to form stones. The more overweight you are, the higher your risk. By age sixty, almost a third of all overweight women have gallstones. If you're obese because you've eaten high-calorie foods with abandon over the years and now decide to go on a crash diet or fast for twenty-four hours or more at a stretch, you'll make matters worse. A stomach that's empty frequently and for long periods of time encourages gallstone formation because there is no stimulus for the gallbladder to contract and keep the bile flowing. So it stagnates and first forms sludge, then stones. If your close blood relatives have gallstones, do not indulge in these fasts.

A diet rich in vegetables and fruit is believed to be protective against gallstones because the soluble fiber they contain interacts with bile to leave it less prone to stone formation. This is not theory; it's fact. Populations whose diet is rich in fiber have a low incidence of gallstones. For example, blacks who live in the heartland of Africa rarely develop them, but those who move to cities, in Africa or elsewhere, have the same incidence of gallstones as Caucasians. That's presumably because of the change in their diet. A similar phenomenon has been observed in Southeast Asia and Japan where, until recently, gallstones were uncommon. With the increasing popularity of the "Western" low-fiber diet, the incidence of gallstones has increased. Japanese who emigrate, especially to the United States, now have the same incidence of gallstones as do Caucasians. The good news is that if you substantially increase your intake of dietary fiber, these stones may even begin to dissolve. See the table on page 116 for the fiber content of various foods.

Eating too much fat and refined sugar, as well as a high cholesterol level in the blood, also predisposes you to gallstones, as do some of the drugs used to lower cholesterol. The latter encourage formation of tiny crystals that ultimately become stones. But if you have to choose between increasing your risk for gallstones and preventing a heart attack, there is no contest!

Most doctors tell their patients with gallstones to follow a very-low-fat or fat-free diet so as not to induce active gallbladder contractions. That means no whole milk and no whole milk products such as cheese, whole-milk yogurt, and cream, as well as butter, eggs, or fatty meats. If the cruciferous vegetables (broccoli, cauliflower, cabbage, and brussels sprouts) or other fruits or vegetables give you gas, as they do many people with (and without) gallstones, you'll need to avoid them too. At the end of this chapter you'll find a list of recommended daily servings of various foods for persons with gallstones. There should be no visible fat in whatever you eat, and you should remove all the skin from poultry. The only fat you should use is monounsaturated olive or canola oil, and even then no more than 1 tablespoon a day, carefully measured. But not everyone can or will comply with such a diet. Take a multivitamin that contains the fat-soluble group (A, D, E, and K).

One of your main dietary goals should be to increase the amount of fiber you consume to a daily total of 35 to 45 grams (see page 119). Try to eat at least five servings daily of fresh fruit and vegetables. If you don't fancy raw vegetables, you may steam them lightly. Eat whole-grain breads such as wheat, rye, or pumpernickel instead of white bread; sprinkle oat bran in your casserole and meatloaf recipes rather than bread crumbs. Use some wheat flour in your baking in addition to white flour. Develop a taste for pasta made with whole wheat. Look for cold cereals that have significant amounts of fiber. For snacks, eat popcorn or low-fat baked wheat crackers instead of high-fat potato chips.

If you've had an acute gallbladder attack and are being carefully observed pending a decision regarding surgery, your doctor may choose to feed you by vein if your gallbladder is really "hot." If your gallbladder disease is less acute, stick to clear liquids such as apple juice, ginger ale, clear, defatted broth, or gelatin, so as not to stimulate the sick organ.

In summary, here's how to reduce your chances of developing gallstones: Choose to be born male; eat a low-fat, high-fiber diet; maintain your normal weight without wild swings up and down the scales; avoid frequent fasts; and keep your cholesterol level low. If you already have stones, follow a low-fat, high-fiber diet, and avoid rushing into surgery.

RECOMMENDED DAILY SERVINGS FOR PEOPLE WITH GALLSTONES

FOOD	SERVINGS	FAT (gm)	CALORIES
Skim milk	2 (8 ounces each)	0	170
Lean protein, such as fish or skinless chicken or turkey	6 ounces maximum	18	300
Vegetables, fresh or steamed	4 plus	0	100
Fruits	3 plus	0	180
Breads, fat-free types only	5	trace	400
Fats, olive or canola oil	1 tablespoon maximum	15	125
Dessert, fat-free types only	1 to 2 servings	0	200
		33	1,475

GOUT

THE PRICE OF THE GOOD LIFE

Do you remember those pictures of eighteenth-century English gentlemen sipping port and soaking a foot in a large basin? They were suffering from gout—a "rich man's" disease—and treating it the only way they could in those days.

Perhaps you thought gout was a thing of the past. Far from it! Gout is the third most common form of arthritis—after osteoarthritis and rheumatoid arthritis, from which it differs in many ways. Osteoarthritis is the result of wear and tear; rheumatoid arthritis is probably caused by some abnormality of the immune system; while gout is due to a metabolic problem—the way the body handles, produces, and gets rid of urates (crystal-containing substances in which certain foods are rich). Uric acid, one form of urate, is a by-product of the body's energy processes, but it's also present in foods with large amounts of purines, which I'll discuss later. Too much uric acid in the blood causes these urate crystals to lodge in the joints, where they are responsible for the severe pain and swelling we call gout. This form of arthritis is also unique in another way. While persons with osteo- and rheumatoid arthritis usually have chronic pain and intermittent flare-ups in one or more joints, gout causes no symptoms between attacks. In the usual scenario, you go to bed feeling fine, and then, sometime during the night, one joint (more than half the cases strike the big toe) begins to hurt like the devil. The pain is so intense you can't even bear the pressure of the bedsheet! The younger you are, the more severe the attack. It may come on for no apparent reason, or after drinking too much red wine, or as a result of some unusual physical or emotional stress, injury, or perhaps overindulgence in rich foods. After a few days, the pain disappears, and you're as good as new—until the next attack.

Gout is essentially a man's disease; only 10 percent of cases occur in women, and rarely before menopause. It also runs in families.

Doctors used to manage gout by prescribing a low-purine diet, and advising their patients to abstain from alcohol and lose weight. This regimen, when adhered to, does reduce the frequency of attacks somewhat, but gout is really a hit-or-miss affair. Colchicine used to be the only medication available to treat a crisis. (If you think "crisis" is too strong a term, you've never had an attack of gout!) But in order for this drug to work, you had to take it every one to two hours until you vomited or developed diarrhea. Only then did the pain subside.

Several newer medications that can, in most cases, predictably prevent and treat gout regardless of what you eat or drink have largely replaced colchicine. The drugs that *prevent* the attacks are allopurinol (which reduces the amount of uric acid made by the body) and sulfinpyrazone and probenecid (which prevent its accumulation by increasing its excretion in the urine). But you've got to take them every single day of your life. The only side effects these agents may give you are a skin rash or disturbed liver function, both of which clear up when the drug is stopped. Whatever happened to colchicine? Doctors sometimes still prescribe it in low doses to help prevent attacks and to aid in the diagnosis, because, aside from one or two other rare forms, gout is the only type of arthritis relieved by this drug.

If an attack of gout should break through this medical shield, it can be effectively controlled by the nonsteroidal anti-inflammatory drugs (NSAIDs). The best one to use for gout is indomethacin (Indocin), which should always be taken after meals and never for longer than necessary. It usually does the job within three or four days. Like aspirin and the other NSAIDs, Indocin can irritate the stomach. Don't use it without your doctor's knowledge, especially if you have an ulcer or are prone to inflammation of the stomach (gastritis). It does require a prescription, so beware of friends bearing gifts of Indocin!

Since these medications are so effective in the prevention and treatment of gout, patients and doctors alike pay very little attention to diet these days. In fact, most medical textbooks don't even refer to diet anymore when discussing this disease. Why deprive yourself of foods you enjoy if a pill works just as well? The rub is that some patients "break through" the preventive-medication regimen and continue to have acute attacks. In such cases, diet *is* important.

If your gout is drug resistant, so that you must be careful about what you eat and drink, keep away from foods that are rich in purines and that raise your uric acid level. The worst ones are virtually every animal organ such as liver, kidney, brain, heart, and pancreas (sweetbreads); goose; such seafood and shellfish as mackerel, anchovies, herring, sardines, scallops, mussels, and roe (caviar); mincemeat, bouillon, gravy; and *supplements* of brewer's and baker's yeast (the amounts of yeast present in other prepared foods or used in baking are too small to cause gout). The following foods contain less purine, and whether or not they will bring on an attack in your case is something you'll have to learn from experience: other fish, poultry, meat, asparagus, dried beans, lentils, mushrooms, dried peas, and spinach.

If you have gout, do not use *diuretic* medications if you can help it (natural substances such as coffee that make you "go" don't count). These drugs raise the level of uric acid by interfering with its excretion from the body and can trigger an acute attack. I have several patients with no previous or family history of gout who suddenly developed symptoms after starting diuretic therapy, either for high blood pressure or fluid retention. Low-dose aspirin can also result in an attack of gout.

Drinking any form of *alcohol* decreases the amount of uric acid you excrete, so too much of any kind can precipitate an attack. However, red wines or "heavy" ones such as Madeira and port are the worst offenders.

Gout used to be called the rich man's disease because it was traditionally identified with fine wines and spirits that only the affluent could afford. There is a "poor man's" gout, too, the result of heavy beer drinking. Yet a third kind, "saturnine" gout, is induced by moonshine made in lead-lined stills. (*Saturnine* does not refer to the planet or to drinking on Saturday night. It's the medical term for lead, which is responsible for the attack.)

Although gout characteristically affects the joints, it can also hurt the kidneys when blood flowing through them leaves its uric acid crystals behind. If these deposits in the kidney affect its function, you must be especially careful with your diet, you must take the prescribed antigout drugs, and you must be sure to drink eight to ten glasses of water a day to dilute your urine and lower the concentration of uric acid passing through your kidneys.

If you're overweight by 20 percent or more, according to the usual tables, or have a high BMI or WHR (see "When You're Overweight," page 344), you must lose weight. Although thin people get gout too, the obese are much more vulnerable. But *never try to lose weight by fasting.* That raises the blood uric acid level and increases the frequency of attacks. In fact, gout is one of the major complications of the more drastic liquid-protein and other weight-reduction diets.

Instead of purine-rich foods, focus on complex carbohydrates such as pasta, rice, potatoes, fruits, and vegetables; go easy on the fat (20 to 25 percent of total calories); and eat protein in moderation (20 percent of your total caloric intake). Drink plenty of fluids to increase the normal urinary excretion of uric acid.

You should certainly take whatever medication your doctor prescribes to prevent gout, but if attacks break through, avoid those foods and the alcohol that can bring them on.

HALITOSIS

THE BAD BREATH YOUR DOCTOR

SHOULD TELL YOU ABOUT,

IF YOUR FRIENDS DON'T!

Your breath will herald your entrance into a small room as effectively as a trumpet, especially if you have recently eaten onions, garlic, or cabbage. Sushi will announce you too, not only because of the fish itself, but the horseradish that usually goes with it. If everybody at home or at work keeps their distance, you'll either have to change your diet or subsist on lots of fresh parsley and strong mints. But don't depend on mouthwashes because the alcohol many of them contain can dry out your mouth and promote bad breath. If you check the label, you'll find that the best-selling brand has an alcohol content of 21.6 percent! If your breath is a problem because of your diet, eat less fat and more fresh fruit and vegetables, which rarely produce an offensive odor (except for those mentioned above).

Persistent bad breath despite a "squeaky clean" diet is called *halitosis*. To help identify its source, keep your lips closed and exhale through your nose. If that smells bad, chances are your halitosis does not originate from your mouth but from elsewhere in the body.

Whether or not your bad breath originates in the mouth depends in large part on the state of your saliva and how much of it you produce. Spit may not be an exotic liquid, but it is a very complex one. It contains enzymes that start the digestive process; it reduces the acidity of what you eat and drink; it helps prevent bacterial overgrowth; free-flowing saliva keeps the mouth clean and lubricated and helps food slide easily into the gut. When you have less saliva, your mouth contains more bacteria, decaying food particles, and accumulated debris—all of which contribute to halitosis. Decreased production of saliva during sleep is the culprit behind "morning breath"; once you get up and going, and the saliva begins to flow again, your breath improves, especially if you brush and floss your teeth. Older persons don't make much more saliva as the day progresses, which is why they are more vulnerable to halitosis.

Sleep and aging are not the only causes of halitosis due to decreased amounts of saliva. Depression; high blood pressure and some of the drugs taken to lower it; chronic alcoholism; an immune disorder called Sjögren's disease; and use of decongestants, diuretics, antihistamines, and most psychiatric medications can all cause dry mouth and halitosis. So will chronic breathing through your mouth. When your mouth is dry for any reason, sucking a lemon drop or a hard sugar-free candy will keep it moist by stimulating the salivary glands. Better still, use a commercially available saliva substitute.

Decaying food lodged between the teeth will produce offensive mouth odors. That is most apt to happen in people with dentures, bridges, or other dental work that traps food particles. Ask your dentist to review with you the principles of good oral hygiene, when and how to brush and floss, and what toothpaste or powder to use.

Other conditions within the mouth that can cause bad breath include abscessed teeth, herpes sores, oral cancers, fungal (yeast) infections, and diseases of the gums and dental cavities. Incidentally, cheese actually prevents such cavities from forming. The most effective ones are cheddar, mozzarella, Edam, Gouda (everyone pronounces it "gooda," but the purveyors of this Dutch cheese will know you're a connoisseur if you ask for "howda"), Monterey jack, Stilton, and Roquefort. Only the latter two have a strong odor of their own.

The most common *nonoral* causes of bad breath are sinusitis (the pus dripping down the back of your throat will not confer a breath conducive to romance), pneumonia (you expect an infection of the lung to result in foul breath), an abscess anywhere in the respiratory tract (nose, throat, tonsils, or lungs), and one particularly nasty chronic disease of the lungs called bronchiectasis. The worst breath I encounter in practice is in patients with lung abscesses and bronchiectasis.

Disorders of the intestinal tract can also cause halitosis. A condition called "chronic atrophic gastritis" will do so, and chronic peptic ulcers may too because of the bacteria in the stomach or duodenum (see page 370). Diverticula of the esophagus (little sacs or pouches where food lodges just after it is swallowed and where it later decays) can result in bad breath too. These pouches often require surgical removal.

Sometimes the cause of bad breath has nothing at all to do with the digestive tract. For example, when the liver fails, the patient's breath smells like rotten eggs; persons whose kidney function is seriously impaired give off a fishy odor; diabetics whose blood sugar is badly out of control have acetone breath, with a very sweet, fruity aroma.

There is an inherited metabolic disorder called trimethylaminuria, or "fish-odor syndrome." Persons who suffer from it lack a digestive enzyme necessary to convert a protein called trimethylamine into an odorless by-product. As a result, trimethylamine is excreted unchanged into the urine, sweat glands, and breath. It has a potent stink, even when diluted to one part per million! The irony of it, however, is that these individuals do not seem to be bothered by their smell! You need *two* trimethylaminuria genes to have the disease. Having only one makes you a carrier, able to transmit it, but free of its symptoms. Since each of your parents can pass only one of these genes on to you, it is necessary that both either have the disease (with two genes) or are carriers (with only one) in order for you to inherit it.

The only way to manage this condition is to reduce your intake of foods that break down into trimethylamine. These include ocean fish, peas, egg yolk, and dairy products. Even then, you won't come up smelling like a rose because choline in the body derived from other foods such as liver, oatmeal, soybeans, and peanuts is also converted to trimethylamine, which persons with this disorder simply can't handle. There's almost no getting away from it, but antibiotics sometimes help a little.

I cannot end this discussion without telling you about a patient I saw some years ago—an intelligent middle-aged woman who came to me in desperation because, for as long as she could remember, even as a child, she had suffered from bad breath. She had been to countless dentists and doctors and undergone every conceivable blood test, chemical analysis, and lung and intestinal X rays without an answer. Parsley, mints, mouthwash, chlorophyll—nothing helped. This stigma had left its mark on her personal and professional life. I didn't know how to help her, but I thought I should first get a whiff of her breath just to see if I could identify some telltale aroma. Guess what? Her breath was as pure as the driven snow. No wonder her workup had been fruitless. She was suffering from a psychiatric disorder in which there is an unfounded conviction that the breath is foul. Had any of her other doctors taken the trouble to confirm her complaint firsthand and gotten a little closer to her, she would have been spared the cost and inconvenience of a complicated medical evaluation and begun on the psychiatric treatment that did ultimately cure her!

In summary, if you have become a social pariah because of halitosis, avoid foods that cause offensive odors. Do the closed-mouth, nose-breathing test described above. If what you exhale from your nose smells fine, but your mouth aroma doesn't, then see your dentist first. If he or she can't find the cause, then consult your doctor.

YOUR HEART

WHAT TO EAT TO KEEP IT HEALTHY

The term *heart disease* is not a single diagnosis. It means that some part of the heart, whose main function is to pump blood to every organ of the body, is not working properly. For example, one or more of its valves may be diseased, a condition one is either born with, or acquires after an infection such as rheumatic fever early in life, or develops later when one or more valves degenerate with age. (Valves direct the flow of blood into, out of, and within the heart itself. When one or more of them leaks or becomes stuck, the blood flows erratically inside the heart, causing it to enlarge and weaken). Heart disease may also reflect damage to cardiac muscle from a viral infection, from long-standing excessive alcohol intake, or from untreated hypertension (see "High Blood Pressure," page 237). But most people think of "heart trouble" in terms of the big daddy of them all—arteriosclerosis, or hardening of the arteries. This process blocks the coronary arteries that feed the heart muscle, reducing the amount of blood, oxygen, and other nutrients it needs to keep efficiently beating.

More than 500,000 Americans die every year of a heart attack caused by arteriosclerosis. Statistically, chances are that you will too. This is the number-one cause of death and disability in men *and* women in the United States. One in five males and one female in seventeen will develop symptoms of this form of heart disease by age sixty. Beyond sixty, men and women develop the disease in equal numbers.

You are especially vulnerable to cardiac death if (1) any of your blood relatives had heart disease (the more there are, the closer their relationship to you, and the younger they were when diagnosed, the greater your risk—but wives, husbands, and mothers-in-law don't count); (2) you smoke cigarettes; (3) you have untreated high blood pressure; (4) your blood "fats" are out of whack (high cholesterol, high triglycerides, high LDL, and a *low* high-density lipoprotein, or HDL—the so-called good cholesterol that carries "bad cholesterol" out of the body); (5) you are diabetic; (6) you are overweight; (7) you are cynical, hostile, and aggressive (components of some type-A personalities); (8) you are physically inactive—just a couch potato; (9) you are male and over forty or a postmenopausal woman.

The more of these risk factors you have, the greater your vulnerability. The good news is that all of them, except your family history, age, and sex, can be controlled or modified. New "miracle" heart drugs, bypass surgery, even heart transplants are all lifesaving—but they come into play only *after* you become sick. The trick is not to need them, and that means *prevention*. I am annoyed when my patients throw in the towel and tell me that their family history is so bad anyway that they have decided to get the "most out of life," enjoy what they can, and "take my chances because nothing I do will make a difference." That's nonsense. Controlling risk factors is not always easy. It takes a firm, ongoing commitment to shun some favorite foods, quit smoking, exercise regularly, manage your stress, treat your high blood pressure, lose weight (and keep it off), and eat right. But none of these, including proper nutrition, is nearly as hard to do as it once was, as I'll discuss later in this chapter.

Blood fats (lipids) are the key constituents of the deposits called plaques that obstruct arteries everywhere in the body, including the heart. One of them, cholesterol, has been singled out as a major player. It has become public enemy number one as far as the heart is concerned. Americans discuss their cholesterol levels as often as they do their weight, their clothes, or their grandchildren.

Cholesterol is an odorless, soft, waxy material normally present everywhere in the body—in the brain, nervous system, skin, liver, gut, heart, skeleton, and even the sex hormones. Everyone needs some cholesterol because it is a vital component of so many biological processes, but you can have too much of a good thing. The liver makes all the cholesterol the body needs from "stepping-stone" molecules. Even if you never had a single bite of cholesterol, you would still never run short! In fact, what is present in the diet is really gilding the lily. High cholesterol levels are statistically associated with an increased vulnerability to arteriosclerosis. That is not to say that everyone with high cholesterol is destined to die of a heart attack. I have many patients in their eighties and nineties with frighteningly high cholesterol levels who are in excellent health. But when you analyze the heart statistics in *populations,* the higher the cholesterol, the greater the incidence of heart attacks. As desirable as it is, however, a "normal" or even low reading is no guarantee against heart disease because so many other risk factors contribute to it.

Believe it or not, until fairly recently, doctors were not sure that lowering people's cholesterol levels did any good. Some researchers were convinced that a high cholesterol level was only a *symptom,* like fever or anemia, and that treating it wouldn't affect the underlying cause. After many years of research, in which scores of thousands of persons were studied, we now have the proof that lowering cholesterol *does* make a difference. For every 1 percent drop in your cholesterol level, there is a 2 percent reduction in the risk of heart attack—regardless of whether that reduction was achieved through diet, drugs, or both. If you drop your cholesterol by 10 percent, you decrease your risk of a heart attack by 20 percent! Those are great odds! What's more, scientists have also been able to demonstrate that reducing the amount of cholesterol in the blood actually shrinks the obstructing arterial plaques.

Given the importance of cholesterol in the scheme of things, everyone should, by age twenty, know his or her own lipid profile, of which cholesterol is one component. This information is important not only to you but to your children. Whether your youngster should have cholesterol tests depends on his or her genetic vulnerability. As a parent, your lipid profile and history of heart disease provide the best answer. I test every teenager (high school graduation is a good time) who has a parent or grandparent with heart disease before the age of fifty-five.

What is a high or dangerous level of cholesterol? What are the safest and most effective ways to lower it? How vigorously should that be done? At what age should intervention begin? How long should you try diet before resorting to drugs? There is general agreement on some of the answers to these questions, but others remain controversial.

If you're over twenty and your cholesterol reading is between 180 and 200 milligrams per deciliter, you're doing fine. Drastic steps to lower it further are unnecessary and possibly undesirable. Cholesterol levels that are *too* low (less than 150 milligrams) may be associated with more cancer of the liver, lung, and pancreas, twice the incidence of cerebral hemorrhage (a stroke in which there is bleeding into the brain), chronic lung disease, and even depression. However, a cause-and-effect relationship is still being debated, and I certainly wouldn't worry about it if you are among the 6 percent of Americans who are lucky enough to have a cholesterol level in that range that is not the result either of dieting or taking medication. Cholesterol readings of 200 to 239 milligrams are borderline high, and anything above 240 milligrams is frankly high. Remember, however, that the risk of a high cholesterol level is compounded by the presence of other risk factors. If you also have high blood pressure, your coronary vulnerability goes up six times. If you smoke, that risk is increased twentyfold!

Your cholesterol reading alone does not tell the whole story. Other important blood fat markers play a role, the best known of which are HDL, LDL, triglycerides, and, more recently, the apolipoproteins.

HDL (high-density lipoprotein) and *LDL* (low-density lipoprotein) are proteins made by the liver to which cholesterol attaches itself. LDL carries 60 to 70 percent of the total cholesterol, and HDL about 25 percent. Both transport cholesterol in the blood for delivery to and use by various organs. Think of HDL and LDL as cholesterol-carrying canoes or barges. How much of your cholesterol is attached to HDL and how much is carried by LDL makes a very big difference in your cardiovascular risk. The cholesterol reading alone only indicates the *total* attached to *both* these lipoproteins. The more HDL and the less LDL you have, the better off you are. When cholesterol carried by LDL approaches a coronary artery, the cholesterol breaks off and is deposited in its wall. This contributes to plaque formation that ulti-mately obstructs the artery. The cholesterol in the HDL "canoe," on the other hand, stays put, does not get out, and remains in the bloodstream where it may help remove LDL. The LDL should be less than 130 milligrams; 130 to 159 is borderline high, and you're at high risk for arteriosclerosis if your LDL is greater than 160 milligrams. The HDL should be more than 45 milligrams. So just knowing the total cholesterol level is not enough. You must also be aware of the HDL and LDL numbers.

Once you have all the numbers, you can obtain the cholesterol/HDL ratio by dividing the *total* cholesterol by the HDL. That ratio should be less than 4.5, and the lower, the better. *Absolute cholesterol numbers without the accompanying lipoprotein data do not tell the whole story!* For example, if your cholesterol is 300, and your HDL is 75, giving a ratio of 4.0, you are better off than if you have a cholesterol of only 210, an HDL of 30, and a ratio of 7.

Many doctors now believe that triglyceride (neutral fat) levels are also a risk factor for heart disease, especially when the HDL is low. It's upper limit of normal is somewhere between 150 and 200 milligrams, but to obtain an accurate measurement, you must fast for at least twelve hours, during which time you may drink only water. Fasting is not required for cholesterol testing, but it is for triglyceride, lipoprotein, and blood sugar determinations.

I saw some sound advice at an airport terminal the other day. There were two billboards. One read STOP. DO YOU KNOW YOUR CHOLESTEROL LEVEL? A second poster carried the following warning: REDUCE YOUR INTAKE OF SATURATED FATS AND CHOLESTEROL. That message is the key to any heart disease prevention diet. Why saturated fat? Because that's what raises cholesterol most, even more so than straight cholesterol! That's why lobster and other shellfish that contain cholesterol but very little saturated fat, are not, as you will see below, nearly as bad for you as a marbled steak.

We have only recently begun to distinguish among the various kinds of fat—saturated, polyunsaturated, and monounsaturated. Most saturated fats are found in animal products, particularly fatty meats, organs such as liver, kidney, or brain, and dairy products such as butter, cream, whole milk, and its derivative cheeses. The most effective way to lower cholesterol is to avoid saturated fats. If you eat meat, make sure it is lean without any visible fat. Marbled steak may be juicy, delicious, and tender, but those white streaks are very rich in saturated fats. If you love barbecued hamburgers, use lean rather than regular ground; try seasoned turkey burgers or soy hamburgers. You can buy a fresh-ground mix of white and dark turkey meat at the supermarket, or better still, ask your butcher to grind white meat only. However, avoid frozen ground meat or poultry products, most of which are loaded with skin and fat. Remove the skin from your poultry before eating it. Remember that most commercially baked products are prepared with cream and whole egg unless otherwise specified. A few of these "bad" saturated fats are also present in some vegetable oils such as coconut oil, palm oil, and palm kernel oil (the stuff they still put in some nondairy coffee creamers, frozen dinners, whipped toppings, cookies, crackers, and cake mixes). Look for them on the label and, to paraphrase one of my favorite songs, "Once you have found them, *always* let them go."

Polyunsaturated fats come from plants and vegetable oils, e.g., corn and safflower (and fatty fish, but more about them later), and are acceptable as long as you don't go overboard and eat too much, and provided they are in liquid form. (See below.) Always read the labels on every salad dressing, because some are high in saturated fats.

The possible impact of too much polyunsaturated vegetable oil on the development of cancer is still unresolved. Once the polyunsaturated fat is rendered solid by the process of hydrogenation (which is what happens to most margarine and peanut butter), producing the so-called trans-fatty acids, you should either avoid it or use it very sparingly because it is bad for the arteries. Again, examine the label on the container (look for the word *hydrogenated*) and buy only those brands that are soft or the tub variety. Even if it is "acceptable," don't eat any more of *any* fat than is necessary to make your food palatable.

The heart-healthiest fat is the monounsaturated variety, specifically canola and olive oil. The latter has been consumed for centuries by people living in the Mediterranean area (Italy, Spain, and Greece), who have a low incidence of coronary artery disease. Personally, I prefer olive oil, especially the virgin or extra-virgin varieties, to any other polyunsaturated oil. Extra-virgin olive oil makes wonderful salad dressing but may smoke or burn when heated. So, for cooking, try canola oil, which cooks well without the strong, distinctive flavor of olive oil that you may not want in every dish. Remember, however, that all fats contain the same number of calories per serving, so while monounsaturated fats may be good for your lipid profile because they lower LDL, each tablespoon contains 135 calories per tablespoon! If you want to limit your total fat to less than 30 percent of your daily calories, use no more than 2 tablespoons of olive or canola oil per day.

Cholesterol is found *only* in animal products. The richest sources are egg yolks, meat, especially animal organs, dairy products, fish, and poultry. You will find none in egg white, fruits, nuts, vegetables, grains, cereals, and seeds.

Page 220 lists foods high in saturated fats and cholesterol. What can you eat and still adhere to a low-cholesterol, low-fat diet? All the fat and cholesterol in an egg is in its yolk, so substitute two egg whites for each yolk in your recipes. All foods of plant origin, such as beans, vegetables, and fruits, are ideal. They contain little or no saturated fats and absolutely no cholesterol. Have at least five or six portions a day, leaving their peel and skins intact to maximize the amount of fiber they provide. Cook them as little as possible to avoid losing their nutrients and natural flavor. Do not cream, butter, or fry your vegetables. Steam them, or braise them in nonfat chicken broth, water, juice, or wine. Bread, pastas, cereals, dried beans, and peas won't raise your cholesterol levels either. And don't worry about their caloric content. They contain fewer calories than foods high in fat (except if you smother them with rich sauces, butter, cream, or cheese)! Remember that weight for weight, *all* fat contains more than twice the number of calories as carbohydrate (or protein, for that matter).

Physicians used to advise against eating shellfish such as clams, scallops, crabs, oysters, and lobsters because of their high cholesterol content, but that's compensated for by the fact that they are very low in saturated fat and rich in polyunsaturated fats, including the omega-3 variety (more about them later). In deciding how much to eat, remember that your total animal protein intake (including fish) should not exceed 6 ounces a day. Caviar, squid, and shrimp are a different story. One tablespoon of caviar contains 95 milligrams of cholesterol, and who can stop after only such a small amount? Ten medium-sized shrimp have 130 milligrams, and there are some 230 milligrams in only 3 ounces of squid. So you should avoid all three if you are seriously trying to lower your cholesterol level by diet. Fish is generally lower in saturated fat than both meat and poultry, and is good for you—provided it comes from uncontaminated waters!

Instead of whole milk and the products derived from it—butter, cheese, ice cream, and cream, which are all full of saturated fat—use the new nonfat formulations of milk, yogurt, sour cream, and cottage cheese. There's even a fat-free cream cheese, and some wonderful yogurt-based, fat-free frozen desserts too.

Soup is good for you, especially if you're watching your weight, because it's filling and can be low in calories. Make sure, however, that it's fat-free. The kind you prepare yourself is best because you know what you put in to it. You'll also find canned, fat-free soups that are rich in fiber and low in salt. But do not be tempted by dehydrated, packaged soups, whose fat content is often high. When eating out, your best bet is clear bouillon or vegetable soup.

How you prepare what you eat, whether it's meat, fish, or poultry, is important. It's okay to barbecue, broil, microwave, steam, pan broil, stir-fry, or marinate in herbs or wine. Avoid deep-frying. When you roast or bake meat, use a rack so that the fat drains off. Refrigerate that fat so it will harden and separate from the rest of the juice. Then moisten the meat with this fat-free gravy. If there's not enough, supplement it with vegetable oil, broth, or bouillon. Boiling water poured over cooked, lean ground beef removes even more of the fat. The remaining beef can be used in stews, sauces, or chili.

Do you remember when oat bran was only for horses? Not any more! It's very popular with humans these days. The truth is that if you eat it regularly, you may obtain a modest drop in your cholesterol of about 3 to 9 percent (depending on how high it was to begin with and how much oat bran you consume). If your reading was 200 milligrams, it may fall to 194; if your level was 266, oat bran can drop it by 9 percent. But to eke out even a slight drop in these numbers, you must eat 50 to 100 grams of oat bran a day. You can consume that amount painlessly by having hot oat bran or oatmeal cereal for breakfast along with an oat bran muffin or two. But remember, many, if not most, commercial oat bran muffins contain lots of calories, as much as 500 or more each. If you decide to go that route, you can supplement your oat bran intake by breading your chicken cutlets with it or via using seasoned pure oat bran in your baking—it makes a tasty crunchy coating. You can also use oats instead of bread crumbs in turkey loaf, or substitute oat bran for white flour.

Prunes, 60 percent of whose fiber is a soluble pectin, will also drop cholesterol levels (they contain iron, potassium, and a small amount of beta-carotene as well). So will dried and canned beans. But pre are your loved ones for a noisy environment!

There have been several reports in recent years that areas of the world where the diet is rich in oily, saltwater fish, such as salmon, sardines, haddock, and mackerel, are remarkably free of coronary artery disease. For example, the coronary death rate among Eskimos living in Greenland is only 3.5 percent, as compared with 50 percent in Denmark. Eskimos consume between 5 and 6 grams daily of the polyunsaturated fats found in saltwater fish, while the Danes (and we) eat less than 1 gram per day. The blood lipid profile of the Eskimo is also much more desirable than ours. Their cholesterol, triglyceride, and LDL levels are lower, and their HDL is higher; their blood clots less easily, and even their blood pressure is somewhat lower. Much of this is attributed to their high consumption of polyunsaturated fish oils.

The preponderant polyunsaturated fats (PUFAs) in our diet are the omega-6 variety, derived mainly from vegetable oils. The PUFAs from fatty saltwater fish and shellfish (notably oysters, mussels, scallops, and clams) are of the omega-3 variety, structurally and biochemically different from omega-6. There are two forms of omega-3; the preponderant one is EPA (eicosapentaenoic acid), the other is DHA (docosahexanoic acid).

To see whether the lower incidence of coronary heart disease in the PUFA-eating populations was, in fact, due to the consumption of these fish, subjects were fed omega-3 fats in various studies. Those who received supplemental EPA and DHA ended up with lower cholesterol and triglyceride levels and higher HDLs. Their blood was also found to clot less easily, presumably because these fats act on the platelets that promote clot formation. Blood pressure was also lower in the treated group and those who had angina pectoris reported less chest pain.

Many doctors agree that omega-3 is good for you. The problem is, we don't know the optimal dose. There is no RDA for omega-3. I recommend three servings a week, 6 ounces each, of these oily fish. The table on page 221 lists the richest sources of omega-3 fatty acids. Fish can be boiled, grilled, poached, steamed, microwaved, or baked, and should be prepared without fat. You can flavor them with a variety of herbs and spices. The use of omega-3 capsules, most of which contain 300 milligrams of fish oil, is still controversial. The usual dosage is 3 grams a day. You're better off getting your omega-3 from fish, not capsules, because the former may contain other beneficial constituents not present in the supplements. What's more, there is as much as 5 milligrams of cholesterol per capsule in some brands of supplement, which adds up to 50 milligrams if you're taking the recommended ten a day. Check the bottle label before you buy, and look specifically for the cholesterol content. I advise most of my diabetic patients not to take omega-3 supplements, but if they do, to limit their daily dose to less than 2 grams a day. Avoid them too if you have untreated high blood pressure, because there is a real risk of stroke in someone who is vulnerable. (There is always the danger of rupture of blood vessels in hypertensive individuals because the increased pressure within the vessels relentlessly strains the vessel walls and weakens them. The blood thinning caused by the omega-3 oils may increase the risk of a brain hemorrhage should a break occur in the wall of the artery. The same precautions, incidentally, apply to aspirin.) Also, if you are pregnant or planning to be, avoid lake whitefish, salmon, mackerel, and canned white tuna for the duration because of the possibility of contamination by mercury and PCBs.

A deficiency of magnesium may contribute to coronary disease, whose incidence is lower in areas where the water is "hard" and contains lots of this trace element. (Magnesium is an important factor in some three hundred human enzyme processes.) Low levels are associated with high blood pressure that may drop when you add magnesium to your diet. (See page 245.) You should suspect too little magnesium on board if you develop leg cramps, muscle twitching or tremors, lack of appetite, confusion, or a rapid heartbeat. But since all these symptoms can result from a variety of other causes, it's best to check your magnesium level with a simple blood test. To make sure you're getting enough, however, eat extra amounts of magnesium-rich foods, especially if you live in a "soft" water area; you drink alcohol regularly and to excess; you are taking diuretics (they cause a loss of magnesium in the urine); or you are on long-term antibiotic therapy with any of the aminoglycosides (neomycin, tobramycin, gentamicin, kanamycin, or streptomycin). Many foods contain magnesium, but the best sources are seeds, nuts, blackstrap molasses, legumes, unmilled cereal grains, and dark green leafy vegetables. See the table on 304 for a more complete list. Diets high in refined sugars, alcohol, and red meat contain less magnesium than those rich in vegetables and unrefined grains. If, for any reason, you're not able to get enough magnesium in your diet to make up for your deficiency, there are supplements in tablet form available by prescription from your doctor. But do not take them if you are pregnant! Whether in your diet or via supplements, magnesium is not a substitute for high blood pressure medication.

Remember all the fanfare in the media about "tired blood" and how iron supplements would cure it? Well, a slight deficiency may actually be good for you! Iron in supplements, or in foods such as red meat, from which it is readily absorbed by the gut, may be associated with a higher risk of heart disease (see page 33).

My mother used to feed me lots of garlic and onions, which, incidentally, belong to the same plant family. She was sure that garlic was the staff of life and would protect me against cancer, heart disease, colds, and, I suspect, girls. She was probably right on all counts and would have been pleased to hear about the woman I read about in a recent journal who insists that the best treatment for her hemorrhoids is a whole garlic clove inserted in the appropriate area! A half clove, and certainly a whole one, eaten daily has been reported to reduce cholesterol levels by up to 10 percent in some individuals. It will also lower elevated blood pressure in susceptible persons. So garlic may be good for you on all three accounts—cholesterol, blood pressure, and hemorrhoids! When I was a child, garlic was not available in tablet form. So if you believed in its healing properties, you paid the price in breath and body odors. Although at least one expert I know insists, as did my mother, that garlic works only if it stinks, the deodorized garlic you can now buy at health food stores is as effective as the real thing. In one study, there was a 6 percent drop in cholesterol after twelve weeks of therapy with 900 milligrams per day taken in capsule form. The active ingredient in garlic that is responsible for these benefactions to mankind is a sulfur-containing compound called alliin.

Onions are also said to lower cholesterol and blood pressure, and decrease the tendency of the blood to clot within the arteries, an effect very much like that of aspirin. I am not aware of any documented studies proving these actions, and, to the best of my knowledge, no specific ingredient responsible for them has yet been identified. But if you like them, and most people do, eat them.

The foregoing dietary advice is for those with a high cholesterol level. If your triglyceride numbers are high (ideally, they should be under 140 milligrams in the fasting state), you need a different diet prescription. In some people, sugars and starches raise the triglyceride level, so if your reading is between 200 and 400 milligrams, you may have to forgo desserts and sweets, and drink no more than 1 ounce of hard liquor, or 2½ ounces of dry table wine, or 5 ounces of beer a day. If your triglycerides are above 400, then you must eliminate all alcohol and fruit juice. You may, however, eat all the vegetables you like, but no more than two servings of fresh fruit daily. (That's because of its sugar content.) For dessert, along with unsweetened fruit, you may have gelatin, angel food cake, or sugar-free sherbet. Sugar-free candy is okay, as are frozen desserts made with aspartame (NutraSweet), but there are currently no sugar-free cakes on the market because aspartame is not heat stable and cannot be used in baking. Your doctor can test you to see whether you require such carbohydrate restriction.

The American Heart Association (AHA) has structured the following general guidelines for heart-healthy eating in a two-step approach. *Step 1* is fairly easy to live with and is recommended for everyone over age two whose cholesterol level is under 220 milligrams and who does not have heart disease or a bad family history of it. The goal of this diet is to reduce the currently high national fat intake by *at least* 15 percent and cholesterol consumption by two thirds. The average cholesterol intake in the United States is between 500 and 750 milligrams a day. The Step 1 diet sets a limit of 300 milligrams daily. Three ounces of meat, fish, or poultry contain 60 to 90 milligrams; one egg has 270 milligrams; and there are almost 400 milligrams in a 3-ounce serving of liver! A simple rule of thumb for controlling cholesterol intake is to limit your animal protein (including fish) intake to no more than 6 ounces per day. Fat currently comprises 40 percent of calories in the American diet, and most of it is saturated. The Step 1 diet allows a *maximum* of 30 percent of your total daily calories from fat of which 10 to 15 percent should come from monounsaturated sources, approximately 10 percent polyunsaturated, and less than 10 percent should be saturated fat. (You'll be getting all the saturated fat you need from your daily animal protein intake, so no additional amounts are necessary.) You can determine these quantities by multiplying the number of calories you eat each day by 30 percent (.30) and dividing by 9, the number of calories in each gram of fat. The resulting figure is the maximum grams of fat you should eat daily. The sources of fat are not always obvious, so check the labels on all packaged food you buy. You can also send away for the U. S. Department of Agriculture's handbook on "Composition of Foods" for practical numbers of grams in household portions. Their "Dietary Treatment of Hyperlipidemia" manual also contains useful information on the ingredients in all packaged foods.

To make up for the reduction of fat, you should increase your carbohydrate intake from the typical American level of 40 to 45 percent of total calories daily to 50 to 60 percent, with an emphasis on complex carbohydrates (vegetables, fruits, dried peas, beans, and whole grains). The remaining 15 or so percent of your calories should come from protein.

The *Step 2* diet is recommended for persons with cholesterol levels ranging between 220 and 275 milligrams per deciliter and/or who have any close blood relatives with premature coronary disease (onset before age sixty-five). It differs from Step 1 in that your total fat intake should be less than 30 percent of total calories, your saturated fat consumption should be less than 7 percent of total calories, and your cholesterol intake should be reduced to below 200 milligrams a day. Carbohydrate and protein intake remain as in Step 1. The Step 2 diet translates into one egg yolk per week (you may have two on the Step 1 diet), no more than 6 ounces of fish, skinned poultry, or the leanest cuts of meat daily, and an abundance of fresh fruits and vegetables.

Step 2 is not the end of the road! There are cases when more stringent restrictions are necessary, as, for example, if you have a bad family history of premature heart disease, your cholesterol levels are above 275 milligrams per deciliter, and your LDL level is greater than 170 milligrams per deciliter. Your doctor may want to go beyond the Step 2 recommendations if your blood fats are not responding to that dietary level. In that event, I advise my own patients to limit their fat intake to less than 20 percent of their total calories, and restrict cholesterol to 100 milligrams a day. That means only 3 ounces of fish or skinned poultry daily and no meat whatsoever. The focus is on dried beans, peas, lentils, egg substitutes, and tofu (soybean curd). Tofu has the consistency of ice cream, is quite tasty, and comes in different flavors. But while it is cholesterol free, it nevertheless has lots of calories. Your coffee should be filtered because boiled coffee is believed to contain substances that raise cholesterol. If you have heart trouble associated with a rhythm disorder, you are better off drinking decaffeinated coffee—but not in unlimited amounts. In one large study, heavy decaf-coffee drinkers had higher death rates from cardiovascular disease. I'm not sure of the reason. Tea raises cholesterol somewhat, and its caffeine may aggravate an existing cardiac arrhythmia.

In my opinion, the Step 1 diet is what all of us should be eating, except that I feel 300 milligrams of cholesterol is too liberal; 200 is more to my liking. I consider the Step 2 diet a way station for anyone at special risk for heart disease or who has already developed it. The table on page 222, prepared by the U.S. Department of Health and Human Services, lists the foods you should choose and reduce in the different American Heart Association diets.

At the present time, only 9 percent of Americans have five or more servings of fruit and vegetables a day. I advise my patients to eat at least seven such servings daily, along with six portions of grain products (e.g., whole wheat bread and breakfast cereals). That may seem like a lot, but a "serving" is quite small. For example, a vegetable serving consists of only half a cup. A serving of fruit is one piece—one apple or one orange (but not just one strawberry), and only half a banana.

Aside from all the tables and charts, and dos and don'ts, there's an art to eating heart-healthy—a way of life, a frame of mind, a pattern of behavior, that can and should become ingrained. I see it all the time in some friends, and, I am happy to say, among my own children.

Even if you are an incurable "snacker," you can do so to your heart's content (accidental pun!) on fresh fruits and vegetables, graham and other fat-free crackers and chips, air-popped popcorn, bread (whole wheat, pumpernickel, rye, Italian, oatmeal, raisin, or English muffins), and a variety of cholesterol-free cakes and cookies. In the past ten years, several other heart-healthy foods (fat-free and cholesterol-free) has become available. They can make any diet interesting, varied, and delicious. You should ask for these products even when eating out, since a growing number of restaurants offer them.

It's important to develop a modus operandi with respect to restaurants if you eat out frequently. What's the point of being "good" at home and then blowing it when you eat out? Most people who do are not lax, they're intimidated—by maître d's, by waiters or waitresses, but, most of all, by not wishing to appear "different." Here are some guidelines for eating out. Avoid those all-you-can-eat buffet bistros. The temptation may be irresistible, but the only bargain you get will be for your pocketbook, not for your weight or heart. When you make your restaurant reservation, ask whether they will prepare the food you want, such as fresh fish and vegetables, in the way you want—broiling instead of deep-frying, for example. When you're dining with friends, you order first, if possible, so that you can set the tone of the ordering and not be tempted by what others choose. It's no shame to order appetizer-size portions, even if you have to pay for the bigger quantity. If you're not sure about the ingredients of a particular dish, don't be afraid to ask. After all, you're entitled to know what you're paying for. Make a habit of ordering fresh fruit for dessert. Many chefs, especially French, are very proud of their sauces—that's what separates the men from the boys in their industry. I remember going to one famous restaurant where they refused to serve my (thin, beautiful, and endowed with a naturally low cholesterol) wife because she wanted a salad for the main course. In order to avoid a confrontation, ask them to put the sauce on the side, then eat as much or as little as you want, depending on how many grams of fat you have left that day. If you're not certain that this particular restaurant serves special food, call ahead to inquire about it.

If you prepare your own food at home, get in tune with and learn all about the low-fat revolution and low-fat cooking. Experiment with herbs and spices to make your culinary creations something you and your family will look forward to eating. You'll find dozens of cookbooks that will convince you that low-fat cooking doesn't mean deprivation. Modify favorite old family recipes to meet your low-fat requirements. For example, instead of sour cream, use low-fat sour cream or nonfat yogurt. Serve smaller portions to yourself, your family, and your guests. They'll appreciate it.

THE VEGETARIAN OPTION

Vegetarianism is currently the rage, and those patients with heart disease or who are vulnerable to it ask me whether I recommend it. According to the Institute of Food Technologists in the July 1991 issue of its journal, *Food Technology,* there are essentially six different types of vegetarianism. The basic diet of all six consists of plant foods. Here are the variations:

1. *Semivegetarian:* dairy foods, eggs, chicken, and fish, but no other animal flesh. This is probably the most popular kind of vegetarianism.
2. *Pesco-vegetarian:* dairy foods, eggs, and fish, but no poultry or other animal flesh.
3. *Lacto-ovo-vegetarian:* dairy foods and eggs only, but no animal (and that means fish too) flesh.
4. *Lacto-vegetarian:* dairy foods, but no animal flesh, or even eggs.
5. *Ovo-vegetarian:* the only animal product consumed is eggs, but no dairy foods or animal flesh.
6. *Vegan:* no animal foods of any kind.

You can see that "vegetarian" does not necessarily mean a low-fat diet. The first four categories all include dairy foods. If any one of them is yours, eat nonfat cheese, nonfat yogurt, egg substitutes or egg white instead of regular cheese, yogurt, and egg yolks. The more restricted your diet, the more essential nutrients you may be missing. So whichever category of vegetarianism you choose, analyze the composition of your diet very carefully. For example, vegans, and even those who avoid animal flesh but eat eggs and dairy products, may become deficient in vitamin B_{12}. This can result in pernicious anemia and severe, irreversible nerve deterioration. This lack of B_{12} is especially dangerous during pregnancy and breast-feeding, in youngsters who are still growing, and in the elderly, who may absorb less B_{12} from their food. The low calorie content and decreased protein content of the vegan diet may be inadequate during pregnancy, and result in low birthweight and impaired growth in infants. Loss of hair and muscle mass is a common complication in adult vegans. So at best, they must be sure to take enough supplements (especially of B_{12}) to meet their needs.

Vegans and ovo-vegetarians, who eat eggs but no dairy food or animal flesh, may develop a lack of vitamin B and calcium too. The latter may cause rickets in children and increases the risk of osteoporosis in women after menopause. Eliminating meat and the iron it contains renders vegetarians vulnerable to iron-deficiency anemia. This is further compounded by the fact that whatever iron they do consume is less well absorbed because of the emphasis on other foods such as soy, protein, bran, and fiber that interfere with iron absorption by the gut. Iron is not the only micronutrient that may be missing in a meat-free diet. Copper, calcium, and zinc may also be deficient. Copper is important in building the body's immunity, in the production of red cells, and in strengthening blood vessel walls. Zinc has myriad functions, including keeping skin, hair, and bones healthy, aiding the development and function of the reproductive organs, maintaining normal taste and smell, synthesizing various proteins and enzymes, helping wound healing, and ensuring the normal functioning of insulin. Its deficiency can cause a host of problems.

Even though vegans and ovo-vegetarians are especially vulnerable to deficiencies of critical nutrients, they can "get away with it" if they consume enough calcium, riboflavin, iron, and vitamin D. Calcium supplements are very important during pregnancy, infancy, childhood, and breast-feeding.

Vegans are really the only vegetarians who are at risk for protein deficiency. Even though almost every animal food, including egg whites and milk, provides all nine essential amino acids (amino acids are the building blocks of protein—see page 12), vegetarians can obtain a complete protein profile in their diet by eating the right combinations of legumes and grains, pasta with nonfat cheese, cereal with nonfat milk, or any rice with beans or lentils every day.

You might also consider eating "substitute meats," protein analogs made from soybeans and that resemble hot dogs, ground beef, or bacon both in appearance and texture. Many of these analogs are fortified with vitamin B_{12}.

IS A HEART CARE PROGRAM FOR YOU?

Some of my patients, mostly those who are "running scared" after a heart attack or whose cholesterol levels are very high (above 300), regularly attend a Pritikin center. This program combines a strict diet and exercise (daily walks) with motivation techniques and close monitoring. Pritikin centers are live-in, and they like you to stay for three weeks, if you can. Their diet makes the American Heart Association Step 2 look like a gourmand's paradise! But most of the "inmates" actually like it!

The Pritikin Diet permits only 10 percent of total calories from fat; cholesterol is restricted to less than 100 milligrams a day, and the protein allowance is under 15 percent. The emphasis is on complex carbohydrates, which comprise over 75 percent of the calories. Salt intake is kept at a reasonable 3 grams daily. (The typical American diet may contain as much as 10 grams.) Although the American Heart Association does not recommend sodium restriction if you don't have heart failure or high blood pressure, I agree with Pritikin. We eat far more salt than we need, and in some cases that may contribute to the development of high blood pressure. You never know you're vulnerable until you develop the disease.

The Pritikin program has two levels. What I have described above is their "maintenance" diet, to which you graduate from the more stringent "regression" diet. The latter consists of eight low-calorie meals a day, consisting mainly of grain, cereal, fruit, salad, potatoes, soup, dried beans, and a "dessert." The "regression" diet is served to newcomers whose blood fats, weight, blood pressure, and blood sugar are out of control. There is no question that most Pritikin clients respond to this regimen and can be upgraded to the "maintenance" diet before they leave for home.

There is not an egg yolk in sight at any Pritikin center; only the whites are used. No organ meats are ever served, and the amount of meat and fish is drastically reduced. The only sugar around is that naturally present in fresh fruits, vegetables, and grain. Don't even *think* of fatty sauces for any dish, none of which are ever fried. The Pritikin team is ingenious in its use of herbs, spices, garlic, onions, and lemon juice. When I last visited one of their facilities, they were allowing one glass of wine per day—under protest! Cigarettes? Smoking? What's that? Never heard of it at Pritikin! Vitamin supplements are not recommended either, the assumption being that their diet provides all you need.

I have found that few of my own patients are able or willing to follow the Pritikin regimen over the long term, mainly because of its rigid fat restriction and the expense. However, if you can stay with it after you come home, away from the camaraderie and dedication of the staff and guests, it will surely keep your weight and cholesterol down. Your blood pressure and blood sugar, if you are diabetic, will also be easier to control, and you may require less medication, or none, to manage these conditions. But expect lots of gas because of the very high fiber content of the complex carbohydrate–rich diet. That problem ultimately resolves itself. The only important abnormality I have observed in some patients coming back from a Pritikin center is a significant elevation of their triglyceride levels. That's the result of the sugar in all the fresh fruit they eat there. If you are planning to visit a Pritikin center, you should have your triglyceride level checked. If it's high, let them know so that they can adjust your diet accordingly.

I recommend Pritikin to my patients whose risk factors are out of control. Only a minority, however, continue to adhere strictly to the program. But even when they do not, they *know* what kind of lifestyle to follow and do so to a greater extent than most people. The most valuable features of a visit to Pritikin are motivation and education.

I knew and admired Nathan Pritikin. He was years ahead of his time; he was derided for years because he was not a doctor and "how dare he give people such radical advice!" Of course, he was right. He followed this diet himself, and after he died (he suffered from leukemia and took his life) I am told that when his coronary arteries were examined, they were found to be remarkably free of arteriosclerosis even though he had suffered from angina pectoris earlier in life.

Until quite recently, Pritikin was the only name prominently identified with a planned, formal risk-reduction program for heart disease. Currently, the Ornish program by Dean Ornish, M.D., is the "talk of the town," especially since a major insurer, Mutual of Omaha, has agreed to reimburse anyone who signs up. The basic dietary principles of the Ornish plan are very much like Pritikin and other regimens that sharply reduce intake of saturated fat and cholesterol, and focus on fiber and complex carbohydrates (except that seeds and nuts are excluded). His is a vegetarian diet—he permits no meat, no poultry, no egg yolk, and no alcohol. Only 10 percent of calories come from fat. But Dr. Ornish, realizing that diet alone is not enough, has broadened his prevention program to include a regimen of moderate exercise, yoga, meditation, and support groups where lifestyle can be reinforced by professionals and other participants. There are those who claim that the Ornish regimen can slow down and even begin to reverse heart disease. In one study of twenty-one patients followed for one year, 82 percent were said to have shown some reduction in the severity of the blockages of their coronary arteries as measured in an angiogram. Despite the fact that some cardiologists and nutritionists think that Ornish is too strict and perhaps even somewhat faddish in his approach (the same criticism that was directed at Pritikin), I predict that satellite centers modeled after his Preventive Medicine Research Institute in Sausalito, California, will spring up throughout the country—especially if more third-party payers agree to pick up the tab.

ALCOHOL AND THE FRENCH PARADOX

A few weeks after I graduated from medical school and just before starting my internship, my parents treated their son, the doctor, to a trip to Europe. My first stop was Paris. Then as now, France, with its wine, women, and song, was the place for a young man on holiday. I had a wonderful time but came back saddened at the obvious French wish to self-destruct. How else could one explain their eating and drinking habits? Even the most humble, modest, and inexpensive restaurant served endless varieties of "forbidden" foods—creamy cheeses, succulent foie gras, thick gravies, marbled meats—all downed with endless quantities of delicious wine, both red and white. Hadn't these people heard about heart disease, or obesity, or cirrhosis of the liver? Didn't anyone care? When I put these questions to my French friends, they invariably responded with a classic Gallic shrug. Today, some forty years later, I know why. The French, despite what they eat, have substantially less heart disease than Americans. So do other countries with similar dietary habits. The answer to the "French paradox" may lie in the wine they drink!

It has been known for some years that there is a higher incidence of heart attacks among teetotalers (that does not mean someone who drinks lots of tea) than in persons who have a couple glasses of wine every day, or a cocktail with dinner, or a bottle or two of beer. Cardiologists were excited at this observation but were hesitant to popularize it for fear of inducing an "if some is good, more must be better" reaction. So it has remained a low-key piece of advice given to selected patients. This protective effect is believed to be due to the fact that alcohol raises HDL, the "good" fraction of cholesterol. I happen to think there is more to it than that. After all, the laying down of plaques filled with cholesterol in the coronary arteries of the heart is a chronic process that takes years to develop. Yet why do persons who suddenly *stop* drinking become vulnerable to a heart attack? That's too rapid a reaction to attribute to an HDL effect alone. Also, alcohol is more protective against *sudden* heart attacks, so whatever protection it confers must also be short acting. Recent research suggests that alcohol works over the long *and* the short term. The long-acting effect is indeed due to a rise in the HDL; the immediate action is on tiny particles in the blood called platelets. Alcohol, whether in wine (red or white), beer, or cocktails, reduces the tendency of these platelets to clump together and form a clot within the blood vessel. Mind you, such clot formation is not always bad. After all, clotting prevents us from bleeding to death when we've been cut. But the clotting *within* the arteries is something to avoid.

A heart attack evolves in two stages. First, fatty material is deposited in the wall of the artery and, as it accumulates, it forms a plaque that progressively narrows the caliber (diameter) of the blood vessel. The final coup de grâce is the formation of a fresh blood clot on the plaque at the site of narrowing that suddenly closes off the vessel and causes the heart attack. So people with angina whose arteries are narrowed, but not totally occluded, experience chest pain on exertion, especially when their arteries go into spasm. They do not, however, suffer a heart attack until they form a clot at the site of the narrowing. So it is hypothesized that alcohol may protect over the long term by slowing down the development of the plaque, and over the short term by preventing the deadly clot formation in the diseased arteries.

What is it in the alcohol that works so admirably? It may be a substance in the skin of the grape (red wine is made with the skin; white wine is not) called resveratrol. The vineyard owners in Bordeaux are so taken with this theory that I understand attempts are being made to synthesize resveratrol and ultimately give it in pill form to protect against heart disease. What a pity that would be! Imagine having a resveratrol tablet with your evening meal, instead of a great wine! I'm skeptical about the whole thing. The Japanese, for example, who also have a low incidence of heart disease, drink mostly rice wine and beer, but very little red wine! There's no resveratrol in rice wine! The whole wine theory may just boil down to the fact that those of us who drink in moderation are a little more relaxed than those who don't, and that this reduced stress is what it's all about.

The bottom line is to drink in moderation. But remember the many important downsides to alcohol in any form—addiction, cirrhosis, behavioral changes, and high blood pressure in some people. Nor is alcohol always good for the heart, especially if you already have a cardiac problem. It can induce disturbances of rhythm (see page 265), and large doses can damage the heart muscle, a condition called cardiomyopathy. Alcohol also deposits its calories around the waist-line—the "beer belly phenomenon." Apart from its cosmetic effect, this particular type of obesity is one of the risk factors for heart disease. So given all the pluses and minuses, should you start to drink now if you never have before? Certainly not if you're pregnant or if there is a family history of alcohol abuse. If you already enjoy and tolerate a daily glass of wine, a cocktail, or a bottle of beer, you may continue to do so.

ANTIOXIDANTS—ARE THEY ALL THEY'RE CRACKED UP TO BE?

Almost every dietary recommendation for the prevention of arterios-clerotic heart disease these days emphasizes the importance of fruits and vegetables—for two important reasons. First, they contain no saturated fat or cholesterol and are rich in fiber. But that's only part of the story. There is also the matter of their antioxidant vitamin content. There is a great and growing interest in antioxidants because many scientists believe that they enhance the immune system and prevent a wide variety of diseases ranging from arteriosclerosis to cancer.

The major antioxidants are beta-carotene (a precursor of vitamin A), vitamin E, and vitamin C. All are present in plentiful supply in many foods such as yellow and green vegetables (broccoli, carrots, tomatoes, spinach, cantaloupes, squash, and sweet potatoes). You will find vitamin E in olive and vegetable oils, some grains, wheat germ, a variety of nuts, leafy green vegetables, dried apricots, and mangoes. Human milk has almost four times as much vitamin E as cow's milk.

It takes a real effort to become vitamin E deficient in America. Vitamin C is present in generous amounts in citrus fruits, broccoli, fresh currants, red and green peppers, and cantaloupe—only a partial list.

According to numerous studies and surveys, persons who consume "enough" antioxidants, preferably in their food, are healthier. The beneficial effect of antioxidants is explained by how the body generates energy and disposes of its end-products. Oxygen is the main "fuel" that sustains most of our biological processes. When these are completed, however, there are residual wastes or by-products to be dealt with. Your stove or fireplace sends its smoke out the chimney; your car has an exhaust pipe. The equivalent waste products of metabolism, especially those associated with oxygen consumption in the body, are *free radicals*. Because our waste-disposal system is not very efficient, these free radicals accumulate in the body. They attach themselves to and damage various substances in the body, notably fat and protein. This union is thought to accelerate cancer, aging, arthritis, and, most recently, disease of the heart and blood vessels. In this latter instance, free radicals act on the LDL circulating in the bloodstream, so that they are more easily deposited in the walls of the arteries, eventually obstructing them. Free radicals also cause the arterial walls to constrict. This spasm, superimposed on the narrowing due to plaque formation, further compromises blood flow within the arteries.

Antioxidants attack free radicals in a fascinating way. They actually penetrate the vulnerable LDL molecule and wait there for the free radicals to come along. When they do, they are either destroyed or otherwise prevented from penetrating the molecule. Antioxidants also circulate in the bloodstream, where they act as scavengers, hunting for and eliminating the "outlaw" free radicals before they can do any harm. So the more antioxidants you have, up to a point, the better.

You can never overdose on antioxidant vitamins from natural foods you eat, but I am not sure the same is true about oral supplements. Still, I prescribe such supplements for my patients with heart disease and those who are at special risk for it *if I am unsure about the adequacy and quality of their diet*. I have never encountered any problem with the doses I recommend—500 to 1,000 milligrams of vitamin C, 400 to 800 IU of vitamin E, and 25,000 units (15 milligrams) of beta-carotene. However, I prefer that my patients to obtain these antioxidants from food, if possible and encourage them to do so. Page 89 lists sources of beta-carotene.

AGE AND THE HEART-HEALTHY DIET

At what age should we begin eating a heart-healthy diet? It's never too early, but it should be no later than two years of age. The best way to teach our children its importance is by example. Although *symptoms* of arteriosclerosis do not usually appear until well into adult life, the coronary arteries begin to show changes as early as the teen years, and these progress with time. So the sooner youngsters develop a taste for and begin to eat several servings daily of fresh fruits and vegetables, complex carbohydrates, fish, skinned poultry, and lean cuts of meat, the better off they will be. Children under age two grow so rapidly that they need more fat than is recommended later in life, but even at this early age, no more than 10 percent of their calories should come from saturated fat. After age two, no more than 30 percent of their calories should be derived from fat (and less is preferable). By ten years, the "average" American boy eats 400 milligrams of cholesterol a day. By age nineteen, that figure rises to 500 milligrams. For some reason, cholesterol intake is not as high in girls who, at age nineteen, consume an average of only 280 milligrams daily.

No one needs more than 300 milligrams of cholesterol per day, even during the years of rapid growth and development. This limitation is not always easily met because of economic and other factors. Many public school lunch programs make no provision for low-fat food substitutes. They often rely on government surplus foods such as whole milk, cheese, and peanut butter—all rich in the very fats one wants to avoid! Some pediatricians worry about restricting the diet of young children in any way. They point to the fact that our kids are healthier, taller, and have greater resistance to disease than those in other countries who are less "well nourished." They fear that altering the diet may undo all that. But what's the point of eating a diet that makes you "tall and healthy" in childhood but kills you early in life?

I believe that youngsters whose parents or grandparents have a cholesterol level greater than 240 milligrams per deciliter, or suffered or died from heart disease early in life, should have their cholesterol, HDL, LDL, and triglyceride levels measured. Their dietary treatment should be *individualized* based on these findings. If the LDL is less than 130 milligrams per deciliter, and the cholesterol below 170, they should be taught healthy eating habits, especially because of their genetic vulnerability. I recommend that any such child over two years of age be started on the Step 1 diet—no more than 30 percent of calories from fat, less than 10 percent of which is saturated, and no more than 300 milligrams of cholesterol a day. Have your child's blood tested every two or three years to make sure the lipid pattern has not changed.

If your child's LDL is above 130, and his or her cholesterol is greater than 200, I again suggest the Step 1 diet. If the results are no better after six months, try the Step 2 diet—saturated fat less than 7 percent of total caloric intake and a daily cholesterol limit under 200 milligrams a day. Children on such a diet should be given supplemental vitamins, minerals, and other nutrients. If necessary, ask for a consultation with a dietician or nutritionist so that you can prepare the tastiest dishes within the limits prescribed.

Should kids ever be given a cholesterol-lowering drug? Only if they have been faithfully following the appropriate diet for one year without effect, and their LDL remains above 190 or the HDL less than 35, and there are other ominous risk factors such as diabetes, high blood pressure, obesity, or a family history riddled with heart disease.

It's easier these days to get kids to eat heart-healthfully. If your child loves a particular food that turns out to be a "no-no," you may be surprised to find a fat-free version in the supermarket. Instead of regular ice cream, try the new fat-free or frozen yogurt products. I honestly can't tell them apart. Add a low-fat snack to your child's lunch box. Take your children shopping with you (for food, that is, not for toys). Teach them how to read the labels and what to look for. Incidentally, this can also serve as a lesson in mathematics!

If it's never too early to begin watching what you eat, is it ever too late? Should older people be "hounded" as insistently as everyone else? That question is addressed by most doctors every day. For example, a seventy-six-year-old man recently asked me whether I thought he should change his diet. He loved red meat, steaks in particular, and had been eating ten eggs a week for as long as he could remember. He was happy and felt well, his last cholesterol level was 210 milligrams, and its ratio to HDL was a borderline 4.8. Having read about the

American Heart Association diet, he wondered whether he should change his ways and follow the Step 1 regimen. Despite everything I have written in the preceding pages, I advised him to continue eating as he had all his life. This is heresy for some of my cardiology colleagues, but my decision was based on my experience, my intuition, and the fact that there are no standards of normality with respect to cholesterol, HDL, and LDL for persons in their seventies and eighties. There are reports that high cholesterol and low HDL can be improved by a combination of diet and drugs, but I am not as yet convinced that doing so has any impact on disease or life expectancy. Apart from the cost and inconvenience of imposing dietary restrictions on healthy older people with normal blood fat levels (I'm not referring to those with heart disease), I worry how it will affect their overall nutritional status. After all, senior citizens often have trouble getting enough calories, vitamins, and minerals anyway—for a variety of reasons (economic, dental, emotional) and we should be careful not to reduce their intake of basic nutrients. For example, aside from their cholesterol content, eggs are an excellent nutrient, and so is milk. Yet both are drastically reduced in the American Heart Association's and every other "heart protection" diet. I tell my patients in their seventies who are in good health, whose cholesterol numbers are normal, that they must be doing something right and to continue doing it, but to drink skim, rather than whole milk. Their genetic profile is protecting them, and that's something on which no doctor can improve.

More often than I care to admit, my best efforts to normalize someone's blood lipids by dietary means fail. Even strict adherence without cheating does not always budge a high cholesterol level. By the same token, I often find excellent cholesterol levels in patients who tell me they pay no attention whatsoever to their diet. How can one explain such disparate observations?

Researchers at the Rockefeller University in New York may have found the answer. They believe that the body deals with cholesterol differently from person to person. In some, after cholesterol is absorbed from the intestine, it goes directly to the liver, which then excretes it into the intestines and out of the body. No matter how much cholesterol such individuals eat, very little gets into the blood, and so their level remains low and their arteries pristine, without any blockage. If you fall into that category, congratulations, you've got it made. Forget any diet. In another group to which one person in five belongs, the liver responds to a cholesterol-rich meal by reducing the amount *it* makes. So here too there's no net increase of cholesterol entering the bloodstream. Then, alas, there is a third category in whom the liver makes large amounts of cholesterol regardless of how little you consume, and dieting has no impact on blood levels. These frustrated people, despite avoiding all cholesterol, continue to have elevated levels. They need cholesterol-lowering drugs. Finally, there are those in whom the cholesterol they eat is delivered directly by the liver to the bloodstream. The less of it they eat, the less accumulates in the walls of the arteries to form the plaques that ultimately cause heart attacks. This is the only group in whom restricting the diet makes a difference. Unfortunately, it is the largest of the four groups!

So try to determine into which category you fall and spare yourself the trouble, frustration, and expense of beating your head against the dietary wall. Here's one way to do it. Eat a normal, balanced diet for four to six weeks. Then have your cholesterol, HDL, LDL, and triglyceride levels measured. If you have a normal pattern, there's no need to follow any particular diet. But if your test is abnormal, adhere carefully to a low-cholesterol, low-fat diet such as the Step 1 or 2 regimen of the American Heart Association. After two months, have yourself checked again. If your cholesterol has dropped by at least 5 to 10 percent, then dieting does make a difference in your case. If there has been no change, concentrate on reducing your intake of saturated fat. That will lower almost everyone's serum cholesterol level. However, you're probably a candidate for medication along with a modest diet such as the Step 1. Discuss these options with your doctor.

YOU'VE HAD A HEART ATTACK! NOW WHAT?

The dietary advice in this chapter has focused on preventing heart attacks in healthy persons and those at special risk. Supposing you've already had a cardiac "event"—you have developed angina pectoris or suffered a heart attack. Is it too late to diet? You may, of course, require a coronary bypass, balloon angioplasty, atherectomy (removal of the plaque or clot in the artery during the angiogram), or laser vaporization—and you should thank your lucky stars that these procedures exist—but diet does remain important, even now. Study after study of persons who have had a heart attack have shown that it is never too late to "eat right," and that, if you do, your outlook is immeasurably better. So the minute you're out of the hospital and the master of your own dietary destiny (with the exception of The New York Hospital, where I work, and the Methodist Hospital in Houston, both of which have designed low-fat, high-calcium heart-healthy diets for their patients, I have found most hospital environments very lax about proper cardiac diets), launch with commitment into a Step 2 diet, eating no more than what is required to maintain a normal weight. You should also have at least three servings of fish per week, and discuss with your doctor the use of a daily aspirin (in addition to whatever cardiac drugs are prescribed) and 400 IU of supplemental vitamin E. In an impressive study of hundreds of men (women should have been included, and will be in future research), eating such a diet reduced the incidence of cardiac *recurrence* or complications by half! This isn't theory. It's fact!

In summary, arteriosclerotic heart disease remains the number-one killer in the Western world—but the numbers are dropping. We are not entirely sure why this is so. Perhaps it's due to earlier, more accurate diagnosis, better medications to keep the blood flowing within the arteries, sophisticated technology and surgery to unblock occluded arteries, fewer adults smoking, improved treatment of high blood pressure, people exercising more, and a changing diet. (Unfortunately, obesity is on the rise, especially among the young.) We are consuming less saturated fat and cholesterol than ever before, and it's beginning to show in the statistics. There are several "lipid" parameters that can predict your vulnerability to heart attack (along with some other important risk factors). Controlling them with the proper diet *can* make a difference. It's easier now than ever to eat and actually enjoy heart-healthy foods, thanks to the profusion of low-fat and nonfat dairy products and substitutes. I have suggested various ways to keep your blood fat profile normal. The rest is up to you. No matter how bad your family history is with regard to heart disease, *you can make a difference by eating a heart-healthy, low-fat diet.*

FOODS HIGH IN SATURATED FAT

Baked goods (made with cream, whole milk, or any oils listed below)
Cured meats/cold cuts
  bacon
  bologna
  salami
  sausage
  other luncheon meats
Fats
  butter
  coconut oil
  lard
  palm and palm-kernel oils
Meats
  beef
  lamb
  meat drippings and gravy
  pork
  veal
Whole milk products
  half-and-half
  heavy cream
  ice cream
  whipping cream
  whole milk
  whole milk cheeses
  whole milk ice creams
  regular yogurt

FOODS HIGH IN CHOLESTEROL

Caviar
Dairy products
Egg yolk
Fish
Meat, especially organ meats (liver, brain, heart, kidney, sweetbreads)
Pâté
Poultry
Squid

RICHEST SOURCES OF OMEGA-3

Anchovies, canned
Bluefish
Herring, Atlantic and Pacific
Mackerel
Salmon, Atlantic and Pacific
Sardines, canned
Trout
Tuna, albacore and bluefin
Whitefish, lake

MODERATE SOURCES OF OMEGA-3

Bass, freshwater and striped
Cod, Atlantic
Flounder
Haddock
Halibut
Perch
Red snapper
Swordfish
Tuna

SHELLFISH SOURCES OF OMEGA-3

Clams, soft-shell
Crab, Alaskan king and blue
Lobster
Mussels, blue
Oysters
Scallops
Shrimp, Atlantic and Japanese

FOODS TO CHOOSE AND DECREASE FOR THE STEP 1*
AND STEP 2 DIETS

FOOD GROUP	CHOOSE	DECREASE
Fats and Oils	Unsaturated oils—safflower, sunflower, corn, soybean, cottonseed, canola, olive, peanut	Coconut oil, palm kernel oil, palm oil
	Margarine—made from unsaturated oils listed above, light or diet margarine	Butter, lard, shortening, bacon fat, hardened margarine
	Salad dressings—made with unsaturated oils listed above, low-fat or oil-free	Dressings made with egg yolk, cheese, sour cream, whole milk
	Seeds and nuts—peanut butter, other nut butters	Coconut
	Cocoa powder	Chocolate
Breads and Cereals	Breads—whole-grain bread, hamburger and hot dog bun, corn tortilla	Bread in which eggs are a major ingredient, croissants
	Cereals—oat, wheat, corn, multigrain	Granola made with coconut
	Pasta	Egg noodles and pasta containing egg yolk
	Rice	
	Dry beans and peas	
	Crackers, low-fat —animal-type, graham, saltine-type	High-fat crackers

FOODS TO CHOOSE AND DECREASE *(Continued)*

FOOD GROUP	CHOOSE	DECREASE
Breads and Cereals	Homemade baked goods using unsaturated oil, skim or 1% milk, and egg substitute—quick breads, biscuits, cornbread muffins, bran muffins, pan-cakes, waffles	Commercial baked pastries, muffins, biscuits
	Soup—chicken or beef noodle, minestrone, tomato, vegetarian, potato	Soup containing whole milk, cream, meat fat, poultry fat, or poultry skin
Vegetables	Fresh, frozen, or canned	Vegetables prepared with butter, cheese, or cream sauce
Fruits	Fruit—fresh, frozen, canned, or dried	Fried fruit or fruit served with butter or cream sauce
	Fruit juice—fresh, frozen, or canned	
Sweets and Modified Fat Desserts	Beverages—fruit-flavored drinks, lemonade, fruit punch	
	Sweets—sugar, syrup, honey, jam, preserves, candy made without fat (candy corn, gumdrops, hard candy), fruit-flavored gelatin	Candy made with chocolate, coconut oil, palm-kernel oil, palm oil
	Frozen desserts—sherbet, sorbet, fruit ice, Popsicles	Ice cream and frozen treats made with ice cream

FOODS TO CHOOSE AND DECREASE *(Continued)*

FOOD GROUP	CHOOSE	DECREASE
Sweets and Modified Fat Desserts	Cookies, cake, pie, pudding—prepared with egg whites, egg substitute, skim milk or 1% milk, and unsaturated oil or margarine; gingersnaps; fig bar cookies; angel food cake	Commercial baked pies, cakes, doughnuts, high-fat cookies, cream pies
Meat, Poultry, and Fish	Beef, pork, lamb—lean cuts *well trimmed before cooking*	Beef, pork, lamb—regular ground beef, fatty cuts, spare ribs, organ meats, sausage, regular luncheon meats, wieners, bacon
	Poultry without skin	Poultry with skin, fried chicken
	Fish, shellfish	Fried fish, fried shellfish
	Processed meat—prepared from lean meat, e.g., turkey ham, tuna wieners	Regular luncheon meat, e.g., bologna, salami, sausage, wieners
Eggs	Egg whites (two whites equal one whole egg in recipes), cholesterol-free egg substitute	Egg yolks (if more than four per week on Step 1 or if more than two per week on Step 2); includes egg used in cooking
Dairy Products	Milk—skim or 1% fat (fluid, powdered, evaporated), buttermilk	Whole milk (fluid, evaporated, condensed), 2% low-fat milk, imitation milk

FOODS TO CHOOSE AND DECREASE *(Continued)*

FOOD GROUP	CHOOSE	DECREASE
Dairy Products	Yogurt—nonfat or low-fat yogurt or yogurt beverages	Whole milk yogurt, whole milk yogurt beverages
	Cheese—low-fat natural or processed cheese (part-skim mozzarella, ricotta) with no more than 6 grams fat per ounce on Step 1, or 2 grams fat per ounce on Step 2	Regular cheeses (American, blue, Brie, cheddar, Colby, Edam, Monterey Jack, whole-milk mozzarella, Parmesan, Swiss), cream cheese, Neufchâtel cheese
	Cottage cheese—low-fat, nonfat, or dry curd (0 to 2% fat)	Cottage cheese (4% fat)
	Frozen dairy dessert—ice milk, frozen yogurt (low-fat or nonfat)	Ice cream
		Cream, half-and-half, whipping cream, nondairy creamer, whipped topping, sour cream

*The Step 1 Diet has the same nutrient recommendations as the eating pattern recommended for the general population. Table derived from *Dietary Treatment of Hypercholesterolemia* by the American Heart Association in cooperation with the American Lung Association. Copyright © 1988 by the American Heart Association.

HEMORRHOIDS

PILES OF FIBER

Joke all you like about hemorrhoids, but remember that *you* will almost certainly have them yourself someday! Why should you be spared when Napoleon and Jimmy Carter were not? I'm no expert on prayer, but I am told that beseeching St. Fiacre may result in relief of hemorrhoid pain—at least among the faithful. But if you decide to pray, kneel, don't sit!

Hemorrhoids are dilated rectal veins that have clotted and become inflamed. Any of the following makes you eligible for membership in the hemorrhoid club: chronic constipation, recurring diarrhea, continual stress, having several babies, frequently lifting heavy objects, sitting around a lot, or standing for long hours at a stretch. You'll further improve your chances of developing hemorrhoids if you're fat, don't eat enough fiber, or tend to become engrossed in a novel while sitting on the toilet. Nearly all of us have some of these characteristics, which is why hemorrhoids are so common.

There are many ways to treat hemorrhoids—surgically (a painful, bloody business that should only be done as a last resort), freezing, infrared photocoagulation, tying them off with rubber bands (easy and effective), frequent soaking in bath or bidet, and topical application of various anesthetic creams, ointments, or suppositories. The best way to prevent them is to eat enough fiber and drink plenty of water. That eliminates straining at stool, a major contributing cause of constipation.

Increase your fiber intake by consuming at least 30 grams of fiber a day, which is much more than most Americans eat. Remember, however, to raise your fiber intake *gradually* over a two- to three-week period, and always drink enough water or fluids—a minimum of 2 quarts daily will prevent the impaction of stool that sometimes occurs when large amounts of fiber are consumed. See page 116 for the fiber content of various foods.

More specifically, your high-fiber diet should consist of at least ¼ or ½ cup of wheat bran or other whole-grain cereals every day. Switch from white to whole-grain bread. Include at least six servings of fruit and vegetables daily, especially those whose skins you can eat (apples and vegetables), whose seeds you can chew (raspberries), and whose hulls you can swallow. Other rich sources of fiber are prunes, dates, figs, and various beans—kidney, baked, navy, and lima, as well as split peas and lentils. Wherever possible, use fresh vegetables in your salads. However, if you prefer them cooked, steam them only lightly to retain as much of the fiber as possible. The longer you steam vegetables, the softer they become. But a steamer is a good investment because you can then add garlic and other herbs to the water to flavor vegetables to your taste.

HEPATITIS

BETTER NEVER THAN LATE!

Have you ever wondered where your soul is located? If you're the sentimental type, you probably think it's in your heart; someone more matter-of-fact might choose the brain. And if you're French, you're probably convinced that it's sitting somewhere in your liver. (The French attribute everything, good and bad, to *"mal de foie"*—"sickness of the liver.") They may be right, because this organ does, in fact, perform myriad functions that maintain the body chemistry on an even keel. It produces antibodies, hormones, and many other different biologicals; it makes substances that keep the blood flowing, yet allow it to clot when necessary; it detoxifies and removes waste products of metabolism. The liver is also a key player in the area of nutrition. Most of what we eat and digest goes directly to it, for storage (as in the case of glycogen, iron, and all the fat-soluble vitamins) or resynthesis (the production of substances such as cholesterol, hemoglobin, and countless proteins that circulate in the bloodstream).

Because it performs so many different and critical roles, when the liver becomes sick, you do too! Some of its ailments are life threatening, many are not. This organ has such great reserves that when you have *mal de foie,* you may feel nothing more than a little lassitude for a few days.

The most common liver disorder is *hepatitis*—an infection or inflammation of the liver. (The suffix "itis" means inflammation or infection, while "hepar" is the Latin word for liver.) There are several different types of *infectious* hepatitis, which can be caused by virtually any virus, fungus, or bacterium. However, the most common by far is acute viral hepatitis due to viruses designated "A," "B," and "C." Although all three can make you miserable, you are virtually sure to recover completely and permanently from hepatitis A. The other two, however, can be more serious.

You "catch" hepatitis A from drinking fecally contaminated water or eating infected food; hepatitis B is usually contracted from "bad" blood or infected needles, and is especially common in male homosexuals, people who share needles for injecting drugs, and health-care workers who accidentally prick themselves with contaminated needles; hepatitis C is almost always acquired from blood transfusions, but it no longer poses nearly as great a threat because donor blood can now be screened for its presence.

Here is the usual sequence of events in a hepatitis A infection: You eat some raw oysters, clams, or other shellfish, or are visiting an area where hygiene is not the strong suit. A few weeks later you notice that your appetite is off; you no longer taste the cigarettes you should have stopped smoking long ago; you may have a little fever. In short, you feel "blah." After about a week or two, things begin to improve, but now you notice that your urine is the color of tea; your eyeballs and skin are yellow. You must be jaundiced! You rush to your doctor, who makes the diagnosis of hepatitis, tells you you don't need medication, and assures you that everything is going to be all right. The yellow hue lasts for a couple of weeks even after all your other symptoms have completely cleared, except that perhaps you're a little more tired than normal. By three or four weeks, your skin and eyes are back to their normal color.

The major symptoms of hepatitis—lack of well-being, poor appetite, jaundice, and fatigue—are common to all three types—A, B, and C. However, they differ with respect to the length of their incubation periods (symptoms of hepatitis A do not develop until three to six weeks after exposure, whereas the other two may "cook" for as long as three months before making you sick) and the possibility of late complications.

Hepatitis A rarely causes death or long-term complications, and most people resume their normal activities in a few weeks, or even sooner. The majority of persons with hepatitis B and C also recover completely, but a small number do not. They remain sick, sometimes very sick, as their hepatitis evolves from the acute stage into a chronic form. In some instances, progressive destruction of liver cells leads to invalidism and death. (Unless, of course, they receive a liver transplant. Several of my patients with severe, chronic hepatitis were lucky enough to receive one, and now lead normal lives.) But let me emphasize that these complications occur in only a minority of people with acute viral hepatitis—most recover completely.

There is no treatment for *acute* viral hepatitis—no antibiotic, medication, or *diet* affects its course in any way. Doctors used to tell these patients to eat virtually no fat, very little protein, and lots of carbohydrates. We now know that that kind of diet will neither harm nor help them. If you have *any* infection, including hepatitis, try to consume as many calories as you can and in whatever form is most palatable to you. The problem with hepatitis, in which your appetite is so poor anyway, is not avoiding certain foods, but getting enough to eat of anything! It's ludicrous to tell someone who is nauseated just looking at food what *not* to eat! You need a nutritionally balanced diet that is appetizing. Small meals and snacks make more sense than larger ones. I recommend a normal fat intake (30 percent of your total calories) and no fried foods, and 20 to 25 percent of calories from lean protein (fish, poultry, and meat) as well as liberal amounts of complex carbohydrate (50 percent of your total calories) for fiber and conversion later to glycogen. And here's a useful tip. If you have hepatitis, what little appetite you have is apt to be greatest in the morning, so that's the time to get most of the calories you need.

One of the first questions someone with hepatitis asks as soon as he or she is beginning to feel better is "When may I have a drink?" Myths die hard, especially old medical ones. There is no evidence of which I am aware that "modest" drinking has a harmful effect in patients with any liver disease *that was not caused by alcohol in the first place*. In my own practice, however, I nevertheless tell my patients not to have any alcohol during the acute phase of their hepatitis as long as their liver blood tests are still worsening. After their condition has stabilized, usually within three weeks, I permit a cocktail or glass of wine with the evening meal—even if some of the liver tests are still abnormal.

In addition to viruses and other infectious agents, hepatitis can also result from injury—by alcohol, cancer, and a host of chemicals, medications, and environmental toxins.

Liver disease caused by alcohol is the fourth leading cause of death among persons between the ages of twenty-five and sixty-four in the United States. Addiction to alcohol is accompanied by serious nutritional deficiency at every stage. That's not only because alcohol is calorie-rich and nutritionally poor, but because it also has a direct toxic effect on the liver. For this latter reason, someone who drinks too much may be a candidate for liver trouble even when his or her diet is "nutritious."

The first evidence of an adverse effect of alcohol is the deposition of fat in the liver. This causes no symptoms; the doctor can neither feel it nor see it, and the diagnosis is made by a sonogram or a CT scan of the abdomen. A fatty liver can clear up if you get on the wagon now. However, if you keep drinking, the fat becomes inflamed, then scars, and after several years can result in cirrhosis of the liver. This is similar to what happens when burned skin is replaced by scar tissue. Although this process can be due to any cause, alcohol is by far the most common culprit, and 15 percent of heavy drinkers die from this form of liver disease. Cirrhosis is not reversible, but eliminating alcohol prevents the formation of more scar tissue. It's never too late to stop drinking.

In summary, there is no specific treatment for acute hepatitis, most cases of which are due to one of three viruses. You will almost certainly recover completely from hepatitis A, which you can get from drinking water or eating shellfish contaminated by sewage; you will also probably recover without complications from viral infection due to hepatitis B (spread largely by use of infected needles and through the stool), and hepatitis C (transmitted through blood transfusions). However, in the latter two, there is the possibility of late complications that can lead to either chronic hepatitis or even cirrhosis (see pages 21 and 22). The good news about any of these forms of acute viral hepatitis is that they do not require any limitation of your diet. If you develop hepatitis, you are more than likely to have a very poor appetite, and you should eat whatever appeals to you. Consume as many calories as you can, just as you would with any infection. Avoid alcohol during the acute phase of the illness, that is, for three or four weeks, but there is no evidence that drinking in moderation after that will do you any harm (unless, of course, you have a drinking problem).

HIATAL HERNIA

DON'T RUSH TO SURGERY

If you were to stand at a busy intersection in your city or town and ask people over the age of fifty whether they have a hiatal hernia, either the police would lock you up or men in white suits would take you away. But before they did, you would probably have a yes answer from over half of the responders.

A brief review of the anatomy of the digestive tract will help you understand what a hiatal hernia is, why it develops, how to prevent it, and what to eat to control its symptoms. The food you swallow enters the esophagus (food pipe), which runs down the interior of the chest and through a hole in the diaphragm (the muscle that separates the abdomen from the chest). Immediately after it enters the abdominal cavity, the esophagus widens to become the upper stomach. The stomach connects to the small intestine, which is followed by the large bowel, which eventually ends as the rectum and anus, where waste products first see the light of day.

Normally, it's a tight fit between the esophagus and the hole in the diaphragm through which it passes because of the action of muscles in the area (sphincters). This opening does not usually permit portions of the upper stomach to slide back up into the chest. But when the sphincter is weak, the hole in the diaphragm enlarges, allowing some of the upper stomach to slip through into the chest cavity. You now have a hiatal hernia! As we get older, muscles everywhere become a little lax, so that hiatal hernias occur in many persons in middle and later life. If, in addition to a portion of the stomach sliding up, some of its contents also spill into the esophagus, the hiatal hernia is said to be accompanied by *reflux*. If stomach acid remains in contact with the esophagus long enough, it causes irritation and esophagitis ("chronic indigestion" or "chronic heartburn").

There are three very common intestinal disorders in the "developed world"—hiatal hernia, diverticulosis (small outpouchings of the large bowel that, when inflamed or infected, can turn into diverticulitis, causing pain, fever, and occasional rupture; see page 155), and gallstones (see page 179). They are all collectively referred to as Saint's triad, which has nothing to do with religion. Dr. Saint, a South African physician, observed in the early 1900s that diverticulosis, gallstones, and hiatal hernias were common in the Western world, but rare in Africa. However, descendants of Africans living elsewhere, for example, in America, develop these conditions as often as do white Americans. The reason appears to be the amount of fiber in the diet. Native Africans consume large quantities of fiber while Americans, at least until quite recently, ate very little roughage and lots of refined sugar. Our "sophisticated" diet has, among other things, led to universal constipation! Straining at stool when you are constipated raises the pressure in the abdominal cavity and in the bowel. When that happens often enough, the bowel becomes distended, portions of its wall become weakened, and the result is the outpouching of diverticulosis. It is easy to see how transmission of this elevated pressure to the sphincter of the esophagus can cause it to loosen up and permit a portion of the upper stomach to slip through the diaphragm, causing a hiatal hernia. Eating more fiber should prevent that from happening. (A low-fiber diet causes gallstones by altering the composition of the bile produced in the liver so that stones form more easily in the gallbladder, where the bile is stored.)

For these and other reasons, doctors recommend a high-fiber diet. Start by simply adding two servings of fresh, raw fruit and two servings of fresh or lightly steamed vegetables to your daily meal plan. Increase your fiber gradually and add it in small doses at each meal to give your body time to adjust. Make these changes over a period of weeks, not in a day or two. Vary the type of fiber you eat. Try different fruits, vegetables, and grains. Add new high-fiber items to your daily intake. For example, use whole-wheat bread to replace white bread, and brown rice instead of white rice. And remember, drink plenty of fluids. Begin with two cups daily and gradually increase it to 4 to 6 cups a day. You'll get more benefits from a high-fiber diet if you drink enough liquids; if you don't, the diet will constipate you. The table on page 120 offers a sample meal plan that provides approximately 43 grams of total dietary fiber, a reasonable objective. For a list of the fiber contents of various foods, see page 116.

So much for preventing hiatal hernia. What's the best way to deal with a hiatal hernia once you have it, especially if it's accompanied by acid reflux and heartburn? There are four steps to follow: (1) To decrease the amount of reflux into your esophagus and to stop your stomach from sliding into your chest, don't lie down, bend over, or strain soon after eating. (2) Wait a few hours after dinner before going to bed. Elevate the head of your bed on six-inch blocks. Gravity will prevent your stomach and its contents from moving up into your chest through the weakened sphincter. (3) Eat frequent small meals rather than fewer heavy ones to decrease the pressure in your stomach. When the pressure in the esophagus is greater than that in the abdomen, reflux is less likely to occur. Drink fluids between meals, not with them, because liquids and food taken together increase the distention of the stomach and promote reflux. Also avoid the following, all of which may cause a decrease in esophageal pressure: nicotine in cigarettes, most liquor, onions, garlic, spearmint, chocolate, caffeine, and fatty foods. (4) Lose weight. A big belly exerts upward pressure on the diaphragm and contributes to reflux. Clothes and belts that are tight around the waist will also aggravate reflux.

To soothe the inflammation of the lining of the esophagus caused by stomach acid, abstain from acidic foods that may further irritate it, as, for example, citrus fruits and juices, tomatoes, and tomato sauce. Use antacids, the best one of which for this purpose, in my opinion, is Gaviscon. Finally, H2 blockers such as Tagamet, Zantac, or Pepcid that stop the specialized cells in the stomach from making acid are also helpful.

In an interesting twist, one of my patients with hiatal hernia and lots of heartburn simply did not respond to these dietary measures. I was puzzled until one day she mentioned that she sleeps on a water bed. The undulating movement of the mattress was increasing her reflux!

The key to the prevention of hiatus hernia and reflux is to eat lots of fiber. Those of us who have already developed the condition can manage its symptoms by the measures I have described: by adding at least 35 grams of fiber to our diets, elevating the head of the bed at night, avoiding irritating foods, using antacids and stomach acid blockers, and losing weight.

HIGH BLOOD PRESSURE

WHO? ME? BUT I'M SO RELAXED!

High blood pressure—hypertension—is called the "silent killer" because it may not cause any symptoms for ten or even twenty years. Don't depend on headaches, dizziness, nosebleeds, nervousness, and fatigue to tip you off to the diagnosis—these are just as common in someone with perfectly normal blood pressure. Your personality also has very little to do with it. Blood pressure may be normal in high-strung individuals and sky high in placid ones. Sure, your pressure will shoot up if you fly into a rage or plunge into a panic, but it will return to normal when the crisis is over. If you have hypertension, however, your blood pressure is always up, even when you're having fun. The only way you'll know for sure whether you have high blood pressure is to have a doctor, nurse, or other health provider put a blood pressure cuff on your arm and tell you. That's something everyone should have done at least once a year.

High blood pressure is a major cause of disability and death in many parts of the world. In this country alone, it affects almost 60 million people, and even children on rare occasions. Above age sixty-five, some 40 percent of whites and 50 percent of blacks (in whom the condition is usually more severe, especially among the young) have significant pressure elevation. The readings, which are expressed in millimeters of mercury (mm Hg is how doctors write it), reflect the pressure under which blood flows through the arteries. Systolic pressure, the top figure, is the pressure in these blood vessels after they receive the wave of blood each time the heart contracts; the bottom reading, called the diastolic, is the pressure in the arteries between beats. There is a common misconception, even among some doctors, that it's only your diastolic pressure that counts, and that if it is normal, the systolic reading doesn't really matter. That's totally wrong. Both the systolic *and* diastolic numbers are important and require treatment if they are elevated.

Your blood pressure changes from minute to minute, depending on where you are, what you are doing, whether or not you have eaten, how you feel, the time of day, whether you are sitting, standing, or lying down—and who's taking it. My patients are often surprised when my nurse invariably obtains readings lower than I do. That's because she is a charming woman, while I wear a white coat. The diagnosis of hypertension should not be made on the basis of a single measurement—by anyone. Get three or four readings before you accept the hypertensive label. And equally important, a normal reading at any time is no guarantee that it's going to stay normal. You've got to keep checking regularly to detect any elevation as soon as it occurs.

Most doctors agree that a reading of 140/90 at any age is borderline and should be carefully monitored. I begin treating my patients when their levels reach 160/95, and start with diet, weight loss, and behavior modification such as biofeedback. If these measures are not successful, then and only then do I prescribe medication.

I can understand why so many people resent taking pills to reduce their blood pressure. The right antibiotic will clear an infection; a painkiller will ease your pain; aspirin will reduce your fever; insulin will lower high blood sugar. But it's an entirely different matter as far as high blood pressure is concerned. Here, you make the "mistake" of letting someone pump up a cuff on your arm, on the basis of which you are told there's something wrong with you—even though you are feeling perfectly well. The pill that's prescribed not only costs money, it makes you sick! You used to sleep like a baby all night, now you have to "go" several times; your previously great sex life is a memory; and you generally feel like a zombie. As if that weren't enough, you have to keep paying to have your pressure checked and rechecked to see whether the medication that's ruined your life is working! If it is, then you are told to continue taking it! Where is the logic? Small wonder that so many patients say, "Hey, who needs this?" They pack it all in and become what we doctors call "noncompliant." Once they stop the drug they bounce right back to their usual state of "good health"—until one day all hell breaks loose.

You see, high blood pressure is not the creation of pharmaceutical advertising; it *is* a major killer and crippler, causing strokes, heart attacks, kidney trouble, leg pain while walking, aneurysms, blindness, and heart failure. If your blood pressure elevation is mild, you may get away without any treatment, but that's something no one can predict. Don't take the chance, especially since there are now medications that will lower your pressure and keep it down without intolerable side effects. All it takes is patience!

Despite the fact that high blood pressure is so common and so deadly, in almost 95 percent of cases we don't really understand why it develops. We can identify certain hormonal changes in the blood, we can measure fluctuating levels of several body chemicals—but we don't know *why* any of this occurs. So in recognition of our ignorance, doctors designate such hypertension as "essential," "idiopathic," or "primary," all of which mean that we haven't a clue as to the cause. In the remaining 5 percent of cases, there are known and usually curable reasons for the elevated pressure—tumors of the adrenal gland (which can be removed), narrowing of the arteries going to the kidney (which can be dilated), disease of one kidney (whose removal restores normal blood pressure), or a congenital constriction of the aorta (the major blood vessel leaving the heart, which can be surgically corrected). Certain medications such as oral contraceptives, steroid hormones, appetite suppressants, nose drops, and antidepressants can also make your blood pressure rise. So if you have newly diagnosed high blood pressure be sure to review *all* your drugs, even those you can buy without a prescription.

Let's assume that your blood pressure was found on several different occasions to be high, perhaps 170/95. That falls into the "mild" to "moderate" category—certainly not "severe" (230/120 would put you in the latter class). You may have worn an ambulatory blood pressure monitor that records your blood pressure automatically every

thirty minutes to one hour (your doctor selects the interval) throughout the day and night—while you are eating, working, sleeping,
arguing, even having sex. This continued recording eliminates the
"white coat syndrome"—the reason my nurse's readings are lower
than mine. Having made the diagnosis of hypertension, your doctor
may want you to have some additional tests, especially if you're under
forty, to make sure you are not one of the 5 percent whose hypertension is curable.

You are now advised to do "something" about your high pressure.
You have the following options to combine as you and your doctor
see fit: (1) Lose weight if you're too heavy. (2) Reduce your salt
intake. (3) Start an exercise program if you have been given the green
light to do so by your doctor. (4) Join a behavior-modification group
to help you handle stress. (5) Reduce your alcohol consumption, if
that's relevant. (6) Take medication, which should be prescribed only
if the other interventions don't work.

If you're too heavy, losing weight is the most important and effective step you can take to lower your pressure. As little as a six- to
twelve-pound drop can make a big difference. The best (and only)
way to lose weight is to reduce your caloric intake by cutting down
your consumption of fat, sugar, and alcohol (see page 344), engage in
regular physical exercise, and in some cases, lower your salt intake as
discussed below.

Salt restriction immediately comes to mind whenever there is a
question of high blood pressure. Doctors differ in their opinions about
its role in hypertension and in the recommendations they give their
patients. Some would have you eliminate it while others permit you
to use as much as you like. Let's take a fresh look at the role salt plays
in high blood pressure prevention and treatment, and how much you
may safely consume.

Salt has a checkered history. Remember what happened to Lot's
wife when she looked back! On the other hand, "salt of the earth" is
a term of approbation; in Greek mythology the Gods loved it! Even
the word *salary* is derived from *salarium*—the salt paid Roman soldiers
for their services. But for the first 99 percent of mankind's existence
on earth, the diet of *Homo sapiens* contained much less salt and considerably more potassium than we eat today, and very little fat. As we
became more "civilized," particularly in the last hundred years, our

diet changed drastically and is now basically one of high sodium, low potassium, and high fat. There is little doubt that several "diseases of civilization," among them high blood pressure, are at least in part the result of these dietary modifications. Populations whose diet has remained high in potassium and low in both salt and fat have less high blood pressure and vascular disease (and fewer malignancies) than we. That observation is somewhat tempered by the fact that they generally have a shorter life expectancy—presumably for other than dietary reasons.

No one needs more than 2 or 3 grams of salt a day, yet Americans consume an average of 5 grams per day, and some eat as much as 10 grams! The World Health Organization conducted a ten-year study of the diets of fifty-five groups of people, ages fifty to fifty-four, living in twenty-two different countries, to see whether there was any relationship between what they ate and the incidence of high blood pressure. Where the diet was low in salt but high in potassium, magnesium, fiber, and omega-3 fatty acids, there was substantially lower blood pressure, fewer strokes, a decreased death rate from heart disease, and a longer life expectancy. Similar examples abound. In Japan, where the consumption of salt is very high, blood pressure is also much more elevated than it is even in this country (although they live longer than we do and are more physically active, according to some). So purely in terms of prevention, I believe it is desirable to reduce the national (and personal) salt intake to somewhere between 2 and 3 grams per day.

So much for prevention. What should you do about your salt intake if you already have high blood pressure? Reducing it makes a real difference in anyone who is salt sensitive (which is only 5 to 10 percent of all hypertensives), especially when combined with weight reduction and exercise. So I recommend a low-salt diet (no more than 2 grams daily) to everyone with high blood pressure together with a no-nonsense warning about weight. If the pressure hasn't fallen after four weeks on this diet, I conclude that the hypertension is not related to salt sensitivity and permit 3 or 4 grams of salt a day, and I prescribe with a blood pressure–lowering drug.

How do you reduce your sodium consumption to 2 or 3 grams a day? It may not be as easy as you think, for one third of the salt in your diet comes from natural sources, one third is added during food processing, and only one third is discretionary. So start with the obvious. If you remove the salt shaker from your table (both at home and at the restaurant) and change nothing else in your diet, your total intake of salt (assuming you eat the "usual" American diet) will drop to approximately 4 grams a day. (Diets and dosages are also sometimes expressed in milliequivalents, or meq. One gram of sodium equals 43 meq, so that 4 grams of salt is the same as 172 meq.) You can drop your salt consumption another full gram a day by not adding any to your cooking or other food preparation. (One level teaspoon of salt contains 2.3 grams of sodium.) Avoid frankly salted foods such as pickles, sauerkraut, herring, buttermilk, anything that is cured, salted, or marinated, and all consommé or broth made with salt. Do not drink commercially softened water, which may be rich in salt (check the label), and beware of the salt content in some brands of tomato juice and vegetable juice. (Juice made from fresh tomatoes in a blender, however, contains only a trace of natural salt. Prepare your Virgin Mary with low-salt tomato juice and use only those brands of Worcestershire sauce that have no sodium.) The table on page 247 lists the most popular drinks and their sodium content. Look at the tremendous variation among them! Most tap water has just a trace of salt, and seltzer water contains none at all, while there are 75 milligrams in a 12-ounce bottle of club soda. How a food is processed can make a tremendous difference to its salt content. For example, 1 cup of fresh corn has virtually no sodium, yet the same amount of canned corn contains almost 500 milligrams! One cup of cabbage has a modest 14 milligrams of sodium, but turn it into sauerkraut, and you'll find 1,560 milligrams in that same cup! A fresh cucumber contains only 9 milligrams, but pickling it adds over 800 milligrams! We tend to equate peanuts with salt, yet 1 ounce of fresh peanuts has but a single milligram of salt. However, after you've roasted and salted them, that same ounce has 119 milligrams! If you need to be careful about how much sodium you consume, be sure to check the label of every food you buy. Some food manufacturers designate canned and frozen items such as soup, vegetables, and even bouillon as containing reduced amounts or "no added salt." But make sure that despite these disclaimers, they haven't slipped in some monosodium glutamate (MSG) or soy sauce! The former contains sodium—e.g., salt; the latter is one of the highest salted foods there is. I know people who scrupulously adhere to a low-salt diet all day, then go to a restaurant and douse their egg roll with soy sauce or dip their sushi into it! Remember too that a food may have more natural salt than is good for you even if none has been added. So, read the label for the amount of sodium per serving and check the number of servings per container for the total salt content. The table on page 248 lists the foods with the highest content of salt, their portion size, and how much sodium they contain.

If your doctor decides that you need not just a low-sodium diet but one that is *very low* in sodium, we are now talking about 1 gram a day! This translates into absolutely no salt at the table, none whatsoever in your cooking, no canned or processed foods, and no food with enough natural salt content that you can taste. Foods with virtually no salt whatsoever include any *unsalted* fat such as margarine, butter, mayonnaise, oil, or other salad dressing; almost any fresh fruit (check the labels on frozen fruit for the presence of salt or sodium sulfite, a preservative); most vegetables, except celery. If you're a bread lover, most bakeries and specialty shops carry low-sodium bread, rolls, and muffins. Your meals need not be bland and boring, given all the wonderful herbs and seasonings now widely available. Try fresh onion, paprika, tarragon, curry powder, oregano, thyme, marjoram, or onion and garlic powders. (But be sure to buy pure garlic, not garlic salt!) Then there are fresh mustard, bay leaf, green and red peppers, fresh tomatoes, sage, and a host of salt-free seasoning mixes. The possibilities are endless. There are several pretty good salt substitutes too, the most agreeable of which, at least to my palate, are Co-Salt, Adolph's Salt Substitute, and Morton Salt Substitute. They all contain substantial amounts of potassium, which, as you will see, is good for high blood pressure, but not if you have any kidney trouble. (Diseased kidneys often cause abnormal retention of potassium, too much of which can have several adverse effects, especially on the heart. So if you have any kidney problem check with your doctor before you use a salt substitute.)

A very-low-salt diet is not always good for you. It can raise the level of insulin and the amount of bad LDL cholesterol in the blood; if you are taking one of the calcium channel blockers such as nifedipine, diltiazem, or verapamil to decrease your blood pressure, a low-sodium diet can render them less effective! So before you become too ascetic and decide that you are going to do without any salt, no matter how great the sacrifice, check it out with your doctor. Such deprivation may be unnecessary and undesirable.

There are other dietary modifications to prevent and lower high blood pressure. Taking enough *potassium* (3,000 to 3,200 milligrams or about 75 meq daily) not only helps prevent the onset of high blood pressure but also protects against strokes. The table on page 251 lists the richest sources of potassium. In a recent study conducted over a twelve-year period, no woman over fifty who consumed lots of potassium—more than 67 meq a day (there are 10 meq in one large glass of orange or grapefruit juice)—suffered a stroke. Those who took less than 40 meq had a stroke rate of 5.3 per 100. Similar results were observed in men. There were no stroke deaths among those who consumed more than 60 meq of potassium a day, but when the intake was less than 50 meq, there were 3.4 stroke deaths per 100 patients. Since the average American diet contains about 60 to 65 meq a day, you do not really need to increase your potassium intake by more than 10 meq a day—or an extra glass of grapefruit juice. That should reduce your risk of stroke by 40 percent regardless of its effect on your blood pressure. Blacks (50 percent of whom over age sixty-five have high blood pressure) who live in the southeastern United States and consume an average of only 30 meq of potassium, less than half the average consumed by the rest of the country, have the highest stroke incidence in the nation. Scots too don't eat much potassium (their average intake is 45 meq a day), and they also have a high stroke rate. (Remember that diuretics—water pills—widely used in the treatment of high blood pressure, cause not only the loss of sodium, which is good, but of potassium too, which is bad. Diuretics are not my favorite blood pressure–lowering drugs for these and other reasons.) Adding potassium supplements to whatever medication you are taking for your high blood pressure can reduce the required dosage of those drugs by 50 percent. Despite all the data mentioned above, the importance of potassium (as well as calcium and magnesium—see below) is not sufficiently emphasized by most doctors, who continue to focus on sodium.

If you conscientiously consume 1,000 milligrams of *calcium* every day, your risk of developing high blood pressure will drop by as much as 40 percent. But you are better off getting it in your food than in supplements. It's especially important for pregnant women, the elderly, black persons, and those who are salt sensitive to have enough calcium to prevent the development of hypertension. On page 242, you will find a list of foods rich in calcium, and how much they contain. Also on page 242 is a list of drugs that increase calcium loss.

Magnesium (which, like potassium, is lost in the urine of people taking diuretics) not only prevents high blood pressure in some people, it's also good for the heart. Whole grains that have not been processed, leafy green vegetables, nuts, fish and seafood, dried fruits, poultry, beef, pork, and lamb are all good sources of this mineral. You should have an intake of 350 to 400 milligrams per day, preferably in your diet, but by supplements if necessary. See the table on page 304 for the magnesium content of various foods.

An extra 500 to 1,000 milligrams a day of *vitamin C* (see page 105 for a list of vitamin C content of foods) may also prevent hypertension.

Alcohol raises blood pressure, even though you may find it relaxing. It is estimated that 5 percent of all cases of hypertension are either due to or aggravated by alcohol. After excessive weight, alcohol consumption is the strongest predictor of elevated blood pressure. I can't tell you what amount is critical because individual response to booze varies so much, but if your blood pressure is up, I suggest you reduce whatever amount you're now drinking and have no more than one or two drinks a day in any event.

The data linking *caffeine* with high blood pressure do not impress me. I do not believe that coffee raises blood pressure (although boiled coffee may increase your cholesterol level). However, for the other reasons mentioned elsewhere in this book, I advise my patients not to consume more than three 5-ounce cups of regular coffee a day.

Cigarette smoking also contributes to the risk of high blood pressure, and there are doctors who refuse to treat hypertensive patients until they have quit.

Vegetarians tend to have lower blood pressure than meat eaters, probably because of their increased fiber intake. Populations in which fiber consumption is high enjoy lower blood pressure. I recommend you try to consume at least 35 grams of fiber daily. For a list of the fiber content of various foods, see page 116.

Some people with high blood pressure respond to *biofeedback* and stress-management techniques, which are certainly worth a try before you start taking medications if losing weight, cutting back salt, getting enough dietary potassium, calcium, and magnesium, reducing your alcohol intake, and exercising have not done the trick.

Regardless of everything you do to lower your blood pressure, you may very well end up needing medication. That doesn't mean you can now gain weight, forget about your diet, and return to a sedentary life. For even if the lifestyle and dietary guidelines I have outlined do not prevent the need for drugs, they will most assuredly reduce the number and dosage required. And side effects of many medications, especially those used in the treatment of high blood pressure, are very much dose related.

We have come a long way in the development and availability of medications for the treatment of high blood pressure. As I stated earlier, no one with elevated readings should ever go through life feeling miserable on medication. There is a right combination of agents for you, but it takes patience and trial and error to find it. From among the plethora of beta-blockers, ACE inhibitors, calcium channel blockers, alpha-adrenergic agents, and diuretics, your pressure can be brought down and kept down without intolerable side effects. Having said that, I must reiterate that you should first try to obtain the same results without drugs.

In summary, whether or not you have high blood pressure, it is a good idea to reduce your salt intake to no more than 3 grams a day. In addition, you may prevent the development of high blood pressure and even stroke by losing weight if you are too heavy, increasing the amount of potassium and magnesium in your diet, consuming enough calcium (1,000 milligrams a day), reducing your alcohol intake to no more than one or two cocktails a day, and adding 35 milligrams of fiber to your meals. I also recommend between 500 and 1,000 milligrams of vitamin C every day from foods, if possible, but from supplements, if not. You are lucky if you live in a community with hard water because it contains calcium and magnesium, both of which seem to lower elevated blood pressure. Always remember that hypertension is a silent disease. Have your blood pressure checked at least once a year, and more often if you have a family history of increased pressure, are black, or are over sixty years of age.

SODIUM CONTENT OF BEVERAGES

BEVERAGE	PORTION	SODIUM (mg)
Beer		
Miller	12 ounces	6
Miller lite	12 ounces	10
Coffee, brewed	6 ounces	4
Juices		
apple	8 ounces	7
orange, fresh	8 ounces	2
tomato, canned or bottled	8 ounces	676
V8, low-salt	8 ounces	47
V8, regular	8 ounces	715
Liquor		
gin	1.5 ounces	trace
rum	1.5 ounces	trace
vodka	1.5 ounces	trace
Milk		
buttermilk	8 ounces	257
low-salt	8 ounces	6
skim	8 ounces	126
whole	8 ounces	125
Soft drinks		
club soda	12 ounces	75
Coca-Cola	12 ounces	8
Diet Coke	12 ounces	75
seltzer	12 ounces	0
tonic/quinine water	12 ounces	15
Tab	12 ounces	27
Soup		
Campbell's beef broth	8 ounces	840
Campbell's chicken broth	8 ounces	784
Lipton Cup·A·Soup, tomato	8 ounces	652
Lipton Cup·A·Soup, vegetable	8 ounces	1,058
Tea brewed for 4 minutes	6 ounces	5
Water		
municipal	8 ounces	7
Perrier	8 ounces	3
Poland Spring	8 ounces	1
San Pellegrino	8 ounces	5

SODIUM CONTENT OF BEVERAGES *(Continued)*

BEVERAGE	PORTION	SODIUM (mg)
Wine		
red	7 ounces	12
rosé	7 ounces	10
white	7 ounces	10

FOODS HIGH IN SODIUM*

FOOD	PORTION	SODIUM (mg)
Bacon	3 slices	303
Bacon bits, imitation	¼ ounce	181
Baking powder	1 teaspoon	426
Baking soda	1 teaspoon	402
Bologna, beef	1 slice	226
Bouillon	8 ounces	82
Catsup	1 tablespoon	178
Cheeses		
blue	1 ounce	396
cheddar	1 ounce	176
cottage, 1% fat	1 cup	918
feta	1 ounce	316
Parmesan, hard	1 ounce	454
Parmesan, grated	1 tablespoon	93
processed Swiss and American	1 ounce	443
Cream of tartar	1 teaspoon	231
Frankfurter		
beef	1	585
turkey	1	472
Milk		
skim	8 ounces	144
protein-fortified skim	8 ounces	126
whole	8 ounces	119
Monosodium glutamate (MSG)	1 teaspoon	750
Mustard	1 teaspoon	65
Olives		
black	10 large	750
green	10 large	926
Peanuts, dry roasted	1 ounce	288
Pickle relish	1 tablespoon	164

FOODS HIGH IN SODIUM* *(Continued)*

FOOD	PORTION	SODIUM (mg)
Pretzels, salted	1 ounce	486
Salami, pork, hard	1 slice	226
Salsa, mild	3 tablespoons	340
Salt	1 teaspoon	2,300
Sauerkraut, canned	1 cup	1,560
Sausage, pork	1 ounce	248
Soy sauce		
low-salt	1 tablespoon	480
regular	1 tablespoon	769
Teriyaki sauce	1 tablespoon	690
Tomato		
fresh	1	11
sun-dried	4 ounces	565
Tomato juice, canned	8 ounces	676
Tomato sauce		
Prego	½ cup	596
Prego no-salt-added	½ cup	21
V8 juice, regular	8 ounces	715

*Note: Processing can make an enormous difference in the sodium content of many foods, as demonstrated below with two foods, corn and cabbage:

	PORTION	SODIUM (mg)
Corn, fresh	1 cup	trace
Corn, canned	1 cup	496
Cabbage, fresh	1 cup	14
Coleslaw with mayonnaise	1 cup	150
Sauerkraut, canned, including liquid	1 cup	1,560

SAMPLE MENU (2 GRAMS SODIUM)*

	PORTION	SODIUM (mg)	CALORIES
Breakfast			
Special K cereal	1 cup	214	123
Skim milk	1 cup	127	86
Banana, sliced	1 medium	1	105
Whole wheat toast	1 slice	159	80
Jelly	1 tablespoon	3	55

SAMPLE MENU (2 GRAMS SODIUM)* *(Continued)*

	PORTION	SODIUM (mg)	CALORIES
Lunch			
Tuna sandwich:			
tuna packed in water	¼ cup	310	70
Hellmann's mayonnaise	1 tablespoon	80	100
cracked-wheat bread	2 slices	280	140
Salad:			
romaine lettuce	½ cup	2	4
tomato	½ cup	7	17
cucumber	½ cup	1	7
olive oil and vinegar	1 tablespoon each	0	127
Fresh peach	1 small	0	40
Snack			
Low-fat coffee or vanilla yogurt	1 cup	149	194
Dinner			
Roasted chicken breast, skinless	4 ounces	84	200
Pasta, cooked	1 cup	3	220
Canned tomatoes	½ cup	196	24
Sautéed vegetables:			
broccoli	½ cup	12	12
carrots	½ cup	19	24
olive oil for sautéing	1 tablespoon	0	125
Fresh blackberries	½ cup	0	37
Nonfat cookies	2 2-inch	50	100
Snack			
Air-popped popcorn	2 cups	0	50
Diet Pepsi	12 ounces	38	0
		1,685	1,940

*No salt added in cooking; no salt added at table.

HIGH-POTASSIUM FOODS

Beans and legumes:
  all varieties dried beans, all varieties dried peas, lentils
Chocolate and cocoa
Coconut
Dried fruits:
  apricots, dates, prunes, raisins
Fresh fruits:
  apricots, bananas, cantaloupes, cherries, honeydews, kiwis, mangoes,
  nectarines, oranges, papayas, peaches, raspberries, tangerines
Juices:
  apricot nectar, orange, prune, tomato, V8
Milk and yogurt
Nuts:
  all varieties
Salt substitutes
Vegetables:
  artichokes, avocados, bamboo shoots, bean sprouts, broccoli, brussels
  sprouts, cabbage, carrots, celery, collards, corn, mushrooms, parsley,
  parsnips, plantains, potatoes, pumpkins, seaweed, spinach, sweet
  potatoes, tomatoes, turnips, water chestnuts, winter squash
Whole grains:
  cereals, bread made from whole-grain wheat, millet, rye, barley, and
  buckwheat, wheat bran

Eat these high-potassium foods in moderation:
Milk—No more than ½ cup per day.
Potato—Mashed or boiled, no more than ½ cup two to three times per
  week.
Protein—Predialysis: no more than 3 to 4 ounces per day; on dialysis, no
  more than 5 to 6 ounces per day (meat, chicken, fish, egg).
Tomato—No more than ¼ cup tomato sauce two to three times per week.
  No sun-dried tomatoes.

POTASSIUM CONTENT OF FOODS

FOOD	PORTION	POTASSIUM (mg)	CALORIES
Cereals and grains			
All–Bran cereal (Kellogg's)	⅓ cup	320	70
shredded wheat cereal	1 ounce	102	102
wheat germ	¼ cup	327	103
rice, white cooked	1 cup	80	264
Dried fruits			
apricots	10 halves	482	83
dates	10	541	228
figs	5	661	238
peaches	10 halves	1,295	311
prunes	10	626	201
raisins	⅓ cup	413	148
Fish, meats, and poultry			
sardines, in oil	2	95	50
beef, extralean, ground broiled	3.5 ounces	313	256
beef, eye round, lean	3.5 ounces	395	175
pork, loin, center	3.5 ounces	420	231
chicken, white, skinless, roasted	3.5 ounces	247	173
Fresh fruits			
apricots	3 medium	313	51
banana	1 medium	451	114
cantaloupe	1 cup	494	57
cherries	10	152	49
honeydew	1 cup	461	60
kiwi	1 medium	252	46
mango	1 medium	322	135
nectarine	1 medium	288	67
orange	1 medium	250	65
papaya	1 medium	780	117
peach	1 medium	171	37
raspberries	1 cup	187	61
strawberries	1 cup	247	45
tangerine	1 medium	132	37
watermelon	1 cup	186	50

POTASSIUM CONTENT OF FOODS *(Continued)*

FOOD	PORTION	POTASSIUM (mg)	CALORIES
Juices			
apricot nectar	8 ounces	286	141
grapefruit, fresh	8 ounces	400	96
orange	8 ounces	496	111
prune	8 ounces	706	181
tomato	6 ounces	400	32
V8	6 ounces	384	37
Milk			
skim	8 ounces	406	86
2% fat	8 ounces	377	122
whole	8 ounces	368	157
Nuts			
almonds, dry roasted	1 ounce	219	167
cashews, dry roasted	1 ounce	160	163
peanuts, oil roasted	1 ounce	183	161
Soybean flour, defatted	½ cup	1192	164
Molasses, blackstrap	1 tablespoon	498	47
Vegetables			
artichoke	1 medium	425	60
broccoli, uncooked	½ cup	143	12
brussels sprouts	½ cup	247	30
cabbage, green, uncooked	½ cup	86	8
cabbage, red, uncooked	½ cup	72	10
carrot, uncooked	1 medium	233	31
celery	7½-inch stalk	115	6
corn	½ cup	204	89
mushrooms, cooked	½ cup	277	21
parsley	½ cup	166	11
parsnips, cooked	½ cup	287	63
plantain	1 cup	716	179
potato, baked with skin	1 medium	844	220
pumpkin, cooked	½ cup	281	24
spinach, cooked	½ cup	419	21
tomato, uncooked	1 small	273	26
turnip	½ cup	106	14
winter squash, all varieties, baked	½ cup	445	39

HYPERACTIVITY

THE SUGAR MYTH

Some children are by nature rambunctious, high-spirited, into everything, bright, and fun. The *hyperactive* child, usually male, also has boundless energy, but that's where the similarity ends. He is irritable, can't concentrate, does poorly in school despite a high IQ, fidgets all day long, and often has temper tantrums. This behavior, which is usually recognized by the time the child is four years old, may continue into the teens and adult life, and may be the forerunner of antisocial or even criminal behavior.

No one knows why some children are hyperactive and others not. Maternal smoking, drinking, drug use, or illness during pregnancy have occasionally been implicated but never proved. The truth is that the cause of hyperactivity remains a mystery.

Once the diagnosis is made—and it's not always easy to distinguish hyperactivity from the effects of chronic stress, depression, or anxiety—the symptoms are usually managed with medication. The classic drug, Ritalin (methylphenidate), doesn't always work. Doctors and parents are loath to medicate children during their formative years and have been trying to manage hyperactivity by dietary means. Many substances have, over the years, been been thought to aggravate symptoms of the disorder, notably food additives, artificial colorings, sulfites, and flavorings. Sugar, especially, and for no reason that is apparent to me, has been implicated. To this day, many parents keep their affected children on a low-sugar diet. But there has never been universal agreement by scientists and experts in behavior that any of these factors plays any role in the causation or aggravation of the symptoms of hyperactivity.

A recent study may help lay some of these food myths to rest. Forty-eight children (twenty-five were preschool age, the rest were six to ten years old), all diagnosed as hyperactive, and whose symptoms, according to their parents, were made worse by eating sugar, were divided randomly into three groups. The first was fed a diet containing large amounts of sugar, the other two were fed no sugar but were given aspartame (NutraSweet, a popular sugar substitute) and saccharine instead. The experiment was continued for three weeks, during which the children were closely observed for any mental or behavioral changes. None was observed. The researchers concluded that neither sugar nor aspartame in the diet has any impact on the symptoms of hyperactivity.

How should a parent of a hyperactive child respond to this study? In my opinion, if you've been feeding him or her a special diet because of what you've heard or read, but have not personally observed any difference, I'd abandon it. (It's a good idea to keep the sugar intake modest anyway.) Hyperactive kids are hard enough to manage without the additional problem of enforcing a diet that does no good. If, on the other hand, in *your* experience with *your* child, you have observed that sugar, aspartame, tartrazine, MSG—or whatever—causes or worsens the symptoms of hyperactivity, continue to withhold them from the diet. After all, this is only one study, albeit well conducted. Future research may prove *you* right, not them.

HYPOGLYCEMIA

NO SUGAR EVEN WHEN YOU NEED IT!

Patients sometimes consult me for a second opinion after they've been told by another doctor, a friend, or an enemy that they have "hypoglycemia." They often say, "You probably don't believe in hypoglycemia, but . . ." I assure them that "believing" in hypoglycemia is not like having faith in God. Of course I believe in hypoglycemia (the medical term for "too little sugar in the blood"), but it is not nearly as common as it is diagnosed. Many persons who think they have it, don't. If you are nervous, are plagued by panic attacks, or experience episodic weakness and tremors, don't accept the "hypoglycemia" label without first undergoing a thorough medical evaluation. A wrong diagnosis, made casually and reflexively, leaves the true cause of these symptoms unrecognized and untreated. I hate to think how many people have been wrongly tagged as hypoglycemic because of symptoms of mitral valve prolapse, thyroid trouble, kidney or liver disease, a tumor of the pancreas, chronic viral infection, or a treatable, underlying psychological problem.

The normal range of blood sugar measured in the fasting state is between 70 and 105 milligrams. If it's 40 milligrams or less, you are, by definition, hypoglycemic. However, symptoms of hypoglycemia can occur at higher levels, as, for example, when the blood sugar drops *quickly* from high to normal levels. But the 40 number is a useful guideline.

The classic symptoms of hypoglycemia are hunger, weakness, a cold sweat, headache, nausea, fatigue, numbness of the face or the extremities, palpitations, lack of coordination, dizziness, confusion, and nightmares. When there is not enough sugar available brain function is impaired. The longer it is deprived of energy (enough sugar), the worse matters become. What may start as slight confusion can end in coma. The best way to prove that these symptoms are due to low blood sugar is to measure it. If it's way down, and you recover after receiving concentrated sugar in one form or another (by mouth, if you're conscious, by vein, if you're not), the diagnosis is clinched.

There are several circumstances in which your blood sugar can drop far (and quickly) enough to cause symptoms; if you are a diabetic, if you're taking more insulin or other sugar-lowering drug than you need; if you eat less than the prescribed dose that the insulin or antidiabetic drug is meant to "burn off"; or exercise so vigorously that you use up too much sugar and therefore have a relative excess of insulin. You'll know you're hypoglycemic when your heart begins to beat rapidly for no apparent reason, or you suddenly become very nervous, hungry, and confused—especially if you've just taken insulin or a sugar-lowering agent. If you're driving a car, pull over—now! To raise your sugar level quickly, you must immediately eat five or six Life Savers or sugar cubes, have 2 to 3 teaspoons of granulated sugar, or drink 4 ounces of ginger ale, 3 ounces of grape juice, or 4 ounces of orange or apple juice. Medications such as *sulfa drugs* and *aspirin,* as well as *alcohol,* can also cause hypoglycemia in diabetics. If you have diabetes, you must remember that you are prone to hypoglycemia and must always carry with you some form of concentrated sugar.

You can also develop low blood sugar if you have kidney or liver disease (both organs help regulate blood sugar levels). Normally, if you go for several hours without eating, the body calls on the liver to pump some of its stored sugar (glycogen) into the circulation. This backup or reserve is what prevents most people from becoming hypoglycemic even after fasting for twenty-four hours or more. There is also a feedback mechanism in the pancreas that prevents it from making insulin when you are fasting and therefore need less. *Anyone who cannot maintain a near-normal sugar level while fasting either has a liver or kidney problem, or is unable to store or release the extra amounts of sugar needed, or has a pancreas that is continuing to make insulin when it shouldn't.*

The most important cause of continuing and inappropriate release of insulin by the pancreas—and hence another cause of hypoglycemia—is an insulin-producing tumor *(insulinoma)*, which does not respond to the usual feedback mechanisms. Alcoholics whose nutrition is impaired to begin with may drop their sugar level sharply when they drink on an empty stomach.

Reactive hypoglycemia, a common type of low blood sugar, is also very much overdiagnosed. Whenever you eat sugar or simple carbohydrates, the right amount of insulin is normally released by your pancreas to convert it into usable energy. When this response is too great, the resulting insulin "overshoot" causes a low blood sugar level. Persons in whom this reaction occurs may be destined to become diabetic sometime in the future. In other words, diabetes, with its high blood sugar (hyperglycemia), is occasionally preceded by years of low blood sugar (hypoglycemia).

Before you accept the diagnosis of reactive hypoglycemia, borrow or buy a home sugar-monitoring device. It's simple to use. As soon as you feel the symptoms coming on, prick your finger and check your sugar level. If it's higher than 60 milligrams, you're not likely to have a low blood sugar problem. It's much more convenient to use such a kit than to depend on your doctor or an emergency room.

The best way for diabetics to prevent the various forms of hypoglycemia is to fine-tune the relationship between insulin dosage, diet, and exercise. If your blood sugar drops too low when your stomach is empty (fasting hypoglycemia), you should be tested for the presence of an insulin-secreting tumor. (This usually requires measuring insulin levels when the blood sugar is low, and obtaining a CT scan or MRI of the abdomen. Such tumors are benign, and must be surgically removed.) If you have reactive hypoglycemia, you can reduce your overproduction of insulin by eating several smaller meals instead of three large ones. You must also avoid highly refined starches, concentrated sugar and anything made with it—candy, honey, jelly, jam, syrup, fruit juice, cakes, cookies, pies, sherbet, and ice cream. These foods are most rapidly absorbed, especially between meals when your stomach is empty and so apt to cause insulin overshoot. Don't feel deprived by this list of prohibited foods. You can still satisfy your sweet tooth with "goodies" made with sugar substitutes such as aspartame (NutraSweet). Just check the shelves of your supermarket (are there any more old-fashioned grocery stores left?), and you will find sugar-free jams, jellies, cookies, cakes, chocolate, pudding, and delicious frozen desserts you won't know aren't the "real" thing. Your diet should be focused on foods that provoke a *gradual* release of sugar into your bloodstream, namely, proteins (make them 30 percent of total calories), complex carbohydrates with a high fiber content— including beans, vegetables, and legumes (40 to 50 percent of calories), fresh fruits and vegatables rather than dried fruit, which is very rich in concentrated sugar, and only enough fat to make your meals palatable. Alcohol also stimulates insulin secretion, so either cut it out or limit it to 1 ounce a day. Limit your caffeine intake because it reduces blood sugar (beware of certain cough and cold remedies, which also may have caffeine added to counteract the effects of drowsiness. See page 45 for a list of foods high in caffeine.)

In summary, although I do "believe" in hypoglycemia, it's a diagnosis I do not make, and one you should not accept, until it's proven. There are several other common conditions such as panic attacks, an overactive thyroid, kidney or liver trouble, various drugs, and insulin-producing tumors that can produce virtually identical symptoms. So before rushing off to change your diet, first make sure of the diagnosis. Once that's been done, and the best way is to actually measure the blood sugar at the height of the symptoms (cold sweat, palpitations, lack of coordination, dizziness), an attack is best treated by eating rapidly absorbed simple sugars to raise your sugar level quickly. If you are diabetic or prone to hypoglycemia for any of the other reasons discussed, always carry with you enough concentrated sugar or candy to abort an attack of hypoglycemia.

INFLAMMATORY BOWEL DISEASE

DRUGS, DIET, AND SOMETIMES SURGERY

Most people think that anyone with recurrent gastrointestinal problems—whether ulcers or recurrent diarrhea—must have an underlying psychological disorder. But although any "condition" can be affected by your state of mind, chronic abdominal symptom are rarely caused by "nerves."

The term *inflammatory bowel disease* (IBD) refers to a group of chronic intestinal disorders that plague millions of men and women throughout the world. They are classified for convenience into two main types—ulcerative colitis and Crohn's disease—which may, in fact, represent several different entities with similar symptoms. The cause of inflammatory bowel disease is poorly understood, its treatment is both difficult and unsatisfactory, and the potential complications vary considerably.

Don't confuse inflammatory bowel disease with irritable bowel syndrome (see page 270). Persons with the latter condition may *feel* miserable, but they are otherwise healthy. They never need an operation to cure them, they are not at risk for a host of serious complications, and they have (but do not always "enjoy") a normal life expectancy. Inflammatory bowel disease, on the other hand, not only impairs the quality of life, it's sometimes a threat to life itself.

Ulcerative colitis eats away the lining of portions of the large bowel; symptoms wax and wane. You may feel relatively well for many months, but then you suddenly become symptomatic again. The disease is two to four times more common in Jews than in non-Jews, and four times more frequent in whites than in nonwhites. Women are affected more often than men, and most cases begin between ages twenty-five and forty-five, although it can develop later in life. As a rule, the later the onset, the more severe the course. Ulcerative colitis also runs in families, so that if you have it, there is a one in three chance that a blood relative does too.

The most common early symptoms of ulcerative colitis are constipation and blood or mucus in the stool. In mild cases, after months or years, intermittent diarrhea develops, with up to five stools a day and cramping lower belly and rectal pain. In most people, the condition remains mild, and affects only the lower part of the bowel. However, in approximately one case in four, the disease progresses—the number of stools is greater, they contain more blood and pus, there is urgency to pass them, the abdominal discomfort is more severe, and you feel tired, lose weight, look sick, and feel sick. A small number of persons go on to the severe form of ulcerative colitis—they become really sick, with fever; constant, loose, bloody stools; fatigue; loss of appetite; and weight loss. This disorder is associated with an increased incidence of cancer of the bowel, probably because of the long-standing inflammation and irritation. Some doctors recommend prophylactic surgical removal of the affected portion of the gut to forestall the appearance of malignancy, especially when the disease is of prolonged duration and the patient is very symptomatic.

Crohn's disease, the other form of IBD, affects the full thickness of the bowel and not just its lining, as does ulcerative colitis. It too strikes Jews preferentially (especially those of middle European origin), and women more frequently than men. It is commonly present in twins and siblings. The symptoms and severity of Crohn's depend on which portion of the bowel it affects, and how severely. Sometimes it is limited to the very lowest part, or is localized to the area near the appendix, or it may affect large portions of the gut, even extending to the mouth and food pipe. So the symptoms of Crohn's disease vary in nature and severity, and include any combination of diarrhea, bloody stools, fever, cramping, and weight loss—not unlike those present in some forms of ulcerative colitis.

Special diagnostic procedures, including a biopsy of bowel tissue, may be necessary to tell these two variants of inflammatory bowel disease apart. Though less likely to develop cancer of the bowel than those with ulcerative colitis, people with Crohn's disease are at somewhat greater risk for doing so than the general population. The main complications are abscess formation, fistulas, malabsorption, and scarring of the bowel, all of which may require surgical treatment.

We do not know the causes of inflammatory bowel disease, but when we finally come to understand them, I doubt that any of the popular psychological theories purporting to explain it will hold water. I predict it will be very much like what happened with lactose intolerance and mitral valve prolapse. Prior to 1963, when we did not realize that so many people lacked the enzyme to digest lactose in their diet, persons who developed gas pains and diarrhea after drinking milk or eating foods prepared with it were thought either to have some food allergy or simply to be nervous. Once we were able to replace the missing lactase enzyme and knew what foods to avoid, the symptoms cleared, and all the psychological explanations were abandoned. The same was true with mitral valve prolapse. Remember all the women with chest pain, palpitations, and anxiety who were assumed to be "high strung" or "unstable" because every test was negative? When the cardiac echo machine was invented and the real cause of their symptoms was discovered, all their complaints suddenly became physical and therefore "respectable." The focus of treatment shifted from psychotherapy to a search for medications to alleviate or control their symptoms.

In the last few years, several new drugs have become available for the treatment of ulcerative colitis and Crohn's disease. They are the hallmark of therapy, and can improve symptoms dramatically in many cases. Unfortunately, they cannot cure or really alter the long-term outcome of these diseases. Even in those few cases where surgery is required to remove severely affected portions of the bowel, the problem remains unsolved because the disease may reappear in remaining areas that were previously unaffected.

Symptoms of IBD develop regardless of what you eat—with *one major exception*. Many of these patients are lactase deficient (see page

295) and improve when they avoid milk and milk products. When dietary lactose is not properly digested because the lactase enzyme is missing, diarrhea, a problem to begin with, becomes worse. I recommend one of the lactase supplements currently available to cover any foods you are eating (and medications you are taking) that contain hidden lactose. Check the label on every packaged food, because milk and its derivatives are present in so many of them. The key words to look for are *whey, casein,* and any term with the word *milk.* The table on page 299 lists the lactose content of various foods. The table on page 300 lists some products to watch out for that you might not suspect contain lactose.

At the height of your symptoms, during an acute attack, it is extremely important to make sure that you get enough fluid. If your IBD is severe, you may even need hospitalization to receive the appropriate medication and intravenous nutrition to rest your bowel. If you are being treated at home and can eat, aim for a high energy intake, 20 calories per pound per day, to include 0.5 gram of protein per pound of body weight (so if you weigh 140 pounds, you would need 70 grams). You may have to eat frequently throughout the day to satisfy these requirements.

People with IBD aren't always able to satisfy their nutritional needs because their appetite is often poor, or their abdominal pain is aggravated by eating, or they lose nutrients because of diarrhea, or they have had extensive bowel surgery. Such people can become dehydrated, malnourished, and deficient in vitamins and minerals such as magnesium, vitamin B_{12}, folic acid, iron, and vitamin D (the latter because two drugs used in the treatment of IBD—prednisone and cholestyramine—interfere with its action). So if you have IBD, ask your doctor about supplemental vitamins and minerals.

The stools of people with IBD, especially ulcerative colitis, sometimes contain abnormal amounts of fat. In such cases, I advise restricting total fat intake to 25 percent of calories, and taking a multivitamin containing zinc, magnesium, calcium, and the fat-soluble vitamins (A, D, E, and K), all of which are lost in the fatty stools. How much of these supplements you need will depend on the frequency and severity of the diarrhea.

There is a complication of Crohn's disease of which you should be aware. This disorder predisposes to kidney stones—specifically those composed of oxalate. This is because bile and other fatty acids are not well absorbed, they hang around the bowel, and promote the absorption of oxalate. So it's a good idea to avoid oxalate-rich foods, especially if you've already had such a stone. The table on page 292 lists some foods rich in oxalates.

There is a myth about inflammatory (and irritable) bowel disease that needs to be dispelled. It seems logical, if you've got diarrhea, gas, and cramping, to reduce your intake of fiber. Wrong! Dietary fiber plays an important part in the management of IBD. However, the type and amount you'll need depend on the nature and severity of your illness, and you should increase it very gradually. Work with your doctor to determine how much fiber you should have. You'll find a list of high-fiber foods on page 116.

In summary, whether you have an irritable bowel or inflammatory bowel disease, you should take whatever medications are necessary to control your symptoms, but nutritional supplements, avoidance of lactose-rich foods, and plenty of fiber are the hallmarks of dietary support.

THE IRREGULAR HEARTBEAT

WHEN HOLIDAYS ARE

BAD FOR THE HEART!

Take it from me—your heart *is* beating right now, even though you are probably not consciously aware of it. Your heart beats regularly, between sixty and one hundred times a minute in most people, but the rate may drop below that if you're an athlete or are very physically fit. It may also beat faster when you have fever, an overactive thyroid, any kind of heart trouble, or anemia, or when you're excited, frightened, emotional, or running for a bus when you're "out of shape."

Most of us are never even aware of a change in our heart rhythm, but we may feel a "skip" or an "extra" beat, a pounding or palpitations, or a sensation of "emptiness" in the chest. In short, we suddenly know that we "have a heart." And it's often scary—because it *is* the heart.

Variations in cardiac rhythm, known as arrhythmias, occur in almost everyone from time to time, depending on what you eat, drink, or smoke; your state of mind; the medicines (and that includes vitamins) you take; whether or not you're tired; or the presence of some underlying disease. Although most arrhythmais are innocuous, you can become dizzy or light-headed, lose consciousness, or even die suddenly if your heart beats very, very rapidly, much too slowly, or totally irregularly.

You are in no position to decide whether or not a change in your cardiac rhythm is important. That's your doctor's call. The onset of *any* arrhythmia, no matter how "benign" you *think* it is, requires an immediate professional evaluation that must include, at a minimum, a detailed medical history, a careful physical exam, and an electrocardiogram. You may also need a chest X ray to determine whether or not your heart is enlarged and/or misshapen; a Holter monitor (in which you wear an instrument the size of a pack of playing cards that records your EKG continuously for a twenty-four-hour period); an echocardiogram (to evaluate the state of your heart valves and muscle); and a stress test to determine whether the flow in the coronary arteries is normal. These procedures, singly or together, will usually determine whether your arrhythmia is normal or reflects some underlying cardiac problem. If they don't provide the answer, more complicated studies may be necessary.

If your arrhythmia turns out to be the type that requires treatment, the first line of therapy is usually medication. Unfortunately, virtually every drug used for this purpose has some side effects, anything from causing a simple loss of appetite to triggering a different, potentially life-threatening arrhythmia. However, what you eat, in conjunction with the medication you take, can sometimes help in the management of some rhythm disorders.

The appearance of any cardiac rhythm "condition" should prompt you and your doctor to review what medications you're taking and at what dosage, how much alcohol you're drinking, whether or not you're using tobacco in any form, your caffeine intake (coffee, tea, colas, and even chocolate and cocoa), and also what you're *not* eating. Trying to lose weight by eliminating rich desserts or reducing your consumption of booze, passing up seconds, leaving something on your plate after every meal even if you are still a little hungry—none of these will induce an arrhythmia. Neither will regular exercise. But crash diets, starving yourself, prolonged fasting—can all cause arrhythmias, and lethal ones at that!

Close medical supervision of a starvation diet is no guarantee of safety. Do not allow yourself to be persuaded to follow any radically calorie-restricted "special diet," even if your diet doctor is "watching you." Physicians used to think that as long as you consumed a minimum of 1,000 calories daily, including protein of "high biological value" (fish, meat, etc.), you were safe. That's not so. What's more, although adding vitamins does lessen the risk of serious trouble somewhat, it does not offer total protection. Starvation diets result in low potassium and magnesium levels that can cause sudden death. And there are other risks too. When you lose a substantial amount of weight in a short period of time, it's not only fat that's "melted." Muscle is also affected, and the heart is a muscle. Any "wasting" of cardiac tissue leaves it more sensitive to certain chemicals, such as adrenaline, that drive it. Too much adrenaline makes both you *and* your heart "nervous." This adrenaline effect is, at least in part, responsible for the arrhythmias that can cause sudden cardiac death.

Tobacco is not a food (though lots of people chew it), and so it theoretically does not really belong in any discussion of diet. But I want to remind you anyway that smoking, particularly cigarettes, can cause almost any kind of "palpitation." I became aware of that personally many years ago (on April 12, 1960, to be precise) when my wife and I were demonstrating a radio-transmitted electrocardiogram, quite revolutionary at the time. I was wearing the battery-operated unit several hundred feet from a monitor that she was operating. Suddenly, while some interested doctors were watching *my* electrocardiogram on the screen, several "extra" beats came into view. My colleagues were concerned and asked my wife where the "patient" was. She found me smoking a cigarette! When I returned to our booth and looked at the monitor, a volley of "extra" beats appeared on the screen every time I inhaled. That was all the convincing I needed. I threw my my half-empty pack of cigarettes into the trash can and have never smoked one since! So if you're experiencing any skipped beats or have palpitations, stop smoking. In fact, don't wait until your heart skips a beat—throw those cigarettes away now.

Can *caffeine,* which is both a food and a drug, disturb the rhythm of the heart? More than four or five cups daily can increase your heart rate and cause rhythm irregularities especially *if you already have a rhythm problem.* So if you are experiencing extra beats, palpitations, or any other arrhythmia, drink caffeine-free coffee, tea, and soft drinks instead. There is no caffeine in seltzer water and regular sodas such as orange, grape, lemon, lime, and ginger ale. Page 45 lists the caffeine content of some of the more popular beverages Americans consume. As you can see, tea has just about half the caffeine content of coffee, but there is very little difference as far as caffeine is concerned among the various caffeinated soft drinks. Note too that the cocoa in chocolate, especially unsweetened baking chocolate, may have as much in 1 ounce, as does a 6-ounce cup of coffee! So check the label of anything you drink (or eat) if you or your heart is caffeine sensitive, including painkillers, cold remedies, and antacids, many of which contain caffeine. But for the record, I believe that up to three cups of coffee a day may actually be good for most people. There's nothing like a cup of hot, fresh brew first thing in the morning to get you going. Coffee helps asthmatics because it dilates the airways. I have also found that one or two cups often increase the amount of exercise patients with angina pectoris can perform before the onset of their chest pain.

Reduced levels of *potassium* and *magnesium* can lead to a variety of cardiac rhythm abnormalities ranging from harmless to life threatening. The most common cause of such depletion is the *diuretic* or water pill, taken for whatever reason (heart failure, fluid retention, high blood pressure). Drinks such as tea that have diuretic properties do not cause potassium or magnesium deficiencies. People with alcohol problems or who take cisplatin (an anticancer drug) or gentamicin (an antibiotic) may also have low magnesium levels. I always suspect low potassium or magnesium in anyone taking diuretic pills who is unusually tired for no apparent reason, or who complains of nocturnal leg cramps. These levels are easily measured in a blood test. If the magnesium is indeed low, I prescribe 250 to 400 milligrams of a magnesium supplement in tablet form. If you have mildly decreased potassium levels, I recommend at least one glass of orange juice and one banana a day. That should be enough to prevent potassium-induced arrhythmias, but if it isn't, there are many potassium supplements available in liquid and tablet form.

Alcohol, especially in large amounts, can induce or worsen a cardiac rhythm disturbance. Regardless of your tolerance to alcohol, "spree" drinking will get you into trouble—even if you have never experienced an arrhythmia before. Since such drinking usually occurs on weekends and holidays, the term "holiday heart" was coined. Emergency-room doctors are kept busy by patients who come to the hospital, usually during a long weekend, with a variety of cardiac rhythm irregularities. Whether it's due to the direct toxic effect of alcohol on the heart, to magnesium deficiency, or, as in starvation, to the release of adrenalinelike substances that overdrive the heart, heavy, sustained drinking can produce a variety of cardiac arrhythmias ranging from fairly innocuous ones to those that can cause sudden death.

So here is how to maintain a normal heart rhythm without drugs: (1) no crash diets; (2) no tobacco; (3) no more than three cups of coffee a day; (4) potassium and magnesium supplements if you're taking diuretics, have a drinking problem, or have low levels for any other reason; (5) alcohol in moderation.

THE IRRITABLE (OR SPASTIC) BOWEL

PLAY "ROUGH" WITH YOUR GUT

The world is full of people with "spastic colon" or irritable bowel syndrome (IBS). Three times as many women as men are afflicted. They go through life plagued by gas, bloating, abdominal cramps, and diarrhea; their stools are too hard one day and too loose the next; and they need to move their bowels so frequently and urgently that their lives revolve around the toilet. They go from doctor to doctor—both traditional and holistic—nutritionists, psychiatrists, gastroenterologists, allergists, hypnotists, acupuncturists—looking in desperation for relief of their symptoms. They are subjected to every conceivable test, all of whose results are normal. Their stools contain the usual amount of fat, and are without blood, parasites, or evidence of other infection; colonoscopy, barium enemas, MRIs, and CT scans all reveal nothing unusual. In the end (no pun intended), they are told they are in "good health," and that they have "nothing more" than an irritable bowel.

Unlike persons with inflammatory bowel disease (IBD; see page 260), if you've got an irritable bowel, despite feeling miserable so much of the time, you actually look healthy. You may be a little underweight, but you're not anemic, and do not run a fever. You'll probably get little sympathy from family, friends, or doctors because you have no objective evidence of "disease." In the final analysis, you are viewed as a victim of an underlying emotional disorder and are told to "snap out of it," and, after a while, may begin to believe this nonsense yourself! But I do not for a moment subscribe to this notion. Many specialists are now convinced that the symptoms of IBS are due to very intense and frequent contractions of the gut muscles, and that the resulting spasms reflect a disturbance of motor function that has nothing to do with anxiety, depression, or neurosis. Whatever emotional problems someone with IBS has stem from their poor quality of life. Psychological support, biofeedback, and other stress-reduction techniques can help you cope with the stress caused by the symptoms of IBS. Since these symptoms—abdominal pain, cramps, gas, bloating, irregular bowel movements—can reflect any number of gastrointestinal disorders, some of which are potentially serious, see your doctor to be certain you don't have Crohn's disease, ulcerative colitis, malabsorption, lactose intolerance, or even cancer. Once these and other disorders have been ruled out, then and only then should the diagnosis of IBS be made. In other words, it's a diagnosis of exclusion.

The treatment of IBS consists of medications to reduce spasm and quiet the bowel, and dietary recommendations. I always start with diet before resorting to drugs. I have my patients with IBS avoid milk and milk products because so many of them have some degree of lactase deficiency. I also recommend lactase supplements. (Lactase is the enzyme that breaks down lactose, a sugar that is a major constituent of milk and its derivative foods. Unless this occurs, the lactose is not digested and becomes fermented by bacteria normally present in the gut. This causes gas, bloating, and cramping. See page 295 and the table on page 299.) Gas-forming foods such as cauliflower, beans, brussels sprouts, onions, and cabbage also aggravate IBS. Meat, fish, chicken, lettuce, popcorn, nuts, and even potato chips don't usually cause abdominal distension, but the effect of any food is unpredictable. The dietary key to improving IBS, however, is eating lots of *fiber*, which makes the stools bulky and waterlogged so that they pass more easily and quickly. Increasing the amount of fiber in the diet results in less straining with bowel movements, and no buildup of pressure within the bowel. Be sure to eat slowly, chew your food thoroughly, and don't sip fluids with your meals. This facilitates air swallowing and increases gas formation. I have also found that a low-fat, high-protein diet seems to improve the symptoms of IBS.

Elsewhere in this book I have detailed the kind and amounts of fiber to eat (see page 116). Plenty of whole-grain fibers and legumes are a must. A high-fiber cereal or hot oatmeal for breakfast is a good way to start the day. To make sure you're getting enough daily fiber, buy coarse miller's bran at your local health food store and have 2 teaspoons three times a day, added to fruit juice, cereal, or soup. As your bowel adjusts, you can gradually double that amount over a period of weeks. Another product that will easily provide the necessary fiber is psyllium, marketed as Metamucil and other brands. Add 1 tablespoon to two glasses of water or fruit juice three times a day. It's very important to drink lots of water on a high-fiber diet. Without it, you may well end up constipated.

Also make a point of having at least six servings a day of fresh fruits and vegetables—especially carrots, oranges, and apples, which contain pectin, a soluble fiber. This is especially helpful if your main complaint is diarrhea rather than constipation. Unlike insoluble fiber, pectin does not impose too much bulk on an already stressed bowel.

Although most people with IBS improve on a high-fiber diet, some do not. In fact, such a diet sometimes aggravates the bloating and abdominal distention and can also cause intolerable amounts of gas. It's much less likely to do so if you start with small amounts of fiber and increase the portions gradually.

If you've got IBS, you'll probably feel better eating smaller meals more frequently. Avoid laxatives or use them very sparingly if you must. Your bowel is sufficiently irritated without them. Antibiotics, especially some forms of erythromycin, can cause a problem in IBS that irritate the bowel.

One final word. "Go" when you get the signal, and eat a normal, balanced diet to maintain good nutrition.

JET LAG

FLY FIRST CLASS, EAT ECONOMY!

The modern jet gets us where we're going so quickly that we think nothing of taking a long weekend several time zones away from home. If it's a pleasure trip, you want to enjoy it; if you're on business, you want to be sharp and think clearly. It doesn't matter whether you lose a couple of days readjusting to the time change if you're going to be away for several weeks, but if your total time budget is only three or four days, you don't want to spend it feeling like a zombie, regardless of your mission.

The human body has a rhythm to most of its functions. We are programmed to sleep when it's dark and awaken when the sun comes up; our temperature is higher every evening than it is in the morning. These patterns all reflect "circadian rhythm," the intricate, programmed ebb and flow of our hormones. When you board a jet in New York at 7:00 P.M., the clock will read 7:00 or 8:00 A.M. some seven hours later when you arrive in Europe because of a five- or six-hour time difference. However, as far as your body is concerned, it's still 2:00 A.M. While you're flying, sitting for hours in a space meant for a five-year-old, your biological timekeeper keeps going. By the time you arrive in the early morning, you're ready for bed. But you haven't spent all that money to be holed up in a foreign hotel, so you drag yourself about, convinced that you're having a good time! That enervation lasts two or three days and is what we call jet lag. No sooner do you begin to adjust to the new time than you're on your way home, and the process starts again at the other end.

Scientists have been trying for years to develop drugs and chemicals to fool the body into thinking night is day and day is night. A breakthrough may finally be in the offing in the form of melatonin, a natural body hormone. Until its proper dosage is determined you can ease the symptoms of jet lag by modifying what and when you eat as you prepare for your trip across several time zones. Here's how to do it.

First, fly during the day whenever possible. That's not always easy because London and Paris are currently the only European destinations to which you can fly in the daytime from the United States. These flights leave around 10:00 A.M. Eastern time (that's 3:00 or 4:00 P.M. in Europe). You arrive in the evening after a six- or seven-hour flight. By the time you've collected your baggage, completed the airport formalities, and reached your hotel in town, it's bedtime. Perfect! You'll have a good night's sleep, and the next morning you should be able to start the day feeling fairly fresh. You may peter out somewhat earlier than usual, but there is not too much jet lag on this kind of schedule.

Second, try the feast-fast-feast dietary recommendations of the scientists at the Argonne National Laboratory (the research and basic sciences center of the U.S. Department of Energy). It may help you to adapt to your biological rhythm more quickly. Here's how it's done.

For three or four days before you leave, get as much sleep as you can and avoid late nights. Three days before departure, is a "feast" day, consisting of breakfast and lunch rich in protein—lots of fish, chicken, eggs (or egg white if you're on a low-cholesterol diet), turkey, nonfat yogurt or low-fat cottage cheese, high-protein cereals, and beans. Dinner should consist mainly of carbohydrates—pasta, potatoes, starchy vegetables, and sweet desserts (assuming, of course, you're not diabetic). Also, and this is important, *do not take any caffeine between 3:00 and 5:00 P.M. on that day.* That means no caffeinated coffee, tea, cola, chocolate, or cocoa. And watch out for the over-the-counter medications that contain caffeine. Check the labels to be sure. The most likely place you'll find it is in cough and cold remedies, to which the caffeine is added to counteract the drowsiness that these agents often induce. (See page 45 for foods containing caffeine.)

The next day, that is, two days before you leave, is a "fast" day, but not quite as rigorous as Yom Kippur or Ramadan. Limit your intake to 800 to 1,000 calories, consisting of salads, clear soup, plain toast, and fruit. To help reduce the number of calories, buy the 40-calorie-per-slice bread now widely available, use fat-free salad dressings, and light fruit jellies and jams. Eat three servings of fresh fruit rather than just the juice, to benefit from the bulk and fiber. Again, no caffeine in the afternoon. The sample menu on page 276 provides an example of a suitable "fast" day.

The day before departure is another feast day—same rules as day one.

On the day of departure you really do fast—nothing but water, of which you can have as much as you like. You may take whatever medications you normally would. If you're going west, young man, that is, toward the Orient from America or to Los Angeles from New York, eat *nothing* until 12 noon and no caffeine the rest of the day. If you're traveling east, for example, from Chicago to Paris, fast all day and drink no coffee or tea after 6 P.M. Try to sleep soon after you board the plane. Forget the movie, the food, and any other distraction the airline provides. Ask your doctor for a short-acting sleeping pill that won't give you a hangover. I used to prescribe a low dose of Halcion, and many doctors still do, but because of reports of amnesia after the use of Halcion, I now recommend Albien, 5 mg; Dalmane, 15 mg; or ProSom, 1 mg, instead. Once you're airborne, *drink no alcohol* whatsoever—even if it's free! Do not eat a full meal. It may look edible, but . . . Stay with fruit, salad, and cookies. Dehydration is a common complication of long flights, so drink lots of mineral or plain water.

What you eat the day you arrive is also very important. When it's breakfast time (regardless of whether you've arrived or are still on the plane), eat a high-protein breakfast. If you know that you will still be airborne at the time, order your breakfast ahead from the airline (you usually need to give at least one day's advance notice to order a special meal). Ask for a vegetarian meal and some low-fat cottage cheese. Eat your breakfast as close to 7:00 A.M. as possible and don't go back to sleep after you've finished. Read or walk about the plane.

After you arrive at your destination later that morning, assume the local mealtime schedule. Do not nap in the morning or afternoon, but retire early that evening.

Although most nutrition scientists are skeptical of all anti–jet lag diets, several of my patients have told me that this feast-fast-feast regimen does help. I have tried it too, and although it doesn't leave me with quite as much energy as I would have had staying home, it does seem to reduce the severity and shorten my symptoms of jet lag. Perhaps it's because of its effect on the enzymes that regulate the amount of sugar stored or released by the liver. In any event, I think it's worth trying. Bon voyage!

SAMPLE MENU TO ALLEVIATE JET LAG—
THE "FAST" DAY

	PORTION	CALORIES
Breakfast		
Fresh cantaloupe	⅓ medium	60
Toast, light, 40 calories per slice	2 slices	80
Low-sugar jelly	2 teaspoons	16
Coffee or tea	1 cup	5
Lunch		
Tuna packed in water	2 ounces	70
Low-fat mayonnaise	1 tablespoon	50
Bread, light, 40 calories per slice	2 slices	80
Fresh apple	1 medium	60
Dinner		
Roasted chicken breast, skinless	3.5 ounces	173
Baked potato with skin	1 small	160
Steamed string beans	½ cup	40
Fat-free dressing	2 tablespoons	20
Fresh strawberries	1¼ cups	60
Snack		
Nonfat sugar-free flavored yogurt	1 cup	100
		974

WHEN YOUR KIDNEYS FAIL

AND YOU'VE GOT TOO MUCH

OF A BAD THING!

Americans are obsessed with the heart, and the French focus on the liver, but does anyone think twice about the kidney? For example, have you ever been asked about your kidneys at a cocktail party and been offered some food or drink to improve their function? Yet virtual strangers have advised you about your cholesterol, haven't they? Everyone knows that the heart pumps blood, the brain controls thought and movement, and the lungs make it possible for you to breathe. But the kidney? Why, all it does is make urine! Don't you believe it. The kidney is an extraordinarily complex organ whose proper function is vital to your health, sense of well-being, and survival.

You may not know or care much about the kidney (there are two kidneys, but they are often referred to in the singular) when it's working properly and free of disease, but, believe me, when you have an attack of kidney stones (arguably the most painful experience there is), or need to "go" every few minutes and it burns when you do, or you see blood in your urine, or are told your blood pressure is high because you have kidney trouble, you will have a newfound interest in and respect for that organ. To understand how the right nutrition can help a sick kidney, you must appreciate its many functions.

As blood circulates through it, the kidney reabsorbs or returns whatever the body needs—blood cells, sugar, proteins, minerals, and water—and *excretes* the waste or end-products of metabolism in the urine it makes. It also *produces* certain hormones and "*detoxifies*" or breaks down and then eliminates various substances that would otherwise accumulate and be toxic to the body. The hormones made by the kidney help control blood pressure (renin), constitute a form of vitamin D that promotes the absorption of calcium from food, prevent anemia (erythropoietin), and regulate blood flow to different areas, much like track switches in a railroad yard, by dilating and constricting blood vessels (kinins). In its detoxifying role, the kidney regulates the blood level of such diverse hormones (other than those it makes itself) as insulin, thyroid, and parathyroid hormones. (The parathyroid consists of four small glands near the thyroid. The hormone it produces controls the amount of calcium moving in and out of bones. Too much results in brittle bones and kidney stones, too little impairs muscular contraction.)

So when your kidneys stop working properly, you can be in serious trouble. When they do, it's very important to determine what went wrong and why, how badly their function is impaired, and how best to control or cure the problem. The diagnostic workup requires a combination of urinalysis, blood tests, kidney X rays, a renal sonogram, and possibly CT scans or MRIs (magnetic resonance imaging) of the kidney area.

The kidney is vulnerable to many different kinds of insult, the most common being infection. Other serious problems include obstruction to the outflow of urine caused by stones stuck somewhere in the urinary system, an enlarged prostate, injury resulting from the use of certain antibiotics, painkillers, contrast dyes used in X-ray procedures, or a variety of other medications and chemical agents; damage from uric acid crystals that have accumulated in the kidney tissue in persons with gout; and the harmful effects of calcium deposits, which form when your blood calcium level is too high or you have long-standing high blood pressure. The first step in the management of kidney disease is to identify and, if possible, eliminate the underlying cause.

Managing the consequences of poor kidney function requires specific approaches, including dietary manipulation. When there is a problem making urine, water, salt, potassium, phosphorus, and protein waste are invariably retained in the body and can accumulate to toxic levels. When erythropoietin (the hormone that controls the formation of red blood cells in the bone marrow) is not produced in adequate amounts, you become anemic; when the detoxifying processes aren't working properly, your insulin levels may need changing. If you're diabetic and have kidney trouble, you may have to modify your insulin dosage or carbohydrate intake; if your calcium levels are too high, you may have to reduce your calcium consumption. (When elevated calcium levels are caused by a tumor of the parathyroid, it must be surgically removed). On the other hand, if the kidneys have retained too much phosphorus, you may need calcium pills to lower the high phosphorus blood level. If you have a high level of uric acid due to gout, you may need medication and/or a low-purine diet to prevent uric acid stone formation in the urinary tract (see page 294 for a list of foods high in purines to avoid).

In most cases, however, when kidney disease is severe and chronic, all major functions are compromised, requiring a standard dietary approach. The major nutritional goals are to slow down the progression of whatever is hurting the kidney, to provide adequate nutrition, and to correct as many abnormalities as possible that have occurred. All this is often easier said than done because if you have kidney disease you probably have very little appetite to begin with, and dietary restrictions may remove what few foods you still enjoy.

When kidney function begins to decline, for whatever reason, the first objective is to reduce kidney workload. From a dietary point of view, that means cutting back on protein intake because it's hard work for the kidney to handle all the protein presented to it in the blood that circulates through it. Experiments in both animals and humans suggest that kidney deterioration is accelerated by a high-protein diet, such as the one we Americans consume. (Although the daily RDA for protein is 63 grams for men and 50 for women, we eat about twice that amount.) The word *protein* may conjure up images of Arnold Schwarzenegger with bulging, firm muscles and strong bones, but too much is not good for you, especially if your kidneys are damaged. How strictly to cut back on your protein depends on the severity of the kidney malfunction. (This traditional view has recently been challenged, but most kidney specialists still believe that people with kidney failure should reduce their protein consumption.)

Proteins are complex molecules composed of carbon, hydrogen, oxygen, and nitrogen, all of which are essential to life. In fact, the word *protein* comes from the Greek word *proteios,* meaning "primary." These building-block molecules join to form twenty-two larger amino acids that, in turn, combine to make up the various proteins that are the basic constituents of muscle, bone, hormones, the hemoglobin molecule in the red blood cells that carries oxygen, and virtually every other tissue in the body. Nine of the twenty-two amino acids are termed "essential," i.e., humans must have *all* of them to survive. (Plants are able to synthesize all necessary proteins from the building blocks available to them. We cannot, and must have specific amino acids—the "essential" ones—in our diet.) Proteins that contain these essential amino acids are designated "high quality," and are present, for the most part, in meat, milk (skim as well as whole), poultry, fish, and eggs. Plant proteins are referred to as "low quality" because they do not contain these essential amino acids. When eaten alone, plants are not nutritionally complete and should always be combined with foods containing high-quality protein. There is nothing pejorative about the designations "high" and "low" quality; they simply reflect the makeup of the protein in question. If you have to limit the protein you consume, you should eat foods with the highest-quality protein and the most nutritious amino acids possible.

If your kidney impairment is "significant," something your doctor decides on the basis of kidney function tests, you should limit your protein intake to about 40 grams daily. One egg and 8 ounces of milk contain 15 grams; 3 ounces of high-quality protein such as fish or chicken provide 21 grams. This amount constitutes only 160 of the 2,000 calories per day you need to fuel the energy processes of your body. The balance must come equally from carbohydrates and fat. Why so much fat? Because you would otherwise have to eat enormous amounts of carbohydrate to fulfill your calorie needs. There are 4 calories in every gram of carbohydrate. To get your 2,000 calories, you'd have to eat 500 grams of carbohydrate, a volume that very few, especially people with kidney disease whose appetite is so poor anyway, will consume. Fat, on the other hand, provides 9 calories per gram, and so is a much more concentrated source of energy.

The carbohydrates you eat should be complex—pasta, beans, and grains (see the table on page 68), rather than simple sugars and candy. Fats, comprising at least 30 percent of total calories, should consist primarily of monounsaturated (olive and canola oils), and as a second choice, polyunsaturated vegetable oils. You'll get all the saturated fats you need in the high-quality animal protein you eat without adding extra amounts. At the end of this chapter you'll find a sample menu with additional choices and combinations for such a 40-gram-protein diet. You will note that twenty jelly beans are permitted despite my saying earlier that simple sugars and candy should be limited. Jelly beans are fat free and, unlike chocolate or candy bars, have neither protein nor fat, and twenty of them provide more than 100 calories.

The healthy kidney regulates how much water you eliminate. (If you're lost in the desert with nothing to drink, it will hold on to all you have and you will make very little urine.) If you have serious kidney disease, you may retain fluid because you've lost the ability to excrete large amounts of water. Your face may become swollen and puffy, and you may have trouble slipping rings on or off your fingers. In these circumstances, limit your fluid intake to three glasses a day. Since diseased kidneys also retain salt, you should have no more than 2 grams of sodium daily. That means no added salt at the table or during cooking, and no salted prepared food (see the table on page 248 for the sodium content of various foods). (There are, however, some forms of kidney trouble in which you *lose* water and salt.)

If your condition worsens, the ability to excrete phosphorous will be compromised. Wheat is the richest source of phosphorous, but it is also abundantly present in eggs, meat, poultry, and processed meats, all of which you should avoid. You may lack calcium because of two different processes. The phosphorus that is not eliminated accumulates in the blood and results in the production of more parathyroid hormone, which, in turn, sucks calcium out of the bones, into the urine, and out of the body. Because kidney disease lowers the vitamin D content of the body, the absorption of calcium by the intestine is also decreased. To compensate for calcium deficiency, you'll need between 1,500 and 4,500 milligrams daily to prevent "softening" of the skeleton. Milk obviously won't do as a source of this calcium because of its high protein content. You'll have to take calcium supplements, the most suitable of which are calcium carbonate and calcium acetate. Calcium lactate, gluconate, or chloride is not as good because they provide less calcium (see page 339). These calcium supplements reduce the absorption of dietary phosphorus, and as the high phosphorus levels drop, so may the amount of parathyroid hormone produced. You may also need vitamin D supplements; your doctor can recommend a dosage based on the calcium, phosphorus, and bone enzyme levels in your blood. Sometimes drugs that bind phosphorus in the stomach to prevent its absorption are required to lower phosphorus concentration.

Potassium retention may become a problem later in the course of kidney disease. Very high levels can result in cardiac arrest. You'll therefore need to avoid potassium-rich foods if your blood levels are too high. Among the top food sources of potassium are fruit (especially bananas), dried fruits, molasses, beef, pork, sardines, wheat, bran, poultry, nuts, soybean flour, and virtually every raw vegetable (see page 251 for a list of high-potassium foods to avoid). The table on page 252 contains a more comprehensive list of foods and their potassium content.

If you become anemic, you might be tempted to consume additional iron. Taking the hormone erythropoietin will control the anemia of kidney disease better than any dietary regimen, but some supplemental iron is usually necessary anyway.

Magnesium, like potassium, is retained by the failing kidney. You can reduce your dietary intake by avoiding antacids and laxatives that contain magnesium. Eat less of the following magnesium-rich foods: seeds, nuts, wheat germ, whole grains, legumes, blackstrap molasses, dark green leafy vegetables, cocoa powder, and chocolate. Fish, meat, and milk also contain small amounts of magnesium.

In addition to these general dos and don'ts, I advise persons with kidney disease to take supplemental multivitamins containing at least 250 milligrams of vitamin C, 400 IU of vitamin E, 1 milligram of folic acid, and the B-complex group containing the RDA of its various constituents.

Before the availability of dialysis and organ transplants, the diet for patients with end-stage kidney disease was mainly palliative—it made them feel a little better in their dying days. Today, however, thanks to new drugs, better and easier techniques of dialysis, and the success of kidney transplantation, the right diet means more than merely going through the motions. It not only slows the processes that are damaging the kidney, it keeps the patient in optimal condition for dialysis or until a transplant is obtained. The basic dietary guidelines for most cases of kidney failure are low protein, high carbohydrate, low magnesium, low potassium, and restricted salt and water.

If, despite all the medication and dietary measures available, your kidney function continues to decline and reaches a point at which the kidney is no longer able to sustain life, you have the choice of a kidney transplant or dialysis. Unfortunately, a compatible kidney, one that your body will not reject, is not always available when you need it. Some of my patients have waited years for a transplant. In the meantime, dialysis is lifesaving. Thousands of men and women now lead almost normal lives between sessions of dialysis or after receiving a transplanted kidney. They can work, play, travel, and, most important, they can enjoy life. Although dialysis is sometimes a way station on the road to a kidney transplant, it is often a permanent solution.

Dialysis machines remove poisonous wastes from the body much as the kidney does. But dialyzing a patient is akin to throwing the baby out with the bath water because, in addition to ridding the body of its toxic wastes, the filtration process also removes precious amino acids (proteins), minerals, and vitamins—all of which must be replaced.

There are two main dialysis techniques—hemodialysis and peritoneal dialysis. The latter sometimes causes infection in the abdomen (peritonitis), not only because it requires the insertion of tubes into the abdomen, but also because the process washes out immunoglobulins, on which normal immune function depends. However, these infections are not difficult to treat. Infection results in some additional loss of protein over and above what is withdrawn during dialysis itself, and replacement of the protein in the diet is important, especially in growing children. The major advantage of peritoneal dialysis is that it can be done at home. This means that you must be "cleansed" four times a day instead of three times a week at a dialysis center. If you lack the means or the setup at home to perform peritoneal dialysis, you'll have to settle for hemodialysis at a kidney center.

Dialysis filters the blood and eliminates its waste. It does not, however, duplicate the hormonal functions of the kidney (see earlier). So insulin, parathyroid, and other hormone levels all become unbalanced during dialysis and must be corrected by dietary manipulation.

If you have been following the restricted diet prescribed for those in kidney failure and "graduate" to dialysis, you can now have more of the protein, carbohydrate, and fat you need to prevent malnutrition. However, there is no one nutritional formula for everyone on dialysis. Each person receiving this treatment requires some limits as to how much and what kind of foods he or she may consume; dialysis makes supplemental vitamins and minerals necessary. This area is so complex that your kidney specialist or team must design a specific diet for you, based on what kind of dialysis you are having, how often, for how long, how much kidney "waste" is withdrawn and what your blood tests show from day to day. For that reason, I can give you only general guidelines concerning what foods need to be monitored, and what nutrients must be replaced.

The body's energy processes require a certain number of calories, which vary from person to person. Sixteen calories daily for every pound of body weight (or 35 to 50 calories per kilogram) is a reasonable goal depending on your age, body weight, and nutritional status. If you weigh 130 pounds, you should eat 2,100 calories daily; someone weighing 160 pounds requires 2,500 calories; and a 200–pounder should have 3,200 calories a day. But if you have advanced kidney disease and your appetite is poor or nonexistent, you may not be able to consume these amounts. When toxic products accumulate between dialysis sessions, eating 2,500 calories a day can be an insurmountable hurdle. At times such as these, you'll need a commercially available nutritional supplement to provide the necessary calories.

What foods should constitute these calories? The amount of protein will vary depending on the severity of your disease, your weight, and the type of dialysis procedure being performed. More is allowed for peritoneal dialysis than for hemodialysis. Determining *your* personal nutritional prescription is a very sophisticated and important skill that is best done by your dialysis team.

Most of the protein you are permitted should come from animal sources (meat, fish, eggs, and poultry), in order to provide the essential amino acids lacking in plant proteins (see earlier). But you also need some of the latter to enhance the palatability and variety of your diet and to give you enough fiber. Since people with kidney failure retain salt and potassium, you may need to restrict consumption of these minerals to 2 grams of each daily. You can easily cut back your sodium to acceptable limits by avoiding salted foods, using no salt in cooking, and removing the salt shaker from your table. Fruits, grains, and vegetables are important sources of potassium, as are meat, poultry, and fish. The table on page 251 lists potassium-containing foods to be avoided. Because of fluid retention, you may not be permitted more than 4 cups of fluid a day. But remember, these are only generalizations, and may not apply in your particular case.

Carbohydrates, both complex and simple, should usually make up 45 to 50 percent of your total daily calories (persons with diabetes should restrict their intake of simple sugars—see page 133). Your diet may be higher in fat than usual (35 to 40 percent of total calories) because fat is a concentrated source of energy, and if you have a poor appetite, it will help satisfy your daily caloric total. Divide this added fat equally between mono- and polyunsaturated forms, since the animal protein in your diet will usually provide about 10 percent of your daily allotment of calories from saturated fat.

If you're on dialysis, you'll need to replace all the vitamins and minerals lost in the dialysis fluid, especially B_1, B_2, B_6, niacinamide, B_3, B_{12}, biotin, magnesium, and folic acid. You will also need supplemental vitamin C, calcium, and zinc. You can restore zinc levels, given the composition of the diet recommended for people receiving dialysis, by eating a complex carbohydrate source such as wheat germ or wheat bran, or from seafood, especially oysters, meat, poultry, popcorn, cheddar cheese, and nuts (see page 151 for a list of zinc-rich foods), or from the zinc present in most vitamin supplements.

People on dialysis retain phosphorus, an excess of which sucks the calcium out of your bones, so you should limit their intake. The table on page 287 lists phosphorus-rich foods.

Remember that you can still lead a long, full life even if you have kidney failure. Dialysis and kidney transplants are practical alternatives, but you will still need to eat properly to ensure their continued success. This means consuming enough calories, limiting the amount of protein you eat (though not nearly as drastically as when you're not having dialysis), supplementing your diet with ample vitamins and minerals, and cutting back on your intake of salt, potassium, and phosphorus. Your health care team must work with you to customize these guidelines to meet your specific needs.

SAMPLE MENU FOR PEOPLE WITH KIDNEY FAILURE
(40 GRAMS PROTEIN)

	PORTION	PROTEIN (gm)
Breakfast		
Cheerios	¾ cup	3
Nondairy creamer	½ cup	trace
Low-protein toast	2 slices	0.4
Margarine	2 teaspoons	0
Jelly	2 teaspoons	0
Coffee	1 cup	0
Sugar	2 teaspoons	0
Lunch		
Omelette:		
egg and egg white	1 each	14
diced zucchini	½ cup	2
olive oil for frying	2 teaspoons	0
Low-protein bread	2 slices	0.4
Applesauce	½ cup	0.5
Jelly beans	20	0
Dinner		
Broiled, diced chicken breast, skinless	2.5 ounces	17.5
Low-protein pasta, cooked	1 cup	0.4
Olive oil, garlic, and herbs for pasta	sprinkle	0
Steamed green beans	½ cup	1.2
Sherbet	½ cup	0
		39.4

FOODS HIGH IN PHOSPHORUS

FOOD	PORTION	PHOSPHORUS (mg)	CALORIES
100% bran flakes	½ cup	354	76
Bran muffin, homemade	1 small	111	112
Cheeses			
American, processed	1 ounce	211	106
cottage, 1% fat	1 cup	302	164
cream (Philadelphia brand)	1 ounce	27	98
cream, light	1 ounce	45	62
mozzarella, regular	1 ounce	105	80
mozzarella, part skim	1 ounce	131	72
Chicken, white meat roasted	3.5 ounces	216	173
Cola	12 ounce	54	154
Eggs, large, boiled	1	86	77
Fish, flounder, cooked	3 ounces	246	99
Lentils, cooked	½ cup	178	115
Milk			
buttermilk	8 ounces	219	99
low-fat, 1% fat	8 ounces	235	102
skim	8 ounces	247	86
whole	8 ounces	227	157
Organ meats			
beef kidneys	3.5 ounces	306	144
beef liver, braised	3.5 ounces	404	161
chicken livers, simmered	3.5 ounces	312	157
goose liver	3.3 ounces	245	125
lamb liver, braised	3.5 ounces	420	220
liver pâté, canned	1 ounce	57	90
Soybean milk	8 ounces	117	79
Yogurt, whole milk, plain	8 ounces	215	139
Yogurt, low fat, flavored	8 ounces	306	119

WHEN YOU HAVE
KIDNEY STONES
WATER, WATER—EVERY DAY!

What do humans and dalmatians have in common? Give up? Most doctors don't know the answer either. Dalmatians and humans are the only mammals with the potential for high uric acid levels in the blood. Too much uric acid can cause gout and kidney stones. I'm not sure why dalmatians develop elevated uric acid levels, but humans do because sometime during our evolution we lost the enzyme that breaks down uric acid into other components.

Every year, half a million Americans rush to their doctors' offices or to emergency rooms in excruciating pain from kidney stones. Most vulnerable are men; Eurasians; anyone living in dry, hot climates, especially in the United States; people who are physically inactive; athletes who fail to replace fluid lost in perspiration after a workout; and persons with gout. For some reason, kidney stones of any kind are rare among Native Americans, blacks, and native-born Israelis. Attacks peak between ages thirty and fifty, and are three times more frequent in men than in women. In short, the determining factors boil down to heredity, age, sex, geography, environmental temperature, and diet.

In the typical attack, there is exquisite, shooting pain down one side of the abdomen, often radiating into the testicle in men, or lodging in the small of the back. It comes in waves, and patients find they have to move about rather than sit still, a phenomenon called "moving irritation." Pain persists until the stone moves to a different location or is passed through the urethra. When that happens, don't flush it down the toilet. Save it for analysis because if you've had one stone, you're very likely to have others of the same composition in the future.

There are four main kinds of stones, but 70 to 75 percent of them contain calcium combined with some other substances, usually oxalate or phosphate. Calcium oxalate stones are the most common. (I know one man with a passion for Bloody Marys who developed recurrent kidney stones because the Worcestershire sauce they contain is very rich in oxalate.) Struvite stones (15 percent) form in persons with chronic urinary tract infections; uric acid stones (8 percent) occur in persons with gout; and cystine stones account for some 4 percent of cases. This last type appears between the ages of ten and thirty and is the result of a congenital abnormality that interferes with the kidney's ability to reabsorb cystine, an amino acid.

When blood coming to the kidney for filtration contains too much of any substance, it crystallizes in the urine, forming sediment and sludge, which can eventually end up as stones. The key to preventing this crystallization process is to drink all the water you possibly can thus diluting whatever substance may form stones and reducing the chances of its solidifying. So if you are prone to kidney stones (and that's virtually everyone), drink more water than you lose in perspiration, sweat, urine, and stool—at least 2 quarts a day. If you have persistent diarrhea or vomiting because of something you ate, from a stomach virus, or from some other intestinal problem, the kidney will reduce its excretion of water to retain enough in the body. This means the formation of less urine, which is more concentrated and thus predisposed to stone formation. To prevent that from happening, make up for the fluids you're losing by drinking enough water.

Until very recently, anyone with a calcium stone was told to cut down his or her calcium intake. The logic was that the more calcium you consume, the more will end up in the urine and thus the greater the likelihood of its forming stones. That sounds reasonable but apparently is not true! Would you believe that the *more* calcium you eat in *food* (but not supplements), the *fewer* calcium stones you will have? That's because the most common kidney stone is calcium oxalate, and it's the *oxalate* and not calcium that's most responsible for stone formation. When your food contains both calcium and oxalate, they compete for absorption by the intestine—and the calcium wins. So the more calcium you eat, the less oxalate gets into the blood and urine from the stomach, and as a result, the likelihood of developing a calcium oxalate stone is reduced. If you have too much oxalate in your urine and a documented history of calcium oxalate stones (both of which facts can be determined by examining any stones you pass and testing a sample of your urine), drink at least 2 quarts of water every day and eat *as much calcium as you like* within reason, that is, no more than 2,000 milligrams a day. (See page 342 for a list of foods and their calcium content.) At the same time, cut down on foods with a high-oxalate content—colas, fresh tea, beer, coffee, cranberry juice, grapefruit juice, as well as spinach and other green vegetables. (Foods with high and moderate oxalate content are listed on page 393.) If you are prone to forming calcium oxalate stones, you *must* avoid high-oxalate foods, you *should* try to cut down on moderate-oxalate foods, but you are probably safe eating the many foods that are low in oxalate such as milk, eggs, cheese, and most meats (but watch out for their impact on heart disease). At the end of this chapter you'll find a sample low-oxalate menu. You should also eat lots of potassium-rich foods because potassium brings water with it to the kidney and helps dilute the urine. That means lots of dried fruit, soybean flour, molasses, wheat, rice, bran, beef, pork, poultry, most raw vegetables, nuts, and sardines. The table on page 252 has a more comprehensive list of foods rich in potassium. Limit your salt intake to 2 grams a day because it results in calcium retention by the body and causes fluid to be retained in the tissues (where you don't want it) instead of passed to the kidneys (where you do).

The guidelines above apply to most normal persons who have a tendency to form calcium oxalate stones. In some individuals, however, the kidneys are unable to reabsorb even very small amounts of calcium. If you have this unusual condition, called a "tubular leak," you'll need to reduce the amount of calcium in your diet as much as possible. There is also an intestinal abnormality in which *too much* calcium, regardless of how much or how little you eat, is absorbed from the gut. This means that more calcium comes to the kidney than it can handle, so calcium stones form. The kidney is also apt to form stones if you consume too much calcium, say, in excess of 2,000 milligrams a day, either as supplements or in the form of antacids.

In certain diseases, the blood contains more calcium than normal. The classic example is *primary* hyperparathyroidism, in which a tumor of the parathyroid glands produces too much parathyroid hormone. Parathyroid hormone sucks calcium out of the bones and into the blood, causing stones to form in the kidney. Don't confuse this over-production of parathyroid hormone with the *secondary* form of hyper-parathyroidism in chronic kidney disease where the parathyroid glands are normal but produce too much hormone. Whereas in primary hyperparathyroidism, you should reduce the amount of calcium in your diet; you should add to it in the secondary variety. The blood should always be checked for hyperparathyroidism in every person with kidney stones.

Excessive vitamin D results in abnormal absorption of calcium from the gut and too much in the urine. This is most likely to happen if you take too much vitamin D in supplements. Do not exceed 400 milli-grams per day unless you are advised to do so by your doctor.

If your thyroid gland is overactive, or if you're taking too much thyroid hormone replacement because you've been told your gland is sluggish, you may end up with an excessive amount of calcium in your urine and stones. Similarly various kinds of cancer can also result in abnormal urinary calcium concentrations.

If you have been confined to bed for any length of time, the calcium lost from your bones gets to the kidneys, where it can form stones.

How does what you eat affect other types of kidney stones? If you have *uric acid* stones (the kind that humans and dalmatians have in common), usually because you have gout, you should neutralize your acid urine with milk and milk products, vegetables (except corn and lentils), and fruits (but not cranberries, prunes, and plums). Cut down on your intake of meat, fish, fowl, shellfish, eggs, cheese, peanut butter and peanuts, sweets, and starchy foods. Coffee and tea are neutral, neither acid nor alkaline, so enjoy them. If these dietary constraints do not appeal to you, you can take sodium bicarbonate or potassium citrate to make your urine less acid. That, together with as much water as you can comfortably drink, will not only prevent uric acid stones from forming, but may well dissolve any that are already present. If you have high levels of uric acid in your blood (which is often the case if you have gout or certain malignancies, or are taking such medications as salicylates and diuretics), reducing these levels will further decrease the likelihood of such stones forming. You can effect such a reduction either by taking a drug such as allopurinol (obviously the easiest way) or by limiting your dietary intake of the foods rich in purines (particularly meats, animal organs, and sardines) listed on page 294.

Cystine stones, which are relatively rare, result from an inherited defect in the kidney that interferes with its ability to reabsorb this amino acid. Excessive amounts in the urine can cause stone formation. The only way to prevent it is to drink water round the clock—two 8-ounce glasses every two hours, day and night! It seems cruel to do so, but someone with cystine stones must be awakened at night in order to guarantee a urinary output of at least 3 or 4 liters a day. There are no other dietary guidelines that make any difference other than to neutralize the acid urine as described above. The key to the management of cystine stones is drinking copious amounts of water—and it's a lifetime proposition.

If you have *struvite* stones because of chronic urinary tract infections, forget about diet and just focus on controlling and preventing these infections.

In summary, if you have any type of kidney stone, you should drink at least 2 quarts of fluid every day. Then follow the specific dietary guidelines above, depending on the composition of your particular stone.

FOODS HIGH AND MODERATELY HIGH
IN OXALIC ACID

Foods to Avoid—High Oxalic Acid Content
Beans:
    all varieties dried, baked, green, wax
Beer, draft
Chocolate, cocoa, and Ovaltine
Fruitcake
Fruits:
    blackberries, blueberries, cranberries, currants, grapefruit, grapes,
    raspberries, rhubarb, strawberries, tangerines

FOODS HIGH AND MODERATELY HIGH
IN OXALIC ACID *(Continued)*

Juices:

Avoid juices made from the above fruits.

Marmalade:

lemon, lime, and orange

Nuts and nut butters

Tea

Tempeh, tofu, soybean crackers

Vegetables:

beets, celery, chives, collards, eggplants, escarole, green peppers, kale, leeks, okra, parsley, spinach, summer squash, sweet potatoes

Wheat germ

Foods to Limit—Moderately High Oxalic Acid Content

Coffee (no more than one cup per day)

Colas (no more than 12 ounces per day)

Corn and corn bread, white corn grits, corn chips, corn tortillas

Fruits:

apples, apricots, cherries, oranges, pears, pineapples, plums, prunes

Sardines

Tomatoes, tomato juice, tomato sauce, tomato paste, catsup, sun-dried tomatoes

Vegetables:

asparagus, broccoli, carrots, cucumbers, lettuce, lima beans, parsnips, canned green peas, turnips

Worcestershire sauce

SAMPLE MENU FOR PEOPLE ON LOW-OXALATE DIET

	PORTION
Breakfast	
Puffed rice cereal	¾ cup
Skim milk	½ cup
Banana	1 medium
Coffee	1 cup maximum

SAMPLE MENU *(Continued)*

	PORTION
Lunch	
Apple juice	4 ounces
Sandwich:	
tuna packed in water	3 ounces
mayonnaise	1 tablespoon
bread	2 slices
Cantaloupe	⅓ medium
Snack	
Plain or vanilla yogurt	1 cup
Peach	1 medium
Dinner	
Grilled chicken breast, skinless	4 ounces
Baked potato with skin	1 small
Margarine	1 teaspoon
Sautéed vegetables:	
cauliflower	½ cup
mushrooms and onions	½ cup
olive oil for sautéing	1 tablespoon
Lemon ice	1 cup

FOODS RICH IN PURINES

Anchovies
Animal organs (brain, heart, kidney, liver, and sweetbreads)
Bouillon
Caviar
Goose
Gravy
Herring
Mackerel
Mincemeat
Mussels
Sardines
Scallops
Yeast (brewer's and baker's)

LACTOSE INTOLERANCE

WHO'S NORMAL ANYWAY?

Is it normal to fill up with gas, to have belly cramps, or to develop diarrhea whenever you drink milk, eat ice cream, or enjoy some soft cheese on a cracker? Most people would say it's definitely not. But that's precisely what happens to most of us on this planet, beginning between the ages of three and fourteen years, but often later in life as well. Your symptoms may be mild or serious, depending on how bad the condition is in your particular case, and how much of these dairy products you eat. The disorder, called "lactose intolerance," is especially common among blacks, Asians, South Americans, Native Americans, Sephardic Jews, and most Caucasians. The only ones relatively unaffected are Scandinavians. So if only 10 to 30 percent of the world can tolerate milk or its products, who's normal, they or the rest of us?

The reason so many people (including three of my four children and myself—but not my wife, as she loves to remind me) do not feel great after drinking milk or eating foods made from it, is that we are deficient in an enzyme called *lactase*. Lactase breaks down dietary lactose (the sugar found in milk) into two simpler sugars—glucose and galactose—both of which are more easily absorbed from the intestine than the parent lactose. When there is not enough lactase around, the intact, undigested lactose is fermented by bacteria normally present in the gut and causes the gas, bloating, cramping, and diarrhea that are the hallmarks of lactose intolerance. There are other enzyme deficiencies which leave other sugars undigested. These are relatively uncommon, but result in similar symptoms. If you have persistent cramping and diarrhea without lactose intolerance, discuss this possibility with your doctor.

There are two solutions to the problem. One is to avoid foods containing lactose. That's not always possible because lactose not only is present in obvious milk derivatives such as ice cream and cheese but it is also hidden in many commercially prepared and baked foods and even medications (see the table at the end of this chapter). The other alternative is to add to your food the missing lactase enzyme, available in tablets or drops under a variety of brand names at all health food stores and pharmacies. In most areas of the country, you can also buy milk pretreated with lactase.

Believe it or not, lactose intolerance was not described until 1963. Initially, it was thought to affect only a small number of Caucasians (whites); we now know that this disorder is widespread and almost universal.

It is interesting to speculate on how lactose intolerance may have evolved over the millennia. Here's one interesting theory. Before dairying was established some ten thousand years ago, adults had no need for the lactase enzyme because the only milk consumed was from a mother's breast, so after weaning, lactase disappeared from the intestinal tract. But with the advent of dairying, milk became part of virtually everyone's diet—at all ages—and the body restored to some of us (the "abnormal" few) the lactase it abandoned thousands of years ago.

But why are so many Scandinavians endowed with enough lactase? The most logical explanation relates to the nature of their climate. Because summers in that part of the world are so short, with relatively little sunlight, the inhabitants don't get enough sun to synthesize vitamin D, which the body requires to absorb calcium from the gut. Lack of calcium causes impaired bone development in childhood and osteoporosis later in life. Now, if in addition to a lack of vitamin D, you also cannot digest, and so avoid eating, the lactose-rich dairy products that contain calcium, you're really in trouble. So, voilà, nature restored the missing lactase to those who needed it most, the frigid-climed vitamin D–deficient Scandinavians, to make it possible for them to consume the calcium they need. Although this theory is a little too pat for my liking, as far as I know, it's the only one around.

How can you tell if you have lactose intolerance? Just drink three full glasses of milk (skim or whole; the fat content makes no difference) and, believe me, you'll know soon enough! But if you actually want to document it, it's most easily done by means of a simple blood test.

Lactose intolerance is not an "all or none" response. Some individuals who have it can handle an occasional glass of milk, an ice cream cone, or a slice of cheese without any trouble. (I have found that some people tolerate chocolate milk better than regular milk.) It's only when they frequently consume larger amounts that they develop symptoms. There is no way of predicting how you will react. Make your own assessment and adjust your diet accordingly.

A lactose-free diet is easier to understand than to live with. It requires avoiding milk and milk products, including skim, dried, evaporated, and condensed forms, not only from cows but from other species as well. Lactose content has nothing to do with how much fat is in the dairy product. Skim or low-fat forms of milk do not help matters. Yogurt contains lots of lactose, as you can see on the table on page 299, but if it has "active cultures" (check the label), it has already been fermented by bacteria and will be easier for you to digest. *Read the labels on every food and drink you buy.* The key words to look for are "lactose," "casein," "whey," "curds," and any reference to milk, be it "milk by-products," "dry milk," "nonfat milk powder," or "milk solids." Note, on the table on page 300, the several improbable sources of lactose, such as some brands of instant coffee and powdered diet drinks. Most bread and cake mixes, including waffles, pancakes, French toast, and biscuits, contain milk, as do several of the better-known dry cereals. Ask your waiter whether the desserts, cookies, or pudding you ordered were made with milk. Chances are that your delicious after-dinner soufflé or the omelet you did not prepare yourself contains milk. Margarine may be cholesterol free, but most brands contain milk products, as do many salad dressings. Fresh fruit is fine, but read the labels on canned and frozen fruits to be sure they have not been processed with lactose. Some are. Meat is lactose free except when creamed or breaded; hot dogs and other sausage products usually contain dried skim milk; vegetables are fine except those to which lactose has been added. If you are very sensitive to lactose, chewing gum may cause symptoms because many brands contain small amounts of lactose. Believe it or not, about 20 percent of all prescription drugs and 6 percent of those you can buy over the counter, including most "placebos" without any "active" ingredients, contain lactose. These small amounts are not likely to affect most people, but they can if you're very sensitive. Candies such as butterscotch and peppermint are likely to have some lactose, as are several nondairy creamers.

One of the problems of being lactase deficient is that the foods you avoid are basically dairy products and therefore important sources of calcium. Decreasing your intake of calcium leaves you vulnerable to osteoporosis later in life. So everyone, especially women who follow a lactose-free diet, should take calcium supplements. See page 342 for a list of foods and their calcium content.

What may a lactase-deficient individual eat? Although you won't find freshly baked products that are lactose free, there are many commercially marketed loaves that are. Always look for the lactose content on the wrapper of any such bread you buy. My family, afflicted as we are by this disorder, has become expert in identifying brand-name products that are lactose free. For example, we discovered that all products made by General Mills, including their frozen fruits, contain no lactose. I especially like their angel food cake, chiffon cake mixes, and graham cracker piecrusts. If you like brownies, as my wife does, their walnut brownie mix is safe too. Other lactose-free delicacies are Nabisco Oreo cookies, Abel's frozen bagels, and Ritz crackers. Feel free to sip Fanta orange soda if you enjoy soft drinks; cereals you can have include Rice Krispies and corn flakes. You may also eat Hershey's special dark chocolate with impunity. This list is hardly comprehensive; let the hunt begin! As you can see, you need not really be deprived of a normal diet if you are aware of all the alternatives. Here is another useful piece of advice: You never know what you will be served when you eat out—at a restaurant or in someone's home. So always carry your lactase tablets or drops with you.

If you're flatulent and uncomfortable and have always attributed it to a nervous stomach, think lactose intolerance. Remember, if you turn out to have it, you are, by definition, normal!

LACTOSE CONTENT OF DAIRY FOODS

FOOD	PORTION	LACTOSE (gm)
Cheeses		
American, processed	1 ounce	2.5
cheddar	1 ounce	0.4
cottage, low-fat	4 ounces	3
cream	1 ounce	0.8
feta	1 ounce	1.2
hard	1 ounce	0 to 3
Muenster	1 ounce	0.3
soft	4 ounces	3 to 6
Cream (whipping, heavy, half-and-half)	1 tablespoon	0.4 to 0.6
Ice cream	1 cup	9 to 10
Milk		
goat	8 ounces	10.9
skim, with added nonfat dry milk solids	8 ounces	11.9
whole	8 ounces	11.4
Yogurt		
regular	8 ounces	10.6
skim with added nonfat dry milk solids	8 ounces	17.4

HIDDEN SOURCES OF LACTOSE*

Bread
Breakfast cereals
Breakfast drinks
Candy
Canned and frozen fruit
Chewing gum
Instant flavored coffees
Instant potatoes
Gravy
Hot dogs
Luncheon meats
Margarine
Medications
Mixes for cakes, biscuits, cookies, pancakes
Nondairy creamer
Powdered diet drinks
Puddings
Salad dressings
Sausage
Soups
Waffles and French toast

*This is a general list. To be certain of the lactose content of any food, check the label. Key words to look for on the label are: lactose, casein, whey, curds, and any reference to milk—milk by-products, dry milk, nonfat milk powder, or milk solids.

LEG CRAMPS

"DANCING" IN THE DARK

Have you ever gone to bed feeling fine, only to be awakened in the night by an insidious, progressive spasm in your thigh, calf, or toes? You try to ignore it, but chances are you end up leaving your toasty, warm bed and hopping about on the floor, doing all kinds of contortions to obtain relief.

These attacks can be prevented by a variety of nondietary maneuvers: Make sure the air-conditioning isn't blowing on your exposed feet; wear socks at night to keep them warm; if you have varicose veins, elevate your legs on pillows or put one-inch blocks under the foot posts of your bed to drain off excessive fluid that accumulates in the feet. The 5-grain tablet of quinine, which you could once buy over the counter, is no longer available because the FDA has determined it is both unsafe and ineffective against leg cramps. Some doctors prescribe 400 or 800 IU of vitamin E daily to prevent these nocturnal leg cramps, but I have never found it to work.

There are several circumstances in which you are apt to develop leg cramps, unless you take dietary measures to prevent them. Vigorous exercise, especially in hot weather, may well cause them (and other muscle cramps) as a result of the salt, and to a lesser extent, potassium and magnesium loss. You can forestall this condition by taking salt tablets or by drinking salt-rich fluids one hour before exercising. Sport drinks are a convenient way to do so. The table on page 306 lists the salt, potassium, magnesium, and caloric content of two commercially available brands (but there are many more) and other beverages. Note that tomato juice is virtually ideal from every point of view. However, be sure to check with your doctor before taking any of these liquids if you have salt-sensitive high blood pressure or are being treated for heart failure. (In the latter circumstance, you are most unlikely to be working up the kind of sweat that is apt to deplete your salt to the point of causing muscle cramps!)

If you are receiving dialysis because your kidneys have stopped working (see page 277), you may develop leg cramps because this procedure removes magnesium from the blood along with the metabolic wastes. The RDA of magnesium for men is 350 milligrams a day, and 280 milligrams for women. But since you are *losing* magnesium during dialysis (you do with diuretics too), you need to replace twice the amount called for in the RDA. You can raise your magnesium intake with the following magnesium-rich foods: seeds, nuts, wheat germ, legumes, whole grains, blackstrap molasses, leafy green vegetables, cocoa powder, and chocolate. (See the table on page 304 for the magnesium content of various foods.) However, it isn't easy for someone with bad kidneys, a poor appetite, and on dialysis to eat as much magnesium as he or she requires. The sample menu on page 305 shows how you can try to do it. However, since only half of the magnesium in food is absorbed by the intestine, the surest way to meet your magnesium needs in these circumstances is to take two tablets of magnesium oxide, each containing 300 or 325 milligrams, or a single 800-milligram pill. You'll know you're taking too much if you develop diarrhea.

If you require daily diuretics for any reason (high blood pressure, heart failure, fluid retention), you are losing extra salt, magnesium, and potassium, and are a candidate for leg cramps. So be sure to consume 2 grams of salt per day, and also supplement your diet with magnesium tablets. Page 249 illustrates a sample daily menu containing a little less than 2 grams of sodium. The table on page 306 lists the sodium, potassium, and magnesium content of several beverages. One glass of orange juice (almost 500 milligrams) and a banana (450 milligrams) every day will usually restore the potassium loss resulting from average diuretic doses. Should more be needed, take 800 milligrams of supplements in liquid, tablet, or capsule form (but always *after* meals because potassium in any form is a gastric irritant).

Pregnant women may experience leg cramps, usually during the second half of their pregnancy, especially if they are in their thirties or have had several children. These symptoms do not portend a threat to the pregnancy, and can easily be corrected by eating more of the magnesium-rich foods listed above. But don't take magnesium *supplements* during pregnancy because they can harm your fetus. Leg cramps at this time may also be due to inadequate calcium and too much phosphorus in the diet. Meat is the richest source of phosphorus. (See page 342 and page 287 for a list of foods rich in calcium and phosphorus.)

If your thyroid gland isn't functioning normally (if it's either hyperactive or sluggish), or if you've had a parathyroid tumor removed surgically, you may have a low blood calcium level. You can relieve the resulting muscle cramps by replacing the missing calcium, either by diet or with supplements, but see your doctor about it first.

Leg cramps are a common complaint in persons of all ages. They are a symptom, not a disease, and may occur in perfectly healthy persons, pregnant women, after vigorous exercise in hot weather without adequate salt replacement, as the result of certain medications such as diuretics, and in a variety of diseases. The first step in their management is to determine the cause and correct it.

MAGNESIUM CONTENT OF FOODS

FOOD	PORTION	MAGNESIUM (mg)	CALORIES
Beans/legumes			
black beans, cooked	1 cup	121	227
black-eyed peas, cooked	1 cup	85	160
broad beans, cooked	1 cup	73	186
chickpeas, cooked	1 cup	78	269
green peas, cooked	½ cup	31	67
kidney beans, cooked	1 cup	80	225
lentils, cooked	1 cup	71	231
lima beans, cooked	1 cup	82	217
split peas, cooked	1 cup	71	231
Cashews, dry roasted	1 ounce	74	163
Cereals			
All-Bran (Kellogg's)	⅓ cup	122	70
Branflakes (Kellogg's)	¾ cup	54	90
Raisin Bran (Kellogg's)	¾ cup	64	120
wheat bran, toasted (Kretschmer)	⅓ cup	180	57
wheat germ, toasted (Kretschmer)	¼ cup	84	103
Peanuts, dry roasted	1 ounce	49	164
Sesame seeds, dried	1 medium	28	47
Soybeans, mature, cooked	1 cup	148	298
Sunflower seeds	1 ounce	100	162
Tempeh	½ cup	58	165
Tofu, raw, firm	½ cup	118	183
Vegetables			
artichoke, cooked	1 medium	72	60
artichoke hearts, cooked	½ cup	33	37
asparagus, cooked	6 spears	9	22
beets, cooked	½ cup	31	26
broccoli, cooked	1 cup	38	44
brussels sprouts, cooked	½ cup	16	30
chicory, uncooked	½ cup	27	21
collards, cooked	1 cup	10	34
corn, cooked	½ cup	26	89
eggplant	½ cup	5	11
green beans, cooked	½ cup	16	22
kale, cooked	½ cup	12	21

MAGNESIUM CONTENT OF FOODS *(Continued)*

FOOD	PORTION	MAGNESIUM (mg)	CALORIES
pepper, yellow	1 large	23	50
potato, baked with skin	1 large	55	220
spinach, uncooked	½ cup	22	6
squash, summer, all varieties, cooked	½ cup	22	18
Swiss chard, cooked	½ cup	76	18
zucchini, cooked	½ cup	19	14

SAMPLE MENU FOR PEOPLE WITH LEG CRAMPS
(700 MG MAGNESIUM)

	PORTION	MAGNESIUM (mg)	CALORIES
Breakfast			
Raisin bran cereal	¾ cup	64	120
Skim milk	8 ounces	28	86
Banana, sliced	1 medium	33	105
Snack			
Kiwi	1 medium	23	46
Lowfat vanilla yogurt	8 ounces	37	194
Lunch			
Black bean salad:			
black beans, cooked	½ cup	60	114
Wishbone Lite Italian dressing	1 ounce	0	14
diced celery	1 stalk	4	6
Whole wheat bread	2 slices	46	130
Roasted chicken breast, skinless	3.5 ounces	27	173
Dinner			
Baked halibut steak	3 ounces	91	119
Baked potato with skin	1 medium	55	220
Spinach salad:			
fresh spinach leaves	1 cup	44	12
regular Italian dressing	1 tablespoon	0	69

SAMPLE MENU *(Continued)*

	PORTION	MAGNESIUM (mg)	CALORIES
Boiled carrots	½ cup	10	35
Boiled peas	½ cup	31	67
Fresh raspberries	1 cup	22	61
Snack			
Orange	1 medium	15	65
Dry-roasted cashews	1 ounce	74	163
Blackstrap molasses	1 tablespoon	43	47
		707	1,846

SODIUM, POTASSIUM, AND MAGNESIUM CONTENT OF SEVERAL BEVERAGES

BEVER-AGE	POR-TION	CALOR-IES	SODIUM (mg)	POTASSIUM (mg)	MAGNESI-UM (mg)
Gatorade	8 ounces	39	123	23	trace
Milk					
1% fat	8 ounces	102	123	381	34
skim	8 ounces	86	126	406	28
Orange juice	8 ounces	248	2	496	27
Thirst Quencher	8 ounces	241	96	26	1
Tomato juice	6 ounces	182	658	400	20

MALABSORPTION

JUST PASSING THROUGH!

Blessed are they with normal digestion and absorption, for they shall be spared the suffering of constipation, diarrhea, bloating, nausea, lack of appetite, and abdominal gas and cramps. Nor shall they emit foul-smelling stools urgently passed (usually in someone else's toilet at the height of a large party with people waiting for their turn in the john) and repeatedly flushed because they float!

A host of diseases and disorders accounts for this array of symptoms, the most common of which are an irritable bowel (see page 270), lactose intolerance (see page 295), the failure of the pancreas to make the enzymes necessary for digestion (see page 353), and inflammatory bowel disease (see page 260). They make the gut hyperactive (as in the irritable bowel) or, as in the case of lactose intolerance, cause the food you eat to become fermented by bacteria in the bowel. Also, when there is a deficiency of digestive enzymes from the pancreas, what you eat is not digested, causing many of these same symptoms. In every one of the above disorders, the bowel itself is intact, but there are problems with its environment, so to speak. However, there are several other conditions in which the intestinal lining itself is diseased and fails to absorb the food you eat. The result is a deficiency of calories, fats, carbohydrates, proteins, and minerals. Children with such impaired digestion are small, poorly developed, and suffer from a variety of symptoms ranging from mental abnormalities to anemia unless the missing nutrients are adequately replaced. Such *malabsorption* is usually the result of an intestinal infection or, as you will see below, a genetic abnormality. Whatever the cause, it can usually be treated successfully, sometimes by diet alone.

A variety of tests may have to be performed to find out why the food you eat is passing through without being absorbed. They include examination of the stool contents, breath analysis (like the cops give drunken drivers), X rays of the stomach and intestines, and often even direct inspection and biopsy of the intestinal lining.

Celiac disease (also called *nontropical sprue* or *gluten-sensitive enteropathy*) is a classic example of malabsorption. It's not very common, and its numbers are declining. Untreated celiac patients are underweight, tired, bloated, anemic, and suffer from chronic diarrhea—all because their food is poorly absorbed. The basic problem is genetic. When gluten, a plant protein, comes in contact with the lining of the intestine, the latter blocks the absorption not only of the gluten, but of virtually every other nutrient eaten with it. How or why this happens is not understood, but totally eliminating gluten from the diet restores well-being within days and soon corrects malnutrition and malabsorption. But a gluten-free diet is not something you adhere to only when you're in the mood to do so. You must follow it rigidly every day of your life come hell or high water. If you do it in a hit-or-miss fashion, you will eventually fail to respond to the change in diet—and that means trouble!

Gluten is the component of wheat that makes the dough of its flour elastic when kneaded. It is also found, though in lesser amounts, in rye, oats, and barley. Although corn and rice contain some gluten too, the quantities are so small that you can eat them safely. Potatoes, soybeans, and arrowroot are gluten-free. The problem is not so much avoiding the obvious gluten-rich foods as it is being aware that they are present where you least expect them—in additives and the fillers in many medications; in the cocktail you enjoy before dinner as well as in beer and whiskey. Most brands of ice cream contain gluten too, as do many dairy products, chewing gum, and even communion wafers! Read the labels carefully on baked and commercially prepared foods. When eating out, inquire about ingredients such as flour and cereal grains that are often used in cooking and baking. The table on page 311 lists the more commonly consumed foods with gluten that you should avoid.

Sprue is an important disease that, happily, can be easily and completely controlled by diet. If you have sprue, it is well worth your while to consult a nutritionist and write to the Gluten Intolerance Group of North America for recipes and brand names of special diet products you can tolerate and enjoy. Their address is P.O. Box 23053, Seattle, WA 98102-0353 and you can also phone them at (206) 325-6980. One of my patients is very enthusiastic about the Red Mill Farms company, which bakes great banana, chocolate, and macaroon cakes that are gluten- and lactose-free. One of my sons (he's lactose-intolerant) contacted them ([718] 384-2150) and tells me their banana cake is as good as anything he's ever tasted—but doesn't cause the gas that the milk-containing brands produce.

A disorder identical to celiac disease, or nontropical sprue, occurs in persons living in tropical climates. Quite logically, it's called *tropical sprue*. It affects not only the residents of these areas, but transients too. American troops in Vietnam and those stationed in Puerto Rico have developed malabsorption that is not genetic, but due to a *bacterial infection* of the gut. Their intestinal lining has the same appearance as in nontropical sprue despite the different cause. Symptoms of tropical sprue may not appear for months after you return home. Once you're diagnosed and treated, your diarrhea, anemia, bloating, and malnutrition will clear up. Therapy is not dietary, as it is in nontropical sprue. You may eat whatever you like. You'll need to take the antibiotic tetracycline or 5 milligrams of folic acid daily for several weeks and a shot of 1,000 micrograms of B_{12} for good measure to cure the disease.

A much more common cause of malabsorption than either type of sprue is hardening of the arteries that supply the intestine. It's the same process that affects the heart, brain, legs, and kidneys, and usually occurs in older persons with other evidence of vascular disease. If you have angina, you're generally comfortable until you exert yourself and create extra work for your heart. It's a similar story in the abdominal form of arteriosclerosis. Your belly pain comes on *after eating* because the gut has to work harder to digest food. That's why these symptoms are called intestinal angina. In addition to abdominal pain, which begins anywhere from fifteen to twenty minutes after eating, you'll also have diarrhea, sometimes bloody. The only effective treatment for intestinal angina (other than major surgery, which may become necessary if a portion of the bowel wall "dies" due to a lack of blood supply), is to impose less of a burden on the small intestine by eating frequent, small meals rather than fewer, larger ones.

Another cause of malabsorption in the Western world is the *gastrectomy* operation in which a substantial portion of the stomach is surgically removed—usually for the treatment of severe gastric bleeding, cancer, or otherwise unmanageable ulcer disease. What with all the new drugs now available for the treatment of peptic ulcers, this operation is now being performed much less frequently. In such cases, there is so little stomach left that food whizzes right through it, too fast for the pancreatic enzymes to digest it. In order to slow down the transit time through and out of the stomach, you need to eat four to six small meals a day instead of the usual three, accompanied by as little liquid as possible. Drink the fluid you need *between* meals.

Malabsorption, or any disorder that causes chronic diarrhea, can lead to malnutrition because of the loss of vital nutrients from the bowel. These must be replaced on an ongoing basis as long as the diarrhea (and the underlying disorder responsible for it) continue. Multivitamin supplements, with particular emphasis on the fat-soluble ones (A, D, E, and K—see page 24) must be taken daily in amounts commensurate with the severity of the diarrhea.

In summary, people with malabsorption suffer from chronic diarrhea because the food they eat is not absorbed. This is the result of some problem with the intestinal lining itself, usually an infection or some other disease process. The most common causes are celiac disease or nontropical sprue (a congenital disorder of gluten sensitivity), tropical sprue (in which the intestinal lining is damaged by infection), the late effects of radiation therapy to the abdomen, arteriosclerosis of the blood vessels supplying the bowel, and gastrectomy in which portions of the stomach have been surgically removed. Treatment of the malabsorption depends on its cause but vitamin supplements, particularly those that are fat soluble (A, D, E, K) should be taken.

GLUTEN-RICH FOODS FOR PEOPLE WITH
MALABSORPTION TO AVOID

Alcoholic beverages:
  ale
  beer
  gin
  whiskey
  vodka
Cereals containing wheat, rye, oats, or barley
Cheeses containing oat gum as an ingredient
Chocolate-covered malted milk balls
Commercial cakes, cookies, pies, and puddings, and some cones for ice
  cream
Dry seasoning mixes
Flours:
  barley
  oat
  rye
  wheat
Grains:
  amaranth
  buckwheat
  bulgar
  kasha
  malt
  millet
  quinoa
  wheat germ
Herbal teas made with malted barley
Hot dogs, luncheon meats, and sausage
Nondairy creamers (check label)
Noodles, pasta, and macaroni made from wheat
Ovaltine and malted milk
Packaged rice mixes
Pie fillings and flour-thickened fruits
Sauces and condiments:
  catsup (check label)
  mustard (check label)
  sauces thickened with wheat flour
  soy sauce

GLUTEN-RICH FOODS FOR PEOPLE WITH
MALABSORPTION TO AVOID *(Continued)*

Soups:
  canned
  dry soup mixes
Wheat starch

MÉNIÈRE'S DISEASE

TOO DIZZY TO EAT?

Many older persons are plagued by tinnitus (noise in the ears), which is usually due to vascular changes in small arteries deep inside the ear. Ménière's disease is a special kind of tinnitus, accompanied by a loss of hearing, dizziness, and vertigo. Dizziness is a vague term. I use it here to describe a feeling of lightheadedness, unsteadiness, or lack of equilibrium. Patients who are *dizzy* will tell me their head is swimming. On the other hand, *vertigo* is associated with a spinning sensation so severe that it is difficult, if not impossible, to maintain balance, often accompanied by nausea and vomiting. Should you have all three symptoms—tinnitus, deafness, and vertigo (the hearing loss is constant, the tinnitus and vertigo come and go), first in one ear and eventually in both—chances are that you have Ménière's disease. To be absolutely sure of this diagnosis, you should be tested for low thyroid function, syphilis, food allergies, or a mild stroke—all of which can mimic Ménière's.

Ménière's is difficult to treat, although some drugs such as Compazine, Antivert, other antihistamines, and sedatives may ease the symptoms a little. However, what you eat and drink can make a difference. You can reduce the frequency of the attacks by *eliminating alcohol and tobacco,* and some people improve after reducing their caffeine intake.

Caffeine is naturally present in coffee, tea, chocolate, and cocoa. It is often added to soda (but not seltzer), nonprescription cold remedies, painkillers, and antacids. So always check the label and select those products without added caffeine. The table on page 45 lists common foods that contain caffeine and that can worsen your symptoms of Ménière's. Also, because these symptoms are largely due to abnormal fluid retention in the inner ear, a limit of 2 grams of salt a day often helps prevent or shorten attacks. Some doctors prescribe low doses of diuretics if these dietary changes alone are not effective. They sometimes help, but foods with natural diuretic properties such as coffee and tea do not. A 2-gram-salt diet is one in which you must avoid frankly salty food, and use none in cooking, in food preparation, or at the table. We usually think of salty foods in terms of herring and lox, but fast foods are an important and unsuspected source of salt. If you eat a Burger King Whopper (it's delicious, mind you), you consume around 600 calories and almost 900 milligrams of salt. Now add to that the almost obligatory medium-sized vanilla shake, and you have an additional 330 calories and over 200 milligrams of salt. What's a burger without french fries? A medium portion will cost you another 340 calories and almost 250 milligrams of salt. So in this quick lunch, in which you have not eaten any "really salty" foods (assuming you've added none to your fries), you've consumed more than 1,300 milligrams of sodium, more than half the permissible amount, not to mention well over 60 grams of fat! The table on page 248 contains a list of sodium-rich foods. You'd think, just scanning it, that there is precious little left to eat. That's not so. You may have up to three servings of any milk product you like (except milk shakes, buttermilk, and many of the processed cheeses, including cottage cheese; remember, however, there are many low-sodium cheese products available); a nice portion (6 ounces) of any animal protein (but make sure it's not koshered); and as many servings of fruit and vegetables as you like (they contain only negligible amounts of salt). Oils contain little if any salt. For a 2-gram-salt diet (see sample menu, page 249), you don't need to bother about salt-free bread. That's usually reserved for more drastic salt-restricted diets.

How much insulin your body makes may also play a role in Ménière's disease. (Insulin is the hormone that controls blood sugar. Too little is associated with one form of diabetes.) An abundance of insulin thickens the walls of blood vessels and constricts them, which may explain why fluid is retained in the inner ear of persons with Ménière's. To prevent an overproduction of insulin, you should reduce your intake of sugar and carbohydrates, forestall allergic reactions, if you can, and avoid steroid hormones, if possible, all of which stimulate the pancreas to make more insulin.

Surgery for Ménière's is a last resort. Although it does eliminate disabling tinnitus and vertigo, it occasionally causes deafness in the affected ear.

MENOPAUSE

FREE AT LAST!

As she enters middle life, a woman's ovaries begin to make less estrogen. By the time you're about fifty, there's so little of it around, your menstrual cycles become irregular, taper off, and finally stop. But menopause is not always a natural phenomenon; surgical removal of the ovaries will also bring it on—and very abruptly!

Many women welcome menopause because it means the end of their periods and freedom from having to use contraception. They are doubly happy if they used to suffer from endometriosis or premenstrual syndrome—both of which disappear at this time. In some women, too, the migraine headaches that plagued them for many years either stop or become milder and less frequent. But for some, this time of life is stressful—a marker of aging and a symbol of diminished femininity and sexuality.

No matter how you perceive it, menopause is often accompanied by a variety of symptoms, both *behavioral* (depression, irritability, mood swings) and *physical* (hot flashes, dryness of the skin and vagina). You also have a new, real vulnerability to diseases and disorders to which premenopausal women are relatively immune. Heart disease, which before age fifty mainly affects males, now strikes women just as often; osteoporosis and easily fractured bones also become a major problem.

It has always seemed logical to me that the best way to deal with the consequences of too little estrogen is to replace what's missing. So I advise my menopausal patients to take estrogen, even if they have no apparent symptoms due to its lack, unless there is some overriding reason for them not to do so, such as some cases of a history of breast, uterine, or ovarian cancer; liver or gallbladder disease; blood clots; or a history of their mother having taken DES, leaving them more vulnerable to gynecologic cancer. Estrogen replacement therapy (ERT) reduces the incidence of heart disease by about 50 percent (especially important if you have a bad family history of arteriosclerosis); it reduces the chances of stroke; and it lessens the severity of Alzheimer's disease. Estrogen also slows the progress of osteoporosis, to which you are more prone if you are white, thin, or a cigarette smoker, drink "too much" (more than two cocktails or two bottles of beer a day), or avoided dairy products (and the calcium they contain) before menopause because you wanted to lose weight or lower your cholesterol. If your doctor okays it, I recommend you start ERT at the very onset of menopause and continue taking it into your seventies. I am not convinced that you need it after that.

The most important *documented* complication of ERT is slowly growing cancer of the lining of the uterus unless, of course, you have had a hysterectomy. But adding another hormone, progestin, to the estrogen for a few days each month sharply reduces that risk. The association between long-term ERT and breast cancer has never been proved to my satisfaction, but to be on the safe side, I advise women who take it to examine their own breasts once a month, have their doctor do it every six months, and get a mammogram every year.

Does calcium *after menopause* help prevent osteoporosis? Many women don't pay attention to their calcium intake before menopause and assume that it's how much they eat after their periods have ended that's important. Wrong! You should have been getting lots of calcium right along, beginning in childhood. At menopause, when estrogen levels decrease, calcium begins to seep out of the bones. Whether they will become fragile and easily broken depends on how much calcium was in your bones when your periods ended. The greater the deposits when you were young, the smaller the risk of osteoporosis (see page 335) later in life. You should have been getting at least 1,200 milligrams of calcium in your diet every day between ages eleven and twenty-four, 800 milligrams between twenty-five and fifty, and you also should have been building up your bone mass with regular weight-bearing exercises such as running and walking. That is not to say you can forget calcium now that your periods have ended. It's particularly important if your diet lacks calcium in substantial amounts. Postmenopausal women on ERT still need 1,000 milligrams a day and all others should have 1,500 milligrams. (See page 342 for a list of calcium-containing foods.)

When foods containing calcium and phosphorus reach the stomach together, they compete for absorption. The more phosphorus there is, the less calcium enters the body, and so the bones are shortchanged. Although this mechanism is not as important as doctors used to think, menopausal women should still avoid too much phosphorus, which is found in foods like meat, poultry, fish, eggs, milk, and cola drinks (see page 287 for other high-phosphorus foods to avoid).

Besides increasing the absorption of calcium from the gut, you also want to stop its loss from the body. Protein, coffee, tea, and salt all tend to suck calcium out of the bones, so use them sparingly. Drink decaffeinated coffee and herbal tea; flavor your food with various herbs, garlic, onions, and lemon juice instead of salt; if you enjoy soup stock made with bones, a little added vinegar will help dissolve the calcium they contain and increase the amount present in the broth itself. We used to think that alcohol also has a negative effect on bone. It does if you're an alcoholic and booze a lot, but social drinkers (women who have eleven drinks or so per week, and men who have sixteen drinks a week) have actually been found to have the thickest bones.

Several drugs promote calcium loss from the body, many of which need to be taken indefinitely. If you are on any of the following, you should supplement your calcium consumption either in your food or in tablets: thyroid hormone (for those with underactive thyroid glands), steroids (if you need them for your asthma or arthritis), lithium (for manic-depressive disorders), tetracycline (an antibiotic used on an ongoing basis for chronic skin or lung conditions), heparin (touted by some to prevent arteriosclerosis if administered regularly), aluminum in antacids, Dilantin (for the treatment of epilepsy and other seizure disorders), and methotrexate (an anticancer drug also widely used to prevent transplant rejection and rheumatoid arthritis).

Calcium isn't the only mineral you need. Magnesium and potassium are important too, but for other reasons. Seven hundred fifty to 1,000 milligrams a day of magnesium will help you relax (a list of the magnesium content of foods appears in the table on page 304); an abundance of dietary potassium, in which fresh fruits and vegetables abound, may reduce the retention of fluid that sometimes occurs after menopause (see the table on page 252 for a list of high-potassium foods).

If you don't get into the sun very much, you will need 400 IU of additional vitamin D. Because almost all commercially available milk is fortified with at least 400 IU per quart, you can meet your requirements if you are a milk drinker (any form—whole, skim, or low-fat). If not, you will find what you need in almost any multivitamin. Check the bottle label just to be sure.

All the above notwithstanding, the *most* important dietary modifications at this time of life should reflect your increased vulnerability to hardening of the arteries. If you already have coronary artery disease, or if your "bad" cholesterol (LDL) is too high and the "good" kind (HDL) too low, or you are taking progestin, have your blood checked at least twice a year. (Progestin can make your blood fats abnormal.) If the ratio between the total blood cholesterol and the HDL is greater than 4:5, regardless of what each of their numbers happens to be, you need to change the way you eat. Say good-bye to those foods that are rich in cholesterol—egg yolk and organ meats such as liver, kidney, sweetbread, brain, and heart. You gourmands should eschew squid, and, the few who can afford it, caviar! You may have 6 ounces of animal protein a day—fish, skinless turkey, and skinless chicken, but as little beef, veal, lamb, pork, luncheon meat, bacon, and sausage as possible. Drastically limit your consumption of butter, lard, hydrogenated shortenings, whole milk, ice cream, and high-fat cheese, as well as palm, palm kernel, and coconut oils. What's left? A myriad of complex carbohydrates—whole grains, lentils, bran, vegetables, and fresh fruit. You can get all the calcium you need from the many nonfat milk products that are rich in calcium and low in cholesterol. You can buy nonfat cottage cheese and sour cream, as well as nonfat yogurt, in several delicious flavors. You'll also find nonfat cheeses and nonfat "butter" spreads galore. If you have lactase deficiency and cannot tolerate the lactose dairy products, there are several brands of commercially available lactase supplements you can add to these dairy products. If you really dislike milk, or are allergic to it, and are not getting enough calcium in your diet, you have the option of taking calcium supplements. Finally, a daily cocktail or two (but no more) may raise your estrogen level slightly, perhaps even enough to ease some of your menopausal symptoms (such modest amounts may also reduce your risk of heart disease). For more information on preventing heart disease, see page 192.

In summary, my prescription for the menopausal woman is to take estrogen if it is safe for her to do so, get plenty of exercise, and follow a diet that contains 1,000 to 1,500 milligrams of calcium a day, supplemented if necessary, and is low in animal fat, protein, and dairy products. (One-quarter cup of skim milk powder contains 100 milligrams of calcium; 1 cup of yogurt has 300 milligrams; there are 300 milligrams in 1 cup of low-fat milk; and eight medium-sized sardines give you 350 milligrams.) If you're intolerant of milk because of a lactase deficiency (see page 295), yogurt is an excellent substitute. You can also buy replacement lactase in various commercial brands. Eat lots of fiber (fruits, vegetables, grains). No more than 30 percent of your calories, at the very most, should come from fat (try to keep that number closer to 20 percent) and cholesterol intake should be limited to 300 milligrams a day (one egg contains almost that amount). Your coffee intake should be no more than three cups a day and your salt consumption should not exceed 2 grams a day. Finally, stop smoking!

MIGRAINE
AND OTHER HEADACHES
NO DEAR, NOT TONIGHT

Every year, Americans pay 18 million visits to emergency rooms or doctors' offices looking for relief from recurring headaches. Common causes of headache are tension and stress, alcohol, arthritis of the spine in the neck area, the side effect of a medication (nitroglycerine and other "coronary dilator" drugs will often do it), fever, high blood pressure, tobacco, too much coffee, something you've eaten, a head injury, food allergy, fluctuations in blood sugar, and, very rarely, a brain tumor. All told, 45 million Americans are headache sufferers; 23 million of whom have migraine.

The term *migraine* is derived from *hemicranium,* the Greek root for "half a head," because the intense, throbbing pain of these headaches is almost always one sided and often focused over one eye. Although there are several types of migraine, the two major ones are designated "common" and "classic." Nine of ten migraines are "common"; they strike without warning and last for many hours or days. The "classic" variety, on the other hand, begins with a fifteen- to twenty-minute prodrome (the symptoms preceding the headache), an "aura," usually visual, with sparkles or stars before the eyes, lightninglike flashes, blurs, or distortions. Occasionally, migraines are "complicated" by numbness and tingling in the face, obvious weakness in an arm or leg, blindness in an eye, or only half the vision in both eyes. Mood change—depression, irritability, or loss of appetite—is also a common accompaniment of all types of migraine. These symptoms are followed by the pain, nausea, and vomiting of the "sick headache" that usually lasts between four and twelve hours.

The incidence of migraine peaks between ages twenty and thirty-five, but it may begin earlier in life. Headache is not its most prominent feature in children, in whom it may present instead as vomiting for no apparent reason, or colic, abdominal pain, dizziness, or car sickness. The typical headaches appear in the teens, continue into adult life, and gradually become less frequent and milder with age.

Migraine runs in families; if you suffer from it, there's an even chance that one or more of your blood relatives do too. Attacks occur as often as every few days or not for months and they can be triggered by a variety of factors. The most common culprit is stress, but precipitants include a change in the weather or a drop in barometric pressure; hunger; fatigue; alcohol (particularly red wine); caffeine; nicotine; certain foods; bright lights; loud noises; specific odors; and sleeping either too much or too little. Female hormones also play an important role in migraine as evidenced by the following observations: Migraine is mainly a disorder of women (80 percent of "migraineurs" are female); headaches often begin at puberty, when large amounts of estrogen begin to be produced; attacks frequently occur with or just before a menstrual period, when estrogen levels drop sharply, or they may have their onset with the use of The Pill; they may stop or become much milder during pregnancy (but are occasionally worse); and they frequently wane with menopause (but continue unabated in some cases).

Until quite recently, the most commonly accepted theory of migraine was that the prodrome was due to *constriction* of the arteries *within* the brain, depriving it of blood. The characteristic one-sided headache that followed was believed to be the result of dilatation or *widening* of the arteries *outside* the brain and in the skull. However, it's more complicated than that. There appears to be an interplay of several processes in migraine—neurological, hormonal, and vascular. Many scientists are now convinced that certain brain chemicals, particularly *serotonin* (a neurotransmitter that facilitates the transmission of nerve impulses), play a key role. For example, they have shown that serotonin levels in the blood drop during migraine attacks, resulting in painful spasm of the blood vessels of the head. Estrogen is believed to be linked to migraine because of its direct influence on serotonin levels in the brain. As mentioned above, stress is the most common trigger for migraines, as it is for tension headaches. But stress relief, on the other hand, can also bring on a migraine, the so-called golfer's headache.

Can a specific food or beverage induce a migraine attack? There's no question that eating or drinking something to which you are allergic can do so. But so will other foods to which you are not allergic, notably those containing *tyramine*. So if you have migraine, avoid such tyramine-rich sources as aged cheeses, chocolate, hot dogs, bacon, and luncheon meats that contain nitrites; ask the waiter at your Chinese restaurant not to use MSG; keep away from fermented foods such as beer, yogurt, sauerkraut, yeast, and brewer's yeast—all of which contain tyramine. I also know some migraineurs who develop headaches after consuming the artificial sweetener aspartame (Nutra-Sweet), or when they're deprived of coffee ("Saturday morning migraine"). But there's another side to the coin. What you eat may *help* with your migraine. Twenty grams (that's a lot) of omega-3 fish oil capsules taken every day can reduce the frequency and severity of your attacks, presumably by altering the balance between prostaglandin and leukotriene production. These substances, made by the body, affect the function of the immune system, which may play a role in the causation of migraine. But remember the caveats I have listed throughout this book with respect to these fish oil supplements. They are not innocuous; large amounts lower vitamin E levels, so you should take 400 IU of that vitamin just to be sure; if you are diabetic or have high blood pressure, check with your doctor about the safety of consuming this much fish oil; and if you have any bleeding disorder, stay away from them. (See page 221 for food sources of omega-3.)

Hunger can also cause headaches, presumably by lowering blood sugar (hypoglycemia), though these headaches are not typical migraines. In a study done at the University of Missouri, 85 percent of seventy-four migraine patients whose headaches occurred either mid-morning or mid-afternoon had abnormal blood sugars. In those who were diabetic, the sugars were sometimes high, but in most, they were abnormally low. If you tend to get your migraine attacks between meals, ask your doctor for a glucose tolerance test. This is how it's done. You have a "fasting" blood test to determine your sugar level after you've had nothing to eat for at least twelve hours. You then drink a solution containing a known amount of sugar, following which your blood is drawn every half hour for five or six hours, and the sugar level measured each time. The information we're looking for is how high your blood sugar level peaks, how soon after you've consumed the drink it does so, and how far it drops. If your pancreas produces too much insulin in response to the sugar solution you drank, your blood sugar will be abnormally low and that's what may be triggering your migraine. In that case, follow a high-protein, low-carbohydrate diet, eating several smaller meals throughout the day rather than the usual three regular ones. (See the chapter on hypoglycemia, page 256.)

There is a variety of drugs to prevent or relieve migraine headaches, and they do work. However, the most impressive one for pain relief in really severe migraine, in my experience, is sumatriptan, still available only by injection in the United States but sold in oral form in Canada and Europe. This drug relieves even the most severe migraine headache within two hours in 80 percent of patients. It should not, however, be used by pregnant women or anyone with angina or coronary artery disease. Preventive treatment is, of course, far more effective and many excellent drugs are available for that purpose (beta-blockers, calcium channel antagonists, tricyclics, and nonsteroidal antiinflammatory agents, or NSAIDs). If you are getting headaches more than twice a week, ask your doctor about these medications.

As happens in so many chronic disorders, a host of "natural therapies" has been recommended for the relief of migraines and other headaches. Acupuncture and relaxation techniques may be very helpful. Some of my patients have responded to various herbal remedies such as meadowsweet, feverfew, ginseng, black horehound, asarum, mahuang, and peony. However, I cannot vouch for their efficacy, or even for their safety, for that matter. Mahuang, for example, is widely used as an aid to weight loss. Thirty-seven people recently required hospitalization in Texas and two may have died because of the ephedrine in this commercially available herb. Ephedrine is a potent drug (considered a narcotic in some states) that speeds the heart and raises blood pressure. So as is the case with any unproven remedy, I'd be very cautious about using any herb without identifying all of its ingredients.

In summary, if you suffer from migraines, avoid those situations, foods, and beverages that you know from experience will bring on an attack. The most common offenders are tyramine-rich foods such as aged cheese, yeast, and processed and nitrite-containing meats, as well as red wine and beer.

Perhaps the best news to emerge from all the recent research in the headache area is the finding that sex often alleviates the pain. That is contrary to the popular (or rather, unpopular) conception. You may want to give it a whirl—see "Diet and Sex" on p. 145. Perhaps the subtitle of this chapter should have read "Yes, dear, tonight!"

MOTION SICKNESS, NAUSEA, AND DIET

IS IT ALL IN THE HEAD, THE EAR, OR THE GUT?

In virtually every one of my earlier books, I have described my wife's disabling vulnerability to seasickness. She becomes deathly ill, not only on the high seas but also on a quiet lake and even in port! Movement that is imperceptible to the rest of the world leaves her nauseated, cold, sweaty, and tremulous. I really do not believe that motion sickness is psychological in origin, and even if I did, I'd never dare say so to my wife! We are both convinced that the terrible nausea is probably due to some abnormality in the balance mechanism of her inner ear.

Thanks to a variety of medications, such as the scopolamine patch, Dramamine, and Compazine, my wife and I are able to enjoy a cruise now and then. I'm not so sure those pressure-point wristbands sold in drugstores really work, but I have bought several anyway for Camilla—just hoping. The package insert says they are used by the British Navy, but it doesn't specify whether it's on land or at sea!

Unfortunately, most anti–motion sickness remedies leave my wife feeling like a zombie. So while I cavort about the boat—eating, swimming, dancing, watching movies, shopping, or playing bingo—she is "resting" in the cabin, grateful just to be left alone. Therefore I am always on the lookout for some nutritional approach without the side effects of medication to help control her symptoms. For years I had heard that gingerroot effectively prevents motion sickness and indeed improves nausea due to any cause. The Chinese have been taking it for this purpose for thousands of years, and it has become popular among Westerners too. The effect of gingerroot was never really scientifically evaluated until quite recently. However, in the last few years, several studies of its use in motion sickness have been carried out—and although the jury is still out as far as I am concerned, some researchers believe that it either prevents or reduces the severity of motion sickness. It is thought to act on the inner ear, nervous system, or stomach. I am not impressed with the data, probably because gingerroot in any of its forms (see below) has had no effect whatsoever on my wife's symptoms. But so many people claim to have obtained relief with it, I suggest you try some and judge for yourself. Never underestimate the power of suggestion, even in motion sickness! But if you do, don't get all confused like one of my patients did recently. She was deathly afraid of becoming seasick on a cruise she wanted very much to take. She read the sparse literature on the subject, consulted me (and I am sure other doctors as well), and ruminated on the matter for weeks before she set sail. When she finally did, the possible remedies—the scopolamine patch, antihistamines, Compazine, and gingerroot—were all a blur. When she finally boarded ship, she taped a piece of gingerroot behind her left ear! It did not work!

The most convenient way to use ginger is to buy the powder in capsules (most contain 500 milligrams) at a health food store. Take two before you board and two more later in the day. If it works, continue this four-a-day dose for the remainder of the cruise. Your pharmacist can also prepare these capsules for you in the same dosage. If you prefer, you can make ginger tea by steeping slices of the fresh root in boiling water or by simply adding a half teaspoon of powdered ginger to a glass of hot water. Don't take the powder dry, however, because it can burn your gullet. Don't worry about calories; 1 teaspoon of ginger powder contains only 6 calories; ¼ cup of the fresh, raw root has 17 calories.

Patients and friends often ask me whether individuals prone to seasickness should try to eat in order to control their symptoms. In other words, does a full stomach leave you less nauseated? As far as I'm concerned, if you can keep it down, eat anything you like, but first take one of the anti–motion sickness medications along with some ginger tea. Some travelers have told me that sipping champagne helps. I have no firsthand experience with this approach because I have never been seasick, nor can I find any reference to it in the literature. Try it if you want to, but don't tell anyone I recommended it.

In the end, if you really want to take a cruise (or to stop being sick in the backseat of a car or in an airplane), your best and most predictable bet is probably the scopolamine patch.

MULTIPLE SCLEROSIS (MS)

A FATTY DIET THAT

MAY ACTUALLY BE GOOD FOR YOU!

Recently, the twenty-six-year-old son of one of my patients was suddenly unable to focus with his left eye. He thought his glasses needed changing, so he had his local optometrist fit him with a new pair. That seemed to help slightly, so he concluded that his left eye was probably "weaker" than the right. A few weeks later, he dropped his fork at a dinner party. Everyone laughed—he'd obviously had too much to drink. But the next morning, when he was cold sober, his coffee cup slipped from his left hand and his fingers began to tingle. A few days later, his right leg felt "awkward" and, as he described it, "out of control," so that he slipped and fell down the stairs. That's when he consulted me.

It wasn't easy for me to tell Mark, his fiancée, and his parents that he had multiple sclerosis (MS). More than one million Americans have this disease, and two hundred new cases are diagnosed every day in this country. MS usually begins between ages twenty and forty. It's more common in women than in men, and there is a familial predisposition. As in Mark's case, symptoms often go unrecognized for months or years.

Mark and his family were distraught by my diagnosis and asked me to be frank with them about the long-term outlook. I explained that, statistically, MS is a chronic disease that shortens life by some five years, and usually impairs its quality, but that there is great individual variability in its course. Although one's mental faculties are typically not impaired, a host of other symptoms frequently develop—bowel, bladder, and sexual function, as well as balance and coordination, are often affected.

The family asked whether there was any cure for MS, or some medication to slow its progress. I gave them a brochure full of useful information prepared by the National Multiple Sclerosis Society in which they read that at this time there is no prevention or cure. I added, however, that there is now a beacon of light at the end of a very long, dark tunnel. Beta-interferon, a naturally occurring body protein that increases resistance, does delay or modify symptoms of the disease and slow its course. Most exciting of all is that it has actually improved the brain scans of some people with MS, especially those who are relatively well between "attacks."

The neurological symptoms of this disease occur unpredictably and in a hit-or-miss manner because MS affects the brain in a peculiar way. Patchy areas of the wrapping or sheath that covers and protects the nerves are lost, leaving stretches of these fibers denuded—much like what can happen to the insulation on electrical wires. This results in the interruption or slowing of transmission of nerve impulses. Symptoms vary depending on which nerves are involved and to what extent, and they also wax and wane dramatically. Someone whose function is severely impaired may suddenly improve and remain relatively well in "remission" for weeks and months. Then, for no apparent cause, his or her symptoms will return, a phenomenon referred to as "exacerbation." Heat, whether in a tub, from the weather, or after exercise, often aggravates symptoms, while exposure to cold tends to improve them.

There are many theories about the cause of MS. *Environmental factors* have long been suspected. Researchers point out that the disease is more common in cold climates, but that those born in frigid climes who move away to temperate zones *before* age fifteen are not at higher risk. However, those who do so later than fifteen are as vulnerable as if they hadn't moved at all. So whatever the causative agent is, it apparently takes root in the first fifteen years of life. One or more viruses are suspect, but none has yet been determined to be the responsible agent. The current consensus is that MS is an *autoimmune disorder,* probably induced by a virus, in which the body's defense mechanisms attack, reject, and destroy perfectly healthy tissues—in this case the nerve sheaths in the brain.

Genetic factors also play a role. If your brother or sister has MS, your chances of developing it are increased by twenty times.

How does the agent that causes MS affect the immune system? No one knows for sure, but some scientists think that fat may be partially responsible. Not all fat, mind you, because, as you will see, one form may actively be protective!

Speculation about the relationship between fat and MS began during World War II when it was noted that the incidence of the disease had fallen in areas where meat and fat consumption had decreased significantly—except among farmers who produced and consumed their own meat and dairy products.

I was in medical school at McGill University when this theory was first being discussed. One of my neurology teachers, Roy Swank, was convinced that the relationship between dietary fat and MS was real, but couldn't prove it over the short term because of the characteristic way the disease waxes and wanes spontaneously. He decided to place a large number of patients on controlled diets and follow them up for many years. So for thirty-four years he has kept track of 144 patients with MS, and from his laboratory at the Oregon Health Sciences University in Portland he reports on and updates their health status. He is convinced, on the basis of his observations to date, that no matter how mild, moderate, or severe their disease, those MS patients who conscientiously follow a diet low in *saturated fat* (found in most meat, whole milk and its derivative cheeses, butter, and palm and coconut oils) and *mono- and polyunsaturated fat* (in vegetable oils) live longer and have fewer symptoms than those who do not. Indeed, the least disabled among them at the start of his studies enjoyed near-normal survival for thirty-four years.

Dr. Swank is apparently not a lone voice in the wilderness. Other researchers also believe that there is some link between animal and vegetable fats and multiple sclerosis, and have taken the theory one step further. They claim that people with MS who avoid the vegetable and "land-based" animal fats, but who also eat large amounts of fatty fish containing *omega-3 fatty acids,* have fewer symptoms and relapses.

These findings deserve serious consideration by anyone with multiple sclerosis. Fats do differ in their chemical structure and biological activity. The omega-6 fatty acids in animal and vegetable fats stimulate the production of prostaglandins and leukotrienes, body chemicals that promote tissue inflammation and contribute to the development of autoimmune disorders. Omega-3 fatty acids, on the other hand, derived from a variety of deep-sea saltwater fish, have the opposite effect; they neutralize the omega-6 group and enhance the efficiency of the immune system. Today's American diet contains fifteen to twenty times more of the "bad" omega-6 than "good" omega-3.

So I advise my MS patients to avoid omega-6 fats and to eat fatty fish. Why? Even if it all turns out to be an unsubstantiated theory, what will they have lost? In fact, that's what I tell most of my patients to do anyway because such a diet may also protect against heart disease. From a practical standpoint, that means eating 5 ounces every day of tuna or any other fish that's *very* rich in omega-3 (see page 221). Moderate amounts of skinned poultry and pasta are okay—but forget red meat and whole-milk dairy products. Your diet should also be rich in legumes, fruits, and vegetables to make up for the calories you're not getting from fat and animal protein, and to provide fiber. How you prepare your food is important too. Avoid the forbidden fats in cooking, and instead bake, broil, grill, microwave, or poach your fish. Marinating foods in lemon juice or herbs, diluted fruit juices, or wine will introduce you to exciting new fat-free tastes. You can also braise your fish and vegetables in defatted chicken or vegetable stock.

If you don't like fish or can't afford to eat it regularly, you can take 2½ grams a day of omega-3 supplements in capsule form, the equivalent of 4 ounces of pink salmon. You'll need seven capsules of Maxepa daily to satisfy that amount. Since omega-3 oils have a prostaglandin effect similar to aspirin and interfere with blood clotting (a good thing for those prone to coronary disease), do not take them if you have a blood disorder. For the same reason, if you have poorly controlled or untreated high blood pressure, it's best not to use them because of the risk of brain hemorrhage. (Avoid aspirin for the same reason.) We used to think that supplemental omega-3 was not well tolerated by diabetics, but more recent studies at Harvard suggest that 2½ grams a day, present in the seven capsules of Maxepa, have no adverse effect in such people.

As with anything else in life, it's not all black and white with respect to the capsules of omega-3 fish oils. Some brands contain as much as 5 milligrams of cholesterol per capsule. If you are trying to keep your cholesterol level down, this is not a good route to follow. Always check the brand of the capsule you're buying. Some, such as Promega, are cholesterol free. Then there is the matter of pesticides. PCB, DDT, and other fat-soluble pesticides may be concentrated in the liver and fatty tissue of fish from contaminated waters. It's a good idea to ask your fish store where their fish comes from, and if there is any question, double-check with your local health department about the safety of those waters.

I have restricted my discussion of MS to what kinds of foods to eat and to avoid that might conceivably influence the course of the disease. But there are other more practical considerations. The neurological complications associated with MS can cause nutritional problems of their own. The ability to shop, to prepare one's meals, and to feed oneself is sometimes seriously compromised, especially in the late stages of the disease. Some persons may even require specially designed utensils with which to eat. It is extremely important, then, to see that your nutritional needs are met; take vitamin and mineral supplements when necessary. If bladder problems are causing increased frequency of urination or incontinence, drink most of your fluids, especially cranberry juice, during the day so as to ensure a good night's sleep.

While pursuing this dietary approach to MS, you should also be looking into the available pharmacological therapies, the most important of which currently is beta-interferon. Unfortunately, this medication is in limited supply as we go to press. If you are in the early stages of the disease, and get frequent "attacks" or exacerbations, contact a neurologist and ask to be put on the waiting list for the next "lottery." Things change quickly, and within six months of signing up, you may well qualify for the drug. It is given twice a week as an injection under the skin, very much like insulin for diabetics. Other medications for MS include steroids to reduce inflammation and various immune suppressants such as Cytoxan.

In terms of other types of therapies, there is interest in the possible benefit of plasma exchange (plasmapheresis), in which the patient's blood is circulated through a filter. The blood cells are separated from the plasma, which is then discarded and the cells returned to the patient. The rationale behind this procedure is that it removes some unidentified substance in the plasma that causes or worsens MS. In another therapeutic approach to the disease, certain blood cells implicated in its causation are selectively destroyed by radiation. Such "total lymphoid radiation" is still experimental, but its effects are being studied in clinical trials. Unfortunately, it has many nasty side effects. Finally, in yet another research procedure, patients are injected with monoclonal antibodies that selectively find and destroy those blood cells thought to play a role in the development of multiple sclerosis. The best way for you to decide which treatment protocol to join is to ask your doctor to contact one or more academic neurological centers where research on MS is being done. Or, you may call the Neurology Branch of the National Institutes of Health in Bethesda, Maryland, which funds and monitors most of this investigational activity.

In summary, the cause of MS remains a mystery. A combination of factors—infection by one or more viruses, the genetic profile, and an immune system gone "haywire"—will probably turn out to be the culprit(s). There are several new and exciting pharmacological approaches to the management of the disease. However, until they are translated into a definite treatment regimen, people with MS should pursue any reasonable course that may have a favorable effect on their disease. A diet low in animal and vegetable fats and rich in fats derived from fish is one such approach. This boils down to eating less than 10 grams of saturated fat per day, lots of legumes, fruits, and vegetables, and 5 ounces of fatty fish daily. This diet protects you, not only against MS, but against cancer and heart disease as well. For more details about this diet read *The Multiple Sclerosis Diet,* written by Roy Swank and published by Doubleday (New York) in 1987.

OSTEOPOROSIS

WHEN YOU GET ALL THE BREAKS IN LIFE

When the emergency room calls to tell me that an older man has been brought in by ambulance, I instinctively assume he's had a heart attack or a stroke. But when the patient is an older woman, I first suspect a broken hip, even though such women suffer heart attacks and strokes at least as often as men do. It's just that by age seventy, more than 40 percent of all women will have fractured at least one bone, usually a hip, spine, wrist, or rib—that's six times more often than it happens in men. Apart from the pain, these injuries cripple and even kill. The condition that causes bones to break so easily and from which one female in four over the age of sixty suffers is called *osteoporosis*.

The term *osteoporosis* ("osteo" is bone; "porosis" means porous) refers to bones that are thin, fragile, and easily broken because they do not contain enough calcium. For someone with this condition, a vigorous cough may fracture a rib; lifting a heavy object (like a grandchild) or taking a bumpy car ride may crack a bone in the spine—so will vigorous dancing. Osteoporotic bones also fracture spontaneously, for no apparent reason. When they do so in the spinal column, it collapses, leaving the affected woman with the familiar "dowager's hump" and considerably shorter. So when we are young, we grow, but as we get older, some of us shrink!

In order to appreciate what can be done to prevent and to treat osteoporosis, you must understand the metabolism of bone. We tend to think of bones as inert structures, probably because we have been conditioned to seeing them in museums. The living skeleton, however, is an active, dynamic organ—as vibrant and "busy" as any other in the body.

Bones are composed of a protein framework; their calcium cover is what makes them hard. (Ninety-nine percent of the body's calcium is present in the bones and teeth.) Bones are pliable and continually being rebuilt and remodeled in response to the mechanical stress to which they are subjected. This flexibility is made possible by the constant movement of calcium, hormones, and other biological substances *into* and *out of* bone through its blood supply. When we are young and growing, or physically active, more calcium is laid down in our bones than is removed from it. But as we approach forty, more calcium begins to be lost than is added.

This flux of calcium between bones and the bloodstream occurs in response to the needs not only of the bone itself, but of other organ systems as well. For example, normal muscle contraction, including that of the heart, and the delicately balanced clotting processes of the blood require calcium. When there is too little available circulating in the blood, the bones oblige by releasing additional amounts. When the demand for calcium becomes excessive and chronic, the bones become calcium poor, fragile, and easily broken.

Why is osteoporosis so much more common in women, especially after menopause? The answer lies in their estrogen levels. This hormone, which is far more abundant in women than in men, puts a brake on calcium loss from bone. When a woman is young and physically active, having babies and caring for them, her need for strong bones is very great and continues even when she is older. Her plentiful supply of estrogen promotes the deposit of more calcium in the skeleton than is lost. But as her hormonal production begins to wane with the approach of menopause and decreases sharply at its onset, her bones lose more calcium than they receive; they become thinner and vulnerable to fracture.

How much calcium is sucked out of your bones or deposited in them is also influenced by how much of this mineral you consume in your diet and how well it is absorbed by the intestine. Peak absorption occurs when you are young and is further increased by estrogen. By approximately age forty-five in women and sixty in men, the absorption process becomes less efficient. Your calcium need is also influenced by how much you lose naturally every day—in the stool, in the urine, and from the skin. That's yet another reason why adequate intake is so important *throughout life*. The table on page 342 lists foods rich in calcium along with their caloric values.

Other factors can also have an impact on the development of osteoporosis and its severity. If you are of slight body build with less muscle mass, you are apt to have less calcium in your bones and are therefore more vulnerable to osteoporosis. Black women, who generally have larger skeletons than Caucasians, are not as prone to developing it. This is an unusual situation in which being petite and thin renders you more susceptible to a disease than being overweight!

Certain drugs, the most important of which are listed on page 342, actively lower the body's calcium level by one mechanism or another. You should have extra calcium in your diet or take supplements if you are on thyroid hormone, steroids, lithium, tetracycline, heparin, aluminum-containing antacids, Dilantin, or methotrexate.

Caffeine, salt, and tobacco also rob the body of calcium by causing the body to excrete more in the urine. Drink decaffeinated coffee and herbal tea; flavor your food with various herbs, garlic, onions, and lemon juice instead of salt; if you enjoy soup stock made with bones, a little added vinegar will help dissolve the calcium they contain and increase the amount present in the broth itself.

Doctors used to think that alcohol had a negative effect on bone. It does if you're an alcoholic and booze a lot, but social drinkers (women who have eleven drinks a week, and men who have sixteen drinks a week) apparently have the thickest bones.

There have also been reports that breast-feeding for longer than six months may result in a decrease of maternal bone mass (presumably due to the calcium in breast milk) (see page 161). This phenomenon may be at least partially reversible.

Osteoporosis is sometimes a complication of other conditions, such as an overactive thyroid, hyperparathyroidism (a condition in which a benign tumor causes the parathyroid gland to secrete too much of a hormone that sucks calcium out of the bones), kidney disease (where excessive amounts of calcium are lost in the urine), and several malignancies (notably multiple myeloma, leukemia, and lymphoma).

Although you are not likely to have osteoporosis and bones that fracture easily before menopause, some very athletic young women do sustain stress fractures while running, jumping, jogging, or engaging in other vigorous sports. The reason their bones crack so easily is that they have less calcium than normal. That's because they are estrogen deficient as a result of having lost so much fat from their body stores, since fat converts some ovarian hormones to estrogen. Other evidence of their estrogen deficiency is their sparse, irregular, or absent menstrual periods. Some athletes deliberately decrease their consumption of dairy products (and thus calcium) in order to lose weight. The combination of body-fat loss, decreased estrogen, and inadequate calcium intake places these young women at substantially greater risk for osteoporosis even before menopause.

Although osteoporosis generally becomes *apparent* after menopause, your vulnerability is determined while you are still young. Too many women believe that eating lots of calcium *after* menopause is what's important. Wrong, wrong, wrong! The best time to get it into your bones is while you're in your teens, when bone mass approaches its peak. A recent study suggests that dietary calcium in early childhood plays a critical role in your later bone history. However, if you've neglected calcium in your diet, better late than never. Here are some dietary guidelines to help you increase your calcium intake, both *before* and *after* menopause.

The RDA for calcium in the first six months of life is 400 milligrams daily; from six months to one year, babies should receive 600 milligrams a day; between one year and eleven years, the goal is 800 milligrams daily. Children and young adults ages eleven through twenty-four should consume between 1,200 and 1,500 milligrams. After age twenty-five, men should have 1,000 milligrams of calcium a day for the rest of their lives, while women ages twenty-five to fifty need 1,000 milligrams daily. After menopause, or if you are pregnant or nursing, you should have 1,500 milligrams per day. Currently, adult women ages twenty-five to seventy-four in the United States consume an average of only 500 milligrams of calcium a day—less than half of what they need!

Note on the table on page 342 that the richest sources of calcium are dairy products (milk, cheese, yogurt), fish and shellfish, and dark green vegetables, except for spinach. (An entire generation of Americans has been brainwashed by Popeye to believe that spinach is rich in iron, which in fact is poorly absorbed, and rich in calcium. Unfortunately, spinach also contains much oxalate, which interferes with absorption of calcium.) An 8-ounce glass of milk contains 300 milligrams of calcium, a quart has 1,200. Some brands of calcium-fortified milk have 500 milligrams per cup. As little as 1 ounce of hard cheese has 200 milligrams of calcium. Note that cottage cheese and cream cheese, ounce for ounce, are not nearly as calcium rich as harder cheeses. Low-fat dairy products such as yogurt and nonfat milk are good dietary sources of calcium as are corn tortillas. Some makers of orange juice sell a calcium-enriched product that has as much calcium ounce for ounce as milk.

The best way to get the calcium you need is from your diet, but if for some reason calcium-rich foods are taboo for you (the dairy sources may have too many calories, fat, or cholesterol, or you may be lactose intolerant), then you must turn to supplements. There is a host of them on the market, in a variety of forms—tablets, powders, and chewable pills—but there are important differences among them. Always read the label on the bottle to see what *kind* of calcium it contains. I recommend calcium carbonate, which is 40 percent calcium, that is, 100 milligrams of calcium carbonate yields 40 milligrams of calcium; by contrast, calcium lactate contains only 13 percent calcium and calcium gluconate is only 9 percent. A very available source is calcium citrate malate, which is not available as a supplement per se, but can be bought in the United States as beverages marketed as Sunny Delight Plus Calcium and Double C Hawaiian Punch.

I used to think, and have previously written, that you can tell whether your calcium supplement is any good by dropping the tablet into 6 ounces of white vinegar, stirring gently, and leaving it there for two hours. If it didn't dissolve in that time, the presumption was that it wouldn't do so in your stomach either. More recent research, however, indicates that what happens in the glass of vinegar does not necessarily correlate with events in your stomach!

Some women patients prefer to get their calcium supplements from over-the-counter antacids. Tums is my favorite because it is almost

100 percent calcium carbonate. You should also look for the aluminum content of any antacid you're taking, not only because of the speculation concerning its role in Alzheimer's disease, but because aluminum interferes with the absorption of calcium from the gut. Bonemeal remains a popular source of calcium among many women, but even though it doesn't contain as much lead as it used to because there's much less lead in the environment and in the vegetation on which cattle feed, bonemeal, oyster shell, dolomite, and various chelates still contain more lead than do laboratory-made calcium preparations. I recommend you stay with the latter. In any event, whatever the source of your calcium supplement, look for the United States Pharmacopoeia seal of approval on the bottle.

To ensure maximum absorption of calcium, always drink a glassful of water with your supplement. Calcium is best absorbed from an empty stomach. So if you are under sixty years of age, you will get more calcium for your dollar if you take it between meals. However, optimal calcium absorption requires acid in the stomach, and since stomach acid content is often diminished in persons over sixty, if you're in this age group, have your calcium supplements *with* meals to take advantage of any acid present in your food. Calcium carbonate can cause constipation, so take it in divided doses. Since more calcium is lost from the body during sleep than in waking hours, take one of these doses at bedtime. Your body needs at least 200 IU of vitamin D daily to absorb calcium, but you are probably receiving that amount if you get between fifteen minutes and one hour of exposure to sunlight a day during the summer months. You do not need supplements if you drink at least one glass of vitamin D–fortified milk daily, or eat a serving of vitamin D–fortified cereal, an egg yolk or two, or a portion of saltwater fish. However, if you think your vitamin D intake is too low, there are many multivitamins and calcium supplements themselves that contain it. Like vitamin A, however, too much vitamin D, say more than 400 milligrams per day, can be harmful.

Replacing the estrogen lost after menopause will also combat osteoporosis. I have discussed in more detail the pros and cons of estrogen replacement therapy (ERT) in the section on menopause. I feel strongly that women who may safely take ERT should do so at menopause (see page 317). In my opinion, the benefits greatly outweigh the risks. There is much more illness, disability, and death from heart disease (whose incidence the use of estrogen reduces by 50 percent) and osteoporosis (which low-dose estrogen helps prevent) than there is from cancer of the breast or uterus. Nor am I convinced of a causal relationship between these malignancies and estrogen, and in any event combining estrogen with progestin virtually eliminates the risk of uterine cancer. But your own doctor knows you better than I do, and you should discuss this question thoroughly with him or her.

Lack of weight-bearing exercise is a key risk factor in the development of osteoporosis. Beginning such exercise early in life helps build bone mass and thickens the calcium deposits in your bones. Walking or jogging is absolutely necessary at all ages, but if your exercise tastes are more exotic, try jumping rope, playing tennis, doing aerobics, rowing, cross-country skiing, using a NordicTrack, or even ballroom dancing. You may love to swim, and it's great for your heart, but it won't do much for your osteoporosis. Neither will yoga. Try to remain active even if you do develop osteoporosis, and be sure to eat 1,000 to 1,500 milligrams of calcium a day to slow its progress. However, avoid sudden movements such as twisting or jumping, which can stress weakened bones.

As we grow older, our intestines actually absorb less dietary calcium. I have discussed elsewhere some of the factors that affect that absorption. You may further optimize the amount of calcium your intestines accept by reducing your phosphorus intake (although nutritionists feel less strongly about this than they used to). Phosphorus, which competes with calcium for absorption, is present in red meats, cola drinks, brewer's yeast, and certain processed foods. (See page 287 for a list of phosphorus-containing foods.) Avoid excessive amounts of these particular foods at and after menopause.

There is no cure for osteoporosis, but several drugs can slow its progress and possibly even restore a little of the lost calcium. These include calcitonin, a hormone produced by the thyroid gland, sodium fluoride combined with calcium, calcitriol (a vitamin D derivative), thiazide diuretics, and perhaps the most effective to date, etidronate (Didronel).

In summary, the best way to prevent osteoporosis is to start increasing the deposition of calcium in the bones early in life. You can help ensure that by getting enough calcium in your food and by doing regular weight-bearing exercises such as running, walking, or jogging.

If your doctor okays it, start estrogen supplements at menopause and continue them for at least ten years. Calcium intake and exercise, though most important before menopause, continue to play an important role throughout life.

DRUGS THAT INCREASE CALCIUM LOSS

Aluminum-containing antacids
Corticosteroids
Dilantin
Heparin
Lithium
Phenobarbital
Phenothiazine derivatives
Tetracycline
Thyroid hormone

CALCIUM CONTENT OF FOOD

FOOD	PORTION	CALCIUM (mg)	CALORIES
Broccoli, raw	½ cup	12	21
Cabbage			
green, raw	½ cup	16	8
red, raw	½ cup	18	10
Collards, cooked	1 cup	30	34
Cheeses			
cheddar	1 ounce	204	114
cottage, 1% fat	1 cup	138	164
cream	1 ounce	23	99
feta	1 ounce	140	75
Gouda	1 ounce	198	101
Muenster	1 ounce	203	104
mozzarella, part skim	1 ounce	183	72
ricotta, part skim	½ cup	337	171

CALCIUM CONTENT OF FOOD *(Continued)*

FOOD	PORTION	CALCIUM (mg)	CALORIES
Milk			
Calcimilk (calcium fortified)	8 ounces	498	102
chocolate milk, 2% fat	8 ounces	284	179
Dairy Ease (lactose-reduced milk), skim	8 ounces	302	86
skim, protein fortified	8 ounces	352	100
whole	8 ounces	290	157
Fish/shellfish			
oysters, raw	6 medium	38	58
salmon, Atlantic, cooked	3 ounces	13	155
salmon, pink, canned, with bone	3 ounces	181	118
sardines, canned in oil, bones included	2 ounces	92	50
Soy milk	8 ounces	10	79
Tofu			
raw	½ cup	130	94
raw, firm	½ cup	258	183
Tortillas, corn	1 tortilla	42	67
Yogurt			
low-fat, coffee	8 ounces	389	194
low-fat, plain, with added nonfat dry milk solids	8 ounces	415	144
nonfat, plain, with added nonfat dry milk solids	8 ounces	452	127

WHEN YOU'RE OVERWEIGHT

NO MORE INTIMATE DINNERS

FOR TWO—ESPECIALLY WHEN

YOU'RE DINING ALONE!

Many Americans view obesity as a disease that's as incurable as cancer, AIDS, arteriosclerosis, multiple sclerosis, rheumatoid arthritis, and diabetes. The common perception in our society is that thin is beautiful, fat is ugly, and obesity is a reflection of gluttony and sloth. Being fat can affect your marital status, your social life, and your pocketbook. Working women who are very overweight earn almost $7,000 less per year than their slimmer counterparts, and their chances of getting married are also decreased by 20 percent. Although fat men are not affected economically, they are less likely to marry. Most people want to lose weight. However, they rarely admit cosmetic or economic motivation. Instead, they invoke the more socially acceptable health reasons. They want to lose weight because it's the healthy thing to do. But is "thin" always healthier?

One American in three is deliberately trying to lose weight, and half of all women are on a diet at some time or other. But despite the many programs designed for that purpose—commercial, hospital based, and doctor directed—27 percent of us remain obese (defined as 20 percent or more above the ideal weight for our height and body type) and we're getting fatter every year! We try diet after diet, and one appetite suppressant after another; we go to fat farms; and we starve ourselves, sometimes to death, in a great national exercise in futility. We may lose a few pounds for a while on one regimen or another, but 95 percent of us regain it all within two to five years—and usually sooner than that. Thanks to high-fashion magazines, TV advertising, and other unrelenting media pressure, millions of us are depressed, frustrated, and angry because we are unable to meet unrealistic goals. I believe that this chronic frustration is much more harmful to our health than weighing a little more than "ideal." The truth is, our dietary obsession is totally unnecessary, and destined to come to naught. Nature has not endowed most of us with the genes that permit us to look anything like our favorite model or movie star. We are also overreacting to the numbers on our scales, confusing cosmetic fantasy with health objectives. Only a relatively small number of persons are "morbidly obese," that is, so excessively fat as to be seriously vulnerable to diabetes, high blood pressure, elevated cholesterol, or arthritic joints.

Your ultimate shape and weight are determined by one or more genes that scientists have not yet identified. But although what you eat will not usually alter your basic body profile permanently any more than it can change the shape of your nose, modifying your eating habits and exercising regularly *can* give you the best weight and figure that nature will allow.

It's normal to gain some weight as you grow older, and doing so is rarely a threat to health. The reason for the extra pounds is in part the decreased physical activity that usually accompanies aging, and the consequent replacement of muscle by fat, which does not burn calories as rapidly as does muscle. Don't embark on a weight-loss program after looking at yourself in the mirror or just because you are heavier than the height and weight tables say you should be. For a true assessment, you need to know your *BMI* (body-mass index) and *WHR* (waist-to-hip ratio). To determine your BMI, multiply your weight in pounds by 700, then twice divide the result by your height in inches. For example, if you're five feet tall and weigh 200 pounds, multiply 200 by 700; that makes 140,000. Five feet equals 60 inches, so dividing 140,000 by 60 gets 2,333, which, divided again by 60, gives you the final figure of 38.9. A BMI of less than 25, regardless of age, places you at the lowest risk of death from all causes (except if you smoke cigarettes, because the lung disease and cancer that they cause have little to do with body weight); a BMI between 25 and 30 reflects mild to moderate overweight and constitutes only a slight risk (except if you have diabetes, high blood pressure, or a very high cholesterol level); a BMI higher than 30 is bad news and requires action! So our hypothetical five-footer who weighs 200 pounds is really in trouble with his BMI of 38.8. No more than a third of all dieting Americans have a BMI greater than 30.

The WHR (waist-to-hip ratio) is even more important than the BMI because it reflects not only the *amount* of fat but also how it's distributed. The latter is largely genetically determined. Here's how to obtain your WHR: With your belly completely relaxed, measure your waist at its narrowest. Divide that number in inches by the widest circumference of your hips, that is, where your buttocks are most prominent. A WHR greater than 0.85 in women and 0.95 in men is fraught with risk. If you've gotten a big beer belly, that ratio is going to be higher than if you're thin at the waist and heavier in the buttocks, which is the case in most "overweight" women. Abdominal fat is worse for you than big buttocks because it has a closer association with the increased insulin resistance and high cholesterol that may lead to diabetes, high blood pressure, and heart disease. So it's better to be pear-shaped than apple-shaped! You are, however, more likely to eliminate a beer belly if you combine exercise with diet. But remember, there are weight limits established by heredity below which you are simply not going to be able to drop.

Playing the yo-yo game is no way to address your weight "problem." Wide swings up and down increase the incidence of heart disease by 50 percent and also raise the death rate from all causes, although not quite as much as we used to think. You are much better off finding a weight plateau and staying there, even if it is somewhat higher than you'd like. As far as your ultimate target is concerned, weighing 20 percent less than the U.S. average for men of your age and height will give you the longest life expectancy. There are no figures yet available for women.

The best way to lose five or ten pounds is very simply to eat only when you're hungry, stop when you're full, avoid snacks, reduce the intake of alcohol with all its empty calories, and exercise every day. Would you believe that 56 percent of all Americans do not engage in any leisure-time physical activity whatsoever? I have been able to control my own weight (more or less) by walking on a treadmill for thirty minutes a day at 3.8 miles an hour at least four times a week. But even after I've worked up a sweat doing so, the computer on my treadmill tells me that I've burned only 200 calories! So how does this help my weight? It does so by raising the basal metabolism, that is, the rate at which my body uses up energy when I am not exercising. Exercise on an ongoing basis sets your thermostat at a higher level.

You're obviously going to have to eat less if you want to lose weight, but the *kind* of calories you consume may be more important than their actual number. *The key to weight loss* is a *low-fat* diet. So emphasize fruits, vegetables, and whole grains, drink low- or even nonfat rather than whole milk, and stay away from hamburgers, ice cream, butter, cheese, luncheon meats, and any food in which you can see the fat. Treat yourself to a low-fat vegetarian meal as often as you enjoy it.

Suppose your BMI is 30 and your WHR is 0.9—both too high. You're worried because your cholesterol is elevated, or you have diabetes, or your blood pressure is up. You want to lose the extra weight to reduce your risk of cardiovascular disease. Good for you! There are several ways to do it. You can go it alone, or you can work with your doctor, or you can sign up at a hospital weight-reduction clinic, or you can try one of the commercial plans. Americans, many of whom are not overweight by any standard except their own, spend more than $33 million on these diet regimens.

Most commercial weight-loss programs consist of various menus with a daily limit of 1,000 to 1,500 calories. Some also offer counseling and companionship because misery loves company. No commercial diet plan I know works for any length of time. If you're interested in reviewing all your options in this area, read the June 1993 issue of *Consumer Reports,* much of which is devoted to an analysis of several commercial diets. In its survey, *Consumer Reports* found that most people prefer Slim-Fast, Dynatrim, and Jenny Craig, and stay with them for about six months. During that time they lose 10 to 20 percent of their starting weight; within six months they regain half of that weight back, within two years they gain two thirds of it back, and within five years they regain 95 percent of the initial weight they lost. If you choose to lose weight on your own, chances are you'll drop about ten pounds and find it easier and less expensive than going commercial. You'll also probably keep it off just as long as if you had signed up with a fancy plan. Another fascinating observation in the *Consumer Reports* analysis was the large number of people who embark on these programs without good reason.

Liquid diet regimens should be followed only under strict medical supervision as a last resort in persons for whom rapid weight loss is urgently required—before major surgery, or as treatment for severe sleep apnea, new onset of adult diabetes, or hypertension that is difficult to control. The usual program consists of 450 to 800 calories daily for about three months taken in a premixed liquid preparation that contains vitamin and mineral supplements. No solids whatsoever are permitted for the duration. The risks of liquid diets are sudden cardiac arrest, gallstones, gout (due to the resulting high uric acid), and psychological stress, not to mention the awful boredom!

The hottest news in the area of weight reduction is the discovery of two natural brain chemicals: one (galanin) triggers a craving for fatty food; the other (enterostatin) suppresses it. The taste for carbohydrate and protein is unaffected by both. There is apparently a method to nature's madness in creating these two proteins with opposite actions. The amount of galanin in the brain increases at puberty in girls to have them eat more fat in anticipation of pregnancy so as to better nourish their fetus. Of course, most women, at least in our society, do not become pregnant during adolescence, but they do put the weight on because of nature's timing! When animals are given enterostatin, they consume 50 to 80 percent less fat. Clinical experiments with these two chemicals may well have begun in humans by the time you read this, but don't hold your breath. It will probably be at least five years before a new diet drug is available.

Here is what I recommend if you seriously want to lose weight. First, see your doctor for a thorough medical evaluation. Discuss with him or her how much of your objective is medically indicated, and how much is motivated by cosmetic goals. You will be screened for the various medical causes of obesity (for example, an underactive thyroid gland will sometimes do it). After you have agreed on the safety, practicality, and desirability of your goals, ask for a referral to a hospital-based weight-loss program supervised by a qualified physician or registered dietician who can structure a 1,000- to 1,500-calorie diet *for you,* one that *you* can follow. You can also contact the local chapter of the American Dietetic Association for the name of a registered dietician who specializes in weight loss. This professional can assess your eating habits, go through a nutrient analysis, and make the appropriate recommendations for safe and effective weight loss. The actual number of calories permitted will depend on your body build and the level of your daily physical activity. A nutritionist can teach you how to substitute one food for another and how to compose portion sizes of the foods you like. You will also learn how to interpret food labels. The fact that no diet-industry program, no matter how good it looks on paper, ever works for any length of time is one of the great unsolved mysteries of medicine. One factor, I am sure, is the fact that none of these programs is tailored to *your* biological makeup. There are behavior-modification programs and clinics at most hospitals to help motivate you so that you adhere to whatever dietary regimen is recommended.

Once you've started a diet that's appropriate for you, you must address yourself to the matter of exercise. One is of limited value without the other. Again, you will need clearance from your doctor about how much exercise it is safe for you to do, and at what intensity. This is not usually a problem for men and women under age forty. You may also want to avail yourself of the services of a trained physical therapist to devise an exercise program that is realistic for you and that you will enjoy. That's the key to keeping at it—liking what you're doing.

In summary, when considering a weight-loss program, first decide what your goals are—and why. Are the reasons cosmetic or health related? Make sure that your target weight is realistic within the limitations of your body build and genetic makeup. Determining your BMI and WHR is a good place to start. Remember that "yo-yo" weight loss and gain appear to be associated with increased cardiovascular disease and overall death rates. Persons who lose only modest amounts of weight do better than those who crash diet. The only menu for permanent weight reduction is regular exercise, ongoing decrease in fat intake, cutting down on alcohol, and a sensible diet that you can comfortably live with over the years.

PAINFUL, LUMPY BREASTS

TO WORRY? TO DIET?

More than half of all adult women have lumpy breasts. You probably became aware of them in your twenties, but they may not have appeared until you turned forty. The breasts (both, as a rule) feel irregular, with areas that are of different consistency to the touch throughout. Don't confuse this with a single lump in one breast. The main symptom of multiple breast lumps is the anxiety they cause, although they may ache just before the onset of your period and improve shortly thereafter.

Lumpy breast tissue, whether painful or not, reflects *normal hormonal fluctuation* and is not a disease. Still, with so much breast cancer around, many women naturally worry that what is now only a benign irregularity may one day become a malignant tumor. This concern is all the more understandable if your mother, sister, or aunt had breast cancer, and your fear is even greater when you hear your doctor refer to your condition as "fibrocystic *disease*." That term should have been replaced long ago by "fibrocystic *breasts*" or "fibrocystic *variations*."

Remember this: The great majority of breast cysts and lumps that come and go are *neither precancerous nor forerunners of breast cancer*. Here's another reassuring observation. Except for the very late stages, cancerous lumps, unlike fibrocystic breasts, are rarely painful, and have no relation to your menstrual cycle. Still, just to be sure, you should have regular mammograms. Your doctor may advise you to have a breast biopsy early on, usually with a needle but sometimes by an incision and removal. But it's not feasible to have a biopsy every time you feel a change. Another mammogram, a sonogram, or a simple needle aspiration may be all that is necessary. "Atypical cells" in the screening biopsy are not often harbingers of malignancy, but if that's what the report reads, you should be reexamined by your doctor every four months, and have a mammogram at least once a year. Don't hide your anxiety. Discuss the implications of your breast findings with your doctor, and be sure you understand them.

If you have painful, lumpy breasts, remember that the best time to do your monthly breast exam is right *after* your period, when your breasts are likely to be the least lumpy. Make note if any of your usual lumps feels more tender or different in some way, and report this to your doctor right away. If you don't know how to do a breast self-exam, ask your doctor or the nurse to show you.

There are several medications that relieve breast discomfort related to the menstrual cycle. The most effective are danazol (a drug that blocks ovulation), bromocriptine (which reduces the level of the hormone prolactin), and various combinations of estrogen and progesterone. Like every medication, these have potential side effects and complications, so always take them under your doctor's supervision.

Can any vitamin or food either provoke or improve fibrocystic breasts? Ask any woman who has them and she'll swear by several effective remedies, notably *vitamin E* or ginseng. In reviewing the studies on this subject done in the past ten years, I was unable to find a single report *proving* that *any* dietary intervention or vitamin supplement works. However, I never argue with success, so if vitamin E helps, take it, of course. The usual dosage is 400 IU per day. As long as you're taking vitamin E, try vitamin B complex supplements too. Anecdotal reports suggest that they may also be helpful.

Methylxanthine in caffeine is one of the main constituents of coffee, and is also present in tea, cocoa, soft drinks, chocolate, and some candies. I have the impression, but no proof, that avoiding caffeine eases the discomfort of lumpy breasts. Whatever improvement I have observed among my own patients may be due to the "placebo" effect and the power of suggestion. Still, I recommend you abstain completely from caffeine, cola, tea, and chocolate when symptoms are troublesome. (For a list of caffeine-containing foods, see page 45.) It may take several weeks before you notice results. In the meantime, be aware that you may experience caffeine withdrawal—and its accompanying headaches—lasting anywhere from a few days to a week or two.

So here's the bottom line with respect to simple "fibrocystic changes" in your breasts: (1) they do not lead or predispose to breast cancer; (2) there are medications that can improve your symptoms; (3) vitamin E and vitamin B complex may have some beneficial effect and there is no harm trying them; (4) abstaining from caffeine-containing foods such as chocolate and cola may help, especially if you expect it to.

PANCREATITIS

ALCOHOL, GALLSTONES, AND BELLYACHES

The pancreas, situated in the midline deep inside the belly, makes insulin and several enzymes that help digest the food we eat. Injury, inflammation, and infection of this organ (pancreatitis) can be acute, lasting only a few days and followed by complete recovery, or it can become chronic, causing recurrent bellyaches every few weeks or months. The chronic form, which is often heralded by repeated attacks of acute pancreatitis, may lead to malabsorption of food and diabetes.

The number-one cause of pancreatitis is *alcohol,* especially more than 2½ ounces every day. Persons with acute pancreatitis often drink three or more times that amount.

One-third of all cases of acute pancreatitis are due to gallstones passing from the gallbladder into the ducts and inflaming the neighboring pancreas. A very high level of triglycerides (a neutral fat) in the blood (usually over 1,000 milligrams per deciliter) can result in pancreatitis too, presumably because this fat irritates the pancreatic cells. Also, since the pancreas lies directly behind the stomach, a peptic ulcer that doesn't heal can eat its way through the lining of the stomach and involve the pancreas. Some drugs, such as diuretics, tetracycline, and estrogen, can inflame the pancreas as can viral infections such as mumps.

Whatever the mechanism, the result of pancreatitis is swelling of the ducts in the pancreas, so that there is obstruction to the normal flow of the digestive enzymes to the intestine. The pancreas becomes engorged and its enzymes back up into its tissues, irritating and inflaming them.

The pain of pancreatitis, felt in the middle of the upper abdomen and radiating through to the back, is excruciating, and is usually accompanied by fever, nausea, and vomiting. Sitting or leaning forward offers some relief. Unlike gallbladder pain, which comes in waves, this pain is steady, and lasts for hours, even days.

The dietary treatment of pancreatitis is simple, but requires close medical supervision. Eat *nothing* during the acute phase! Most attacks are severe enough to require a stay in the hospital, where you'll receive all nutrition intravenously and have your fluids replenished. You'll get the painkillers you need and, when the attack is over, you'll be able to start drinking clear liquids, gradually returning to a normal diet.

If attacks keep recurring, more and more of your pancreatic tissue will be damaged and its normal digestive functions progressively impaired. When that happens, much of the food you eat won't be sufficiently "broken down" (digested) to be absorbed because of the lack of the necessary enzymes. It will pass out through the stool almost intact. Digesting fat is the biggest problem. When the pancreatic enzymes are not available, the stool is loaded with fat—diarrheic, foul smelling, and difficult to flush down the toilet because it floats! That's not only embarrassing if you're using someone else's bathroom, it has serious nutritional implications too. Fat leaving the body in this way takes with it the fat-soluble vitamins—A, D, E, and to some extent K—resulting in their deficiency (see page 24).

If you have chronic pancreatitis, the most important single thing you can do is to stop drinking alcohol—completely and permanently. Some persons with chronic pancreatitis become diabetic because the diseased pancreas cannot make enough insulin. They then usually require insulin or sugar-lowering drugs. The next step is to replace whatever enzymes the pancreas can no longer make. Take them before and during each meal, the dosage depending on how much is naturally available from your body. There are several of these enzymes on the market, but the ones I have used most are Viokase, Pancrease, and Cotazym. Their new formulation in enteric-coated microspheres makes it possible to deliver large amounts with fewer side effects. Although one to three of these capsules before meals and with snacks go a long way toward replacing what's missing, it's not the same as having a normal pancreas. So challenge your pancreas as little as possible with the food you eat, but be sure to get adequate nutrition. You will have to determine just how much of each nutrient you can handle. Don't try to replace all the fat you're losing in the stool because the pancreas simply can't deal with it. The supplemental enzymes can go only so far. An upper limit of 15 percent of calories from fat, mostly from mono- and polyunsaturated fats, is a realistic goal (you'll get animal fat in the protein allotment). The enzymes that digest protein are also in short supply in chronic pancreatitis. As with fat, it will take a process of trial and error to see how much meat, poultry, and fish you can handle comfortably. However, I recommend you limit your *animal* protein intake to 25 to 30 grams daily, or 3 to 4 ounces of lean animal protein such as skinless chicken or fish. I emphasize animal protein because it provides the essential amino acids lacking in vegetable protein, and the latter will be obtained in the carbohydrate allotment described below.

What does this leave you to eat? Carbohydrates, lots and lots of complex carbohydrates prepared without added fat—vegetables, fruits, beans, pasta—the kind of diet that vegans follow. These foods do not require the pancreatic enzymes for digestion, so they must make up the bulk of your diet. Be sure to take a multivitamin containing the fat-soluble vitamins (A, D, E, and K) as well as B_{12}, which is sometimes lacking in people with chronic pancreatitis.

The table on page 356 lists the foods to avoid and those you may eat if you have chronic pancreatitis. You're better off with several smaller meals than fewer larger ones. The table on page 358 is a guide to how much of each kind of food you should consume daily. It reflects a 15 percent fat content and 1,500 calories. If you need more calories, you may eat extra bread and fruit. If your blood level of triglycerides is very high, say, in the hundreds, then omit fruit juice, and limit your intake of fresh fruit to two or three servings per day. Do not have any fat-free sugared desserts. Eat those made with aspartame (NutraSweet) instead. However, they will all be frozen because there is no way to get the aspartame into desserts that have been baked. In short, this is the kind of diet prescribed for diabetics.

There is an interesting twist to the management of this disorder, one that is still controversial, but promising. Elsewhere in this book I have made several references to oxygen-free radicals—the end-products of many energy processes. Oxygen-free radicals are thought to contribute to most of mankind's health problems, ranging from the aging process to cancer to coronary heart disease. And now comes the interesting observation that pancreatitis too may be initiated or aggravated by these metabolic "bandits." Animal experiments in which the pancreas was deliberately injured in order to induce pancreatitis have shown that when animals are pretreated with antioxidants that neutralize free radicals, the degree of damage is minimized. I am not aware of any clinical trials in which large numbers of persons with chronic pancreatitis have been given these antioxidants, but I can tell you this: If I had the problem myself, I would take the following antioxidants—25,000 IU of beta-carotene (15 milligrams), 800 IU of vitamin E, and 1,000 milligrams of vitamin C every day. They may turn out not to have any beneficial impact on chronic pancreatitis, but then what will you have lost?

In summary, chronic pancreatitis is usually the result of excessive alcohol intake or intolerance to it. In some cases, it is due to gallstones or chemical substances or medications that damage the pancreas. Nutritional management consists of total abstinence from alcohol, reducing your fat intake, decreasing the amount of protein you consume, eating mostly complex carbohydrates, and replacing the missing pancreatic enzymes. I also recommend the supplemental antioxidants beta-carotene, vitamin E, and vitamin C.

FOODS TO AVOID AND INCLUDE FOR PEOPLE WITH PANCREATITIS

AVOID	INCLUDE
Avocado	Bread
Bread, waffles, croissants made with cheese and/or eggs	fat-free French
Candy made with nuts, butter, or cream	fat-free Italian
	light, 40 calories/slice

FOODS TO AVOID *(Continued)*

AVOID	INCLUDE
Cream soups	Candy
Creamed vegetables	hard candy
Desserts	jelly beans
cakes	Cereals, nonfat
cookies	Desserts
ice cream	frozen desserts, nonfat
pastries	frozen yogurt, nonfat
pies	fruit gelatin
Doughnuts	fruit ices
Egg yolks	meringues
Fish packed in oil	Egg whites
Meat	Fat-free vegetable soups
bacon	Fish
beef	canned in water
luncheon meats	fresh
sausage	Fresh fruit
veal	Jelly and jam
Peanut butter	Nonfat milk products
Whole milk products	nonfat cottage cheese
butter	nonfat cheeses
cheeses, whole milk	nonfat yogurt
half-and-half	skim milk
heavy cream	Pasta
whipping cream	Poultry
whole milk	skinless chicken
yogurt, regular	skinless turkey
	Rice
	Soups
	defatted broths
	fat-free vegetable
	Vegetables, plain, including potatoes

DAILY SERVINGS OF FOOD FOR PEOPLE WITH PANCREATITIS

FOOD	PORTION	FAT (gm)	CALORIES
Breads/grains/pasta	6 servings	0	480
Desserts, fat-free	1 serving	0	200
Fruits	4 servings	0	240
Oil	2 teaspoons	10	90
Protein	4 ounces	12	200
Skim milk	2 to 3 cups	0	170 to 255
Vegetables	5 servings	0	125
		22	1,505 to 1,590

PARKINSON'S DISEASE

WHEN "GOOD" FOOD AND "HEALTHY"

MULTIVITAMINS CAN HARM YOU!

Doctors do not communicate with their patients the way they used to—and should. Computerized history taking and sophisticated technology have largely replaced the one-on-one, in-depth exchange that was formerly the hallmark of the doctor-patient relationship. The change has been justified in the name of cost-effectiveness. I happen to be old-fashioned. In my opinion, the only doctors who can properly diagnose their patients without asking the right questions and without taking the time to listen to the answers are veterinarians. The following experience emphasizes how true this is.

Several years ago a man with long-standing Parkinson's disease came to me for a routine cardiac examination. He looked awful! His Parkinson's had become very bad. He was drooling and shaking terribly, and could barely get up from his chair. I asked him what medications had been prescribed for his Parkinson's, and I was satisfied that he was taking them as directed. I phoned his neurologist to discuss whether there was anything more to be done. She assured me that the deterioration was "par for the course" and reflected the "natural" history of the disease.

I reviewed the events of the previous few weeks with the patient and his wife and asked whether he had recently had a fever or infection. (Sometimes an unrelated illness can worsen Parkinson's disease.) No, he had not. "Are there any other symptoms I should know about?" I asked. "Well," said his wife, "my husband has begun seeing things that aren't there—like little people on the branches of the trees outside our bedroom. He is also depressed and isn't sleeping too well." "Anything else?" "Not really," the patient himself interjected, "except that I am much more tired than usual, and my appetite is lousy." "The vitamins I've been giving him haven't helped either," added his wife. "They are really strong too. I was sure they'd pep him up." I asked for the name of the vitamin preparation, looked it up, and found that it contained B_6, which some multivitamins do. Vitamin B_6 neutralizes levodopa—the most commonly used anti-Parkinson's drug at that time, which this man was taking regularly! Two weeks after he discontinued the B_6, his symptoms improved considerably. If I hadn't taken the time to elicit this rather ordinary bit of information, his symptoms would have worsened progressively.

Many persons take an over-the-counter multivitamin almost as a matter of course. They feel that the small amounts of vitamins they contain (usually no more than the RDA) can do no harm and—who knows?—may even correct a minor nutritional deficiency of which they may be unaware. But when they're sick, even with something as benign as a cold, or need more energy, or are depressed, they may resort to megavitamins. The difference is that the latter contain much higher doses than do run-of-the-mill multivitamins. For example, the usual dose of vitamin C in a multivitamin ranges from 50 milligrams to 500; someone who feels a cold coming on may take 2,000 milligrams or more. Once symptoms start, they may increase the dosage to as much as 5,000 milligrams. *Those* are megadoses! Megavitamin preparations are also apt to contain additional substances and more trace elements in greater amounts than the usual multivitamin. Megadoses can have mega–side effects. In this particular case, because it was "only a vitamin" and not a "real" medicine, my patient's wife didn't think to tell me that she was giving it to her husband until I asked. Most patients with Parkinson's disease now take levodopa together with carbidopa (Sinemet). *The adverse reaction to vitamin B_6 does not occur when the levodopa is present in this combination.* Some patients, however, still take their levodopa "straight." If you are among them, check the label on your multivitamin bottle to make sure it doesn't contain B_6. The words to look for, besides B₆, are pyridoxine, pyridoxal, and pyridoxa-mine. You should also cut back on your *dietary* intake of this vitamin. The small amount of vitamin B_6 you need (the RDA is 2 milligrams a day for men and 1.6 milligrams for women) is easily obtained from many foods. If you have Parkinson's disease and are on levodopa, consult the list of foods on page 364. A single 3½-ounce portion of braised beef liver contains 0.91 milligram of B_6 and a medium baked potato has 0.7 milligram. Together, these will satisfy the minimum daily requirement and cost you only 381 calories. Three ounces of any whole-grain cereal will also suffice. Do not be *too* stringent in avoiding B_6. Too little will leave you anemic (you'll know when you are because you'll feel cold and tired, and your friends will tell you you look pale) and your skin will become dry, itchy, and scaly.

To appreciate how diet affects Parkinson's disease, you need to understand how this disorder affects the brain. There are some 1.5 million persons with Parkinson's disease in the United States. The usual onset is between the ages of fifty and sixty-five (although I have two such patients in their forties). Men are more often affected than women, and more whites than blacks. The classic symptoms are the characteristic tremor; the shuffling, lurching gait; the eyes that stare and never blink; the rigid limbs; and the expressionless, almost mask-like face. These are all due to the loss of certain pigmented nerve cells (substantia nigra) in the brain that produce a chemical called *dopamine*. These cells are linked by special fibers to another part of the brain (the corpus striatum) that controls movement, posture, balance, and walk-ing. Dopamine is needed for impulses ("messages") to reach the corpus striatum. When the nigra cells that produce it are damaged or destroyed, there is a deficiency of dopamine, the corpus does not receive its signals, and the symptoms of Parkinson's develop. Their severity depends on how much and how quickly dopamine produc-tion has dropped. That differs from patient to patient, which is why the disease is severe and rapidly progressive in some and mild in others.

No one knows what kills the pigmented dopamine-producing brain cells in Parkinson's disease. Since there are no clear-cut genetic factors, the most popular current hypothesis is that the disease is due to an environmental toxin that some people cannot handle. There is no obvious cause in at least 85 percent of cases, but typical symptoms can occur temporarily in persons taking certain tranquilizers such as Compazine, Mellaril, Haldol, Prolixin, and Stelazine. Unlike "natural" Parkinson's, these disappear when the offending drug is discontinued.

There is no way to replace the missing dopamine because of the "blood-brain barrier," which prevents the drug from getting into the brain from the bloodstream. This barrier protects the delicate brain tissues from a variety of toxic agents circulating in the bloodstream, but it's too bad that dopamine is on that "banned" list.

Some thirty years ago it was discovered that an amino acid, levodopa, which *can* cross the blood-brain barrier, is converted to the missing dopamine once it enters the brain. The problem is that it cannot be injected. It must be taken orally. Unfortunately, when it reaches the stomach, enzymes there quickly convert most of it to dopamine, where it does no good. Dopamine prevents Parkinson's only when it is present in the brain. To get enough levodopa into the brain and converted *there* to dopamine, very large doses are required, and these usually cause intolerable side effects. Another landmark discovery improved matters greatly. It was found that when a drug called carbidopa is added to levodopa, the enzymes do not convert the latter to dopamine in the stomach, leaving more of it to enter the brain. The combination of levodopa and carbidopa (marketed as Sinemet) contains 75 percent less levodopa than the pure preparation of the latter drug, thus minimizing its side effects. Sinemet is currently the cornerstone of treatment for Parkinson's disease. *Remember, vitamin B$_6$ has no adverse effects on levodopa as long as it's combined with carbidopa.* So if you have Parkinson's, and because of a nutritional deficiency must have extra B$_6$, be sure to take your levodopa as Sinemet.

When levodopa, either alone or in combination with carbidopa, is taken for anywhere from two to five years, its beneficial effects begin to lessen. Some patients develop the "on-off" phenomenon: Either they suddenly "freeze" in their tracks no matter what they're doing— walking, eating, or just getting out of a chair—or their movements become aggravated, gross, and uncontrollable. They may also hallucinate, as did the patient I described earlier.

Taking "time off" from these drugs, referred to by doctors as a "drug holiday," may improve the on-off phenomenon. Decreasing the dosage of the levodopa will usually abate the excessive movements and hallucinating, but then all the other manifestations of Parkinson's may get worse! Several medications are often helpful. They include

Artane, Cogentin, antihistamines like Benadryl, amantadine (an anti-viral drug), pergolide (Permax), bromocriptine, and Parlodel. A new drug, Eldepryl (deprenyl), shows promise in slowing the loss of dopamine.

You can also try *dietary* manipulation. Here's how it can help. Levodopa is an amino acid, that is, a protein. When taken by mouth together with any other protein, both compete for absorption by the intestine. Because there is a limit to how much protein the gut can absorb in any given digestive session, less levodopa "makes it" to the brain. The same competition for admission among amino acids occurs across the blood-brain barrier. (Nature does not play favorites with its amino acids.) So if you are experiencing the "on-off" phenomenon, the trick is to leave the field clear for the levodopa when you're taking it during the day. That means limiting the protein in your diet between breakfast and dinner to a total of about 7 grams. In that interval, you should avoid eating beef, fish, chicken, lamb, shrimp, veal, beans or legumes, and dairy products, especially cheese. What *can* you eat? The sample menu on page 366 will give you a good idea of how to proceed. Note that you can meet the daily RDA for protein at dinner with just 4 ounces of high-quality protein in fish, chicken, or lean beef. I have recommended juice rather than fruit because many Parkinson's patients have difficulty chewing and swallowing fruit. However, if you are able to do so, you can substitute an apple (which contains only 0.3 grams of protein), or three fresh apricots (1.5 grams), or an orange (1.4 grams). Notice too that by the end of lunchtime you will have consumed only about 6 grams of protein. There is a low-protein pasta available at most markets, but you may have to ask for it. This menu provides a total of about 43 grams of protein for a twenty-four-hour period, which I do not recommend you exceed. You should perceive a noticeable difference in your symptoms of Parkinson's disease within one week after this limitation and redistribution of your protein intake.

I also advise patients with Parkinson's, especially those who shake very badly, to avoid alcohol and caffeine (see the table on page 45 for a list of caffeine-containing foods and beverages), both of which often aggravate the tremor.

Apart from this specific dietary advice, use common sense. Don't attempt a thick New York steak if you have a bad tremor or trouble chewing or swallowing. It's much easier to eat soft, semisolid, or blenderized foods frequently and in small portions during the day.

These are exciting times for people with Parkinson's disease. A great deal of promising research is being conducted at a feverish pace. The most promising areas are the introduction of Eldepryl in its management (this drug makes it possible to delay therapy with Sinemet and to use smaller doses) as well as the implantation of fetal tissue that can make the necessary dopamine. But knowing what to eat and when to do so can make a difference right now.

VITAMIN B$_6$ CONTENT OF FOODS*

FOOD	PORTION	VITAMIN B$_6$ (mg)	CALORIES
Avocado	½ medium	0.24	153
Banana	1 medium	0.66	105
Beans/legumes			
black beans, cooked	1 cup	0.12	227
chickpeas, cooked	1 cup	0.23	269
green peas, cooked	½ cup	0.17	67
kidney beans, cooked	1 cup	0.21	225
lentils, cooked	1 cup	0.35	231
lima beans, cooked	1 cup	0.30	217
navy beans, cooked	1 cup	0.30	259
soybeans, cooked	1 cup	0.40	298
split peas, cooked	1 cup	0.09	231
Beef/pork			
beef kidney, cooked	3.5 ounces	0.52	144
beef liver, braised	3.5 ounces	0.91	161
ground beef, extra-lean, broiled	3.5 ounces	0.27	256
beef round, lean, roasted	3.5 ounces	0.38	175
pork center loin, broiled	3.5 ounces	0.47	231
pork tenderloin, lean, roasted	3.5 ounces	0.42	166

*Note: Check labels to determine if a food has been enriched with B$_6$. The key words to look for are pyridoxine, pyridoxal, and pyridoxamine.

VITAMIN B₆ CONTENT OF FOODS* *(Continued)*

FOOD	PORTION	VITAMIN B₆ (mg)	CALORIES
Bread			
wheat	1 slice	0.03	61
white	1 slice	0.01	64
whole wheat	1 slice	0.05	155
Brewer's yeast	1 tablespoon	16	40
Cereals			
All-Bran (Kellogg's)	⅓ cup	0.50	70
Branflakes (Kellogg's)	¾ cup	0.50	90
Cheerios	1¼ cups	0.50	110
Extra-Fortified Oatmeal (Quaker)	1-ounce packet	2	95
Raisin Bran (Kellogg's)	¾ cup	0.50	120
wheat bran	½ cup	0.39	65
wheat germ, toasted (Kretschmer)	¼ cup	0.16	103
Chicken			
breast, no skin, roasted	½ breast	0.51	142
light and dark meat, no skin, roasted	3.5 ounces	0.47	190
Fish			
flounder, cooked	3 ounces	0.20	99
herring, Atlantic, cooked	3 ounces	0.30	172
mackerel, cooked	3 ounces	0.43	114
pollack, Atlantic, cooked	3 ounces	0.28	100
salmon, Atlantic, cooked	3 ounces	0.80	155
swordfish, cooked	3 ounces	0.32	132
tuna canned in water	3 ounces	0.30	99

VITAMIN B₆ CONTENT OF FOODS* *(Continued)*

FOOD	PORTION	VITAMIN B$_6$ (mg)	CALORIES
Grains/Flour			
brown rice, long-grain, cooked	1 cup	0.28	216
white rice, long-grain, cooked	1 cup	0.19	264
whole wheat flour	1 cup	0.41	407
Potato, baked with skin	1 medium	0.70	220
Tofu			
raw	½ cup	0.06	94
raw, firm	½ cup	0.12	183

SAMPLE MENU FOR PEOPLE WITH PARKINSON'S DISEASE

	PORTION	PROTEIN (gm)
Breakfast		
Cream of wheat cereal	½ cup	2
Apricot nectar	8 ounces	0.9
Low-protein toast	unlimited	—
Jelly or jam	unlimited	0
Butter or tub margarine	unlimited	0
Sugar or sugar substitute	unlimited	0
Nondairy creamer (for cereal and coffee/tea)	1 cup	0.5
Decaf coffee or herb tea	1 cup	0
Lunch		
Cream of cauliflower soup	1 cup	1.5
Low-protein pasta with herbs	unlimited	—
Olive oil, for pasta	1 tablespoon	0
Lettuce salad, chopped or diced	1 cup	1
Olive oil, for salad	1 tablespoon	0
Caffeine-free soda	12 ounces	0
Snack		
Apple juice	6 ounces	0

SAMPLE MENU *(Continued)*

	PORTION	PROTEIN (gm)
Dinner		
Grilled chicken breast, skinless	4 ounces	28
White rice	½ cup	2.0
V8 juice	6 ounces	1.3
Steamed carrots	½ cup	0.9
Fruit ice pop	2 ounces	0
Snack		
Low-fat flavored yogurt	½ cup	4.5

PEPTIC ULCERS

YOU MEAN I'M INFECTED,

NOT NERVOUS?

The complete turnabout in doctors' understanding and management of peptic ulcers should be required reading for every medical student and practitioner. It is a humbling experience. We doctors can be so dogmatic, so authoritarian, so "know-it-all," so often intolerant of skepticism concerning any therapy that has the official seal of approval from the "establishment." Yet every now and then, it turns out that some medication we have been prescribing routinely, or advice we have been giving with the best of intentions and based on "incontrovertible" scientific evidence, is completely wrong! So it's important for doctors (and patients too) always to remain critical, to take nothing for granted, to welcome intelligent challenges to traditional approaches, and to be receptive to new ideas.

Until very recently, ulcers were believed to have a "psychiatric" cause—the plague of nervous people. "My boss (or husband or wife) is driving me up the wall. Unless I change jobs (or get a divorce), I'm going to have an ulcer." Guess what? That's all hogwash! Of course, you may have sleepless nights, or feel anxious or depressed because of your work or home situation, but neither your boss nor your spouse can give you an ulcer. If you do develop one, it will probably not be from frustration or other emotion.

But surely diet is important, isn't it? Won't that hot chili and all the other spices and acids you eat and drink erode your stomach lining? Surprise! They won't! For years we believed that what we ate either produced ulcers or at least made them worse. Patients with severe stomach ulcers were sometimes even fed rectally to rest their upper intestinal tract! There were other fallacies too, some of which persist to this day. Here are a few of the more popular ones: (1) "Ulcer patients should eat frequently." Although some patients do feel better doing so, it's a very individual matter and frequent small meals do not agree with every ulcer patient. (2) "Drink lots of milk." Wrong thing to do! The protein in the milk stimulates acid production in the stomach, making matters worse! (3) "Avoid spicy foods." Nonsense! Although, as you will see below, some foods should be used sparingly, they do not include the traditional villains.

The term *ulcer* refers to a break in the internal lining of any organ in the body. Ulcers form in the mouth, skin, vagina, that is, in virtually every lining or tissue in the body. *Peptic* refers to its occurrence either in the stomach itself or in the first portion of the small intestine that immediately follows it — the duodenum. Think of the upper gastrointestinal tract as a J-shaped organ, most of which consists of stomach, except for the end of the loop that is the duodenum. Before it is determined exactly where on the J an ulcer is located, it's referred to as "peptic." If it turns out to be in the stomach, it's called "gastric"; when it involves the uppermost portion of the small intestine, it's "duodenal."

Men have twice the incidence of duodenal ulcers as women, and the numbers peak for men between the ages of forty-five and sixty-four years. In women the disease is most frequent after age fifty-five. You're more likely to develop an ulcer if you have chronic lung disease, cirrhosis of the liver, or rheumatoid arthritis, or if it runs in your family.

Cancers rarely, if ever, form in the duodenum, but they do in the stomach where they can mimic the appearance of an ulcer. That's why every stomach ulcer must be biopsied and then carefully reexamined at three- to four-week intervals until it is completely healed. (Some "gastric" ulcers are probably cancerous right along, but the diagnosis is missed.)

We used to put all the blame for peptic ulcers on too much stomach acid. It was believed that the mucus covering the stomach lining could resist normal amounts of acid but not high concentrations. So for decades treatment consisted *solely* of antacids to neutralize excessive gastric acid. You must have some stomach acid to develop an ulcer, but it needn't be too much. In fact, most persons with ulcers have normal stomach acid content, but their problem is that *any* quantity can erode their stomach lining (mucosa). *Whether or not you develop an ulcer depends on the ability of the mucosa to resist the corrosive action of acid in any amount*—large *or* small, and that resistance is due to a variety of different factors. (Gastric acid is made by special cells found only in the stomach, and it spills over into the neighboring duodenum. The small intestine beyond the duodenum is not vulnerable to acid ulceration.)

With conventional treatment, 80 percent of ulcers will recur within six to twelve months; almost all flare up again within two years. We never really understood why they kept coming back, despite all the available drugs and diets. The reason is obvious today! Many "run-of-the-mill" duodenal ulcers, and some gastric ones too, are due to infection by a bacterium called *Helicobacter pylori*. Nearly 40 percent of healthy people harbor this organism in their upper intestinal tract, and it is present in 50 to 90 percent of patients with duodenal ulcers and gastric ulcers. But you've got to look for it. One way to do so (with 95 percent accuracy) is to take a biopsy of the ulcer area with the small forceps at the end of a tube (endoscope), which is passed down the food pipe. But there are now equally dependable breath and blood tests that will identify the presence of the organism too.

In my own practice, I prescribe bismuth, antibiotics (tetracycline or amoxicillin), and Flagyl for ten to fourteen days to anyone with a peptic ulcer and documented *H. pylori* infection. But treating the infection alone is not enough. The mucosa must also be protected by reducing the amount of gastric acid in the environment that can penetrate it, and that's done by a variety of methods. Drugs for this purpose include the H2 blockers, which stop the stomach cells from making acid in the first place (there are many from which to choose but the prototypes are Zantac, Tagamet, and Pepcid); Prilosec (omeprazole); antacids to neutralize whatever acid is present; and sucralfate, a drug that coats the ulcer and helps protect it from further damage by acid in its environment.

Is *H. pylori* catching? The fact that it's contagious would explain why several members of one family often have the disease, and why it is so common in areas of poor hygiene. But we don't know how or by what route it is transmitted.

Although the discovery of the H2 blockers and the availability of new and more powerful suppressors of acid secretion such as Prilosec have made diet less important in the management of peptic ulcers, there are specific foods and chemicals you should avoid that stimulate the acid-producing cells in the stomach. Others that neutralize whatever acid is present and perhaps even enhance the resistance of the lining itself should be favored. Let's look at some of them.

Salt (among Asians, soy sauce is the main culprit) and refined sugar may be bad for people with ulcers. I advise my ulcer patients to stop smoking, cut down salt intake (see page 248 a list of foods and beverages high in sodium), and reduce the amount of sugar in their diet. It may surprise you to learn that, in the interval between ulcer attacks, alcohol *in moderation* does not harm the stomach lining nor does milk protect it. You can decrease your chances of ever developing an ulcer by eating at least two slices of bread and at least 25 grams of fiber every day. Details of such a diet are described on page 120. Basically, it involves substituting white bread with whole-grain bread, eating whole-grain pasta whenever possible, starting your day with shredded wheat or bran or cooked oatmeal instead of corn flakes, and consuming at least three servings of fresh fruit *and* raw vegetables every day.

Remember how you worried about preparing a bland diet for a dinner guest who had an ulcer? The truth is that bland diets do not help ulcers at any stage. Indeed, at least one study has shown that they are associated with a higher rate of recurrence than normal diets. By the same token, spicy foods, even peppers (black, red, and chili) will neither cause nor aggravate an ulcer. Indeed, eating peppers every day may be protective! However, any foods or spices that, in your experience, provoke or worsen your symptoms should be avoided.

If you're having an *acute* attack of ulcers, there are certain dietary guidelines to follow. Do not drink coffee, *regular or decaffeinated,* both of which stimulate the production of stomach acid; do not consume any alcoholic beverages, especially beer or the 80-proof variety. Inasmuch as most bland diets have little or no fiber, they may actually be detrimental, since fiber is protective to the entire intestinal tract. I am amazed at how often hospitals, even today, continue to feed patients "ulcer diets"—frequent feedings of milk, cream, and eggs throughout the day. They will put pounds on you and raise your cholesterol, but will do nothing for your ulcer. The theory that such feedings neutralize stomach acid is all wrong. Whatever buffering effect they have is offset by the increase in stomach acid secretion that they stimulate. Even though frequent feedings do you no good, overeating at a meal distends the stomach and worsens ulcer symptoms. Ulcer patients used to be told to have a snack at bedtime in order to neutralize stomach acid and prevent it from eroding the stomach during the night. Wrong again! You're better off not having any food after your evening meal because that stimulates the production of more acid. Take a swig of liquid antacid instead. Cigarettes and ulcers don't mix because tobacco is a powerful stimulus to stomach acid secretion. People with ulcers usually avoid fruit juices because of their citric acid content. The word *acid* frightens them. Although three or four glasses of orange or grapefruit juice at one sitting may give you an upset stomach, citric acid has no effect on an ulcer one way or another. The cardinal rule for people with peptic ulcers is to avoid any food or liquid that they know from previous experience causes them distress.

The incidence of peptic ulcers has decreased significantly in the past few years and one of the reasons may be the increasing substitution of saturated fats by vegetable oils. Vegetable oils contain linoleic acid, a precursor of prostaglandin, which protects the lining of the intestinal tract. The reason aspirin and the NSAIDs (nonsteroidal antiinflammatory drugs) cause bleeding when used regularly and frequently is not so much because of irritation of the mucosa due to direct contact, but rather as a result of their antiprostaglandin action. Another possible reason for the decreasing incidence of peptic ulcer is the increased consumption of dietary fiber.

Are there any foods that, if eaten regularly, will prevent ulcers? I'm not sure. Bananas are said to thicken the lining of the stomach, making it more resistant to erosion by acid. Powder from unripe plantains, a member of the banana family, is also said to be protective against gastric, but not duodenal, ulcers.

The yeast in yogurt is bactericidal, that is, it kills the *Helicobacter* within forty-five minutes after contact. But to completely eradicate the organism, you still need antibiotics. Since yogurt remains in the stomach and duodenum for at least forty-five minutes, have a cup (make sure it contains active cultures) three or four times a day if you have a peptic ulcer. And here's something that just occurred to me. You may be able to kill two birds with one stone by eating *banana* yogurt!

In summary, potent antacids and medications that block the production of gastric acid effectively treat ulcer *symptoms*. *However,* it's extremely important to eradicate any documented underlying infection by *Helicobacter pylori,* which is often the primary cause of this disease. Contrary to "time-honored advice," you should avoid milk, cream, and bedtime feedings, all of which stimulate the production of gastric acid. During the acute stage, keep away from cigarettes, alcohol, and coffee, both regular and decaffeinated. Add bananas or plantain dishes to your diet, and eat a cupful of yogurt three or four times a day for a couple of weeks. Your diet should be rich in fiber, and for all kinds of other good reasons, low in salt and refined sugar. A combined medical and dietary approach should shorten the course of your ulcer and reduce the frequency of its recurrence.

PORPHYRIA

A SWEET SOLUTION

A thirty-seven-year-old woman came to see me the other day with a whole list of seemingly unrelated complaints. For example, in the past few months she'd had attacks of pain in her belly that were occasionally so severe she thought she would die; at other times, they hardly bothered her at all. When I asked her to show me where it hurt, she said there wasn't any one place in particular. Sometimes the spasms were in the middle of the abdomen, but she'd also felt them high up or low down. Frustrated, I asked on which side they occurred. Either the right or the left. Did these attacks come on after eating? Not necessarily. Had she noticed any change in her bowel habits? No. Two other statements also puzzled me: Her appetite had remained intact, and she had not lost any weight.

The young woman's symptoms didn't ring a diagnostic bell. I felt a little better about not being able to help this patient when she admitted that I was the fifth doctor she had consulted in as many months. The other four had put her through the wringer with every imaginable test—abdominal sonograms, CT scans, and MRIs—and she'd given enough blood to supply a blood bank. To make her point, she handed me a thick manila folder full of test results that I reviewed very carefully. They were all normal!

We went over her symptoms again—this time in greater detail. I have made more diagnoses over the years by listening to patients than from putting them through all kinds of expensive tests. The only other symptom I was able to elicit was occasional slight fever, never higher than 101 degrees, and rarely lasting longer than a few hours. That was it as far as her story was concerned.

It was now time for the physical exam. Her temperature was normal, and so were her heart, lungs, and lymph glands. Her blood pressure was slightly elevated, but that was to be expected because I was a new doctor, and she was very worried. I paid special attention to her abdomen, which was tender wherever I pressed on it—high up, low down, left side and right. However, I couldn't feel any lumps, and her liver, spleen, and kidneys were not enlarged. Her gynecologic exam was also normal. When I was through, I drew blood that I planned to have extensively tested and asked her to leave a urine specimen. I promised to call my patient as soon as all the results were in. Frankly, at this point, I was stumped, but there was something about her story that rang true. I was convinced that she *was* sick! We said good-bye, and she took her specimen cup to the bathroom, and then went home.

When one of my patients leaves a urine specimen, my lab technician collects it from the bathroom and tests it immediately. Urine is best examined when it's fresh. However, instead of using the patients' toilet, which is where the technician would normally have found her specimen, this woman went to the staff bathroom. Her urine specimen sat there unnoticed until the next morning, when a technician went to wash her hands. She took one look at the container and rushed it to me. The reason for her excitement was that this specimen was not the usual yellow color. It was black! Suddenly I had my diagnosis!

Porphyria is the only condition in which urine left standing overnight turns black. All this woman's bizarre complaints now made perfect sense. I couldn't wait to give my patient the good news. I phoned her at home and shouted, "Mrs. Jones, this is Dr. Rosenfeld. I think you have acute porphyria." A stony silence was followed by, "That's not the opinion for which I consulted you," and she hung up. We've laughed about her response many times since after she told me that she thought it inappropriate for me to have told her at the time that she had a "cute" anything! (A doctor friend of mine had a similiar reaction from a woman when he informed her that she had "acute angina.")

Porphyria is a congenital disorder, an "inborn error of metabolism," which occurs in five to ten of every 100,000 people. It creates a problem with an enzyme system that, among other functions, controls pigment formation in the body. (That's the reason some of these patients have skin rashes too.) However, porphyria can also come on after exposure to a variety of different substances, most commonly barbiturates, sulfa drugs, griseofulvin, Dilantin (used for the prevention of seizure disorders), methyldopa (a blood pressure–lowering medication), several antidepressants, and certain antibiotics. Exposure to unusual stress can also do it, as will a crash diet or fasting for a day or more. The disease has many faces. It can affect virtually any organ, but favors the skin, liver, or nerves. This particular patient had random abdominal pain because of nerve involvement in that area.

The most common form of the disease is called "acute intermittent porphyria" (which is what my patient had). These individuals can go for years without any symptoms and then suddenly an attack occurs "out of the blue." Very often, however, "out of the blue" turns out to have been the result of one of the medications mentioned above or a change in eating habits. We don't really understand what triggers these attacks, but if you or other members of your family are known to have the disease, do not fast or embark on a stringent diet. If you experience strange belly symptoms or shooting pains in various parts of your body, think of porphyria. Don't be shy about suggesting the diagnosis to your doctor, either. I'd have welcomed a clue from my patient! If in addition to random bursts of pain you also have high blood pressure and an occasional low-grade fever, and someone else in your family has similar symptoms, then the possibility of porphyria is a very real one indeed. The clincher is the appearance of dark urine, most apparent after it has been left standing for several hours.

There is currently no cure for porphyria, but there are medications to help its symptoms. Given the progress being made in gene therapy, it's more than likely that a permanent solution will be found in the foreseeable future. But in the meantime, eating a very-high-carbohydrate diet, between 300 and 600 grams a day, can help prevent acute attacks. You're better off focusing on complex carbohydrates rather than simple sugar (especially if you are diabetic). Such a diet requires eating frequently, and means 4 calories for every gram. The sample menu below indicates what you'd have to consume daily to satisfy an intake of at least 300 grams (the low end of the scale for porphyria) of complex carbohydrate. Note that this diet includes seven servings of fruit, 3 cups of skim milk (to keep the fat content and calories to a minimum), and ten portions of complex carbohydrate such as bread, pasta, and cereal. There will be times when you simply do not feel like eating that much, in which event you will need concentrated sugar drinks to provide the necessary amount of carbohydrate. But man cannot live by sugar alone. You'll need a little fat and some protein as well, depending on your energy requirements. Six ounces daily of lean protein such as fish or chicken, and 1 or 2 tablespoons of olive oil should be enough. One final caveat. This regimen will reduce the frequency of your porphyria attacks, but you run the risk of gaining weight unless you embark on a regular exercise program to use up all those extra calories.

SAMPLE DAILY CARBOHYDRATE INTAKE FOR PEOPLE WITH PORPHYRIA (300 GRAMS)

FOOD	PORTION	CARBOHYDRATE (gm)	CALORIES
Bagel	1 large	61.8	250
Apple juice	8 ounces (2 servings)	29	116
Pasta, dry	4 ounces	83.6	420
Banana	1 medium (2 servings)	30	120
Grapes	15	15	60
Shredded wheat cereal	2 ounces	45.2	204
Raisins	⅓ cup (2 servings)	39.2	148
Skim milk	3 cups	36	270
		339.8	1,588

WHEN YOU'RE PREGNANT

TWO MUST EAT BETTER THAN ONE

Women hear so much these days about what *not* to consume when they're pregnant—no alcohol, no tobacco, no coffee—that they may forget how important it is to eat the *right* foods in the *right* amounts to better their chances of having a healthy baby! I must confess to a sense of guilt in writing this section, because I know that some of my recommendations are beyond the reach of many underprivileged women in this, the richest nation on earth. What follows in these pages will make a difference only if every pregnant woman receives prenatal care, can obtain (buy or be given) the proper nutrition to help nourish her growing fetus, and understands the importance of doing so. I also want to emphasize that these are general guidelines; I encourage every pregnant woman to work with her doctor to develop an eating plan that's best for her.

Eating for a healthy pregnancy should start *before* conception. That's often easier said than done because many pregnancies aren't planned. Some women are not aware that they are pregnant until well into the second month. If they were on a diet, not paying particular attention to their nutrition, and not taking any prenatal vitamins, their fetus may be short-changed. What you eat before your pregnancy and during its first twelve weeks helps determine how well your child's immune system develops, how healthy he or she will be, and, indeed, can even help prevent a miscarriage. So if you are trying to start or enlarge your family, don't diet. Forget about your waistline for now. Once you're pregnant, that measurement will become academic anyway.

Even if you are convinced that *fasting* now and then is good for you because it eliminates accumulated toxins (I am not personally aware of any evidence that this is so), never fast while pregnant! No matter how well nourished you are, even if you are fat with seemingly inexhaustible energy reserves on which to draw, fasting for only twenty-four hours can lower your blood sugar and increase its ketone level (ketones are toxic by-products of fat metabolism)—both of which can hurt the fetus. If you are a religious Jew and feel guilty about violating the fast on Yom Kipper, or are Muslim and celebrating Ramadan, a letter from your obstetrician to your rabbi or mullah should get you off the hook and allow you to continue a proper, uninterrupted nutrition plan for you and your baby.

Years ago, obstetricians used to advise patients to limit their total weight gain during pregnancy to fifteen pounds in an attempt to lower the incidence of toxemia (the high blood pressure that develops in some women in the third trimester). They arrived at that figure by allowing seven and a half pounds for the baby, and two pounds each for the amniotic fluid, larger uterus, engorged breasts, and increased volume of blood in the body. I also suspect they wanted the mother to give birth to a small baby in order to ensure an easier delivery for her, the baby, and themselves! But pregnant women who gain less than twenty pounds are more likely to give birth to low-weight infants who don't do as well in the long run. So the guidelines have been changed. Putting on enough weight during pregnancy is normal, natural, and necessary to provide enough nutrition, not only for your own metabolism, which is working overtime, but to sustain the fetus and promote its growth. Doctors now advise a three- or four-pound weight gain in the first trimester and three or four pounds per month during the rest of the pregnancy, for a total of twenty-five to thirty pounds. But remember, these are only suggestions—not hard-and-fast rules—and there is room for flexibility. For example, if you were overweight before you became pregnant, your limit should be twenty to twenty-five pounds; if you were thin to begin with, a weight gain of as much as thirty-five pounds may be desirable; if you are "growing" twins, your target weight gain should be thirty-five to forty-five pounds. Where does all this weight go? The baby accounts for about eight pounds; the rest is in your enlarging breasts and uterus, the extra body fat upon which you will draw when nursing, retained fluid, the placenta, and the amniotic sac.

Pregnancy usually requires 300 extra calories per day, every day. That generally means 2,500 calories daily for women under thirty-five years of age, and 2,000 if you are older than thirty-five. But these numbers are only guidelines and will vary with your body build, the rate at which you are gaining weight, and your level of physical activity.

Make sure that your daily menu includes (1) six or more servings of fruit and vegetables (a serving of fresh fruit usually consists of one piece, say an apple or a pear, but only half a banana; a serving of canned fruit or fruit juice without added sugar is ½ cup; a serving of raw vegetables equals 1 full cup, but only ½ cup if cooked); (2) seven or more servings of whole-grain or enriched bread, grains, and cereal (one slice of whole-grain bread or 1 ounce by weight is a serving; a serving of hot cereal consists of ½ cup, but if it's cold and ready to eat, you'll need ¾ cup); (3) four or more servings of milk or milk products, with 1 cup of milk or yogurt equaling a serving; (4) four or more servings of meat, poultry, fish, eggs, nuts, dried beans, and legumes (a serving of beans, peas, or lentils is generally ⅓ cup; a serving of meat, poultry, or fish is 1 ounce; and 1 egg is equal to 1 serving). You should consume a minimum of 1,500 milligrams of calcium, easily obtained in 4 cups of milk daily—skim, low-fat, or whole, as well as yogurt—which will also provide 32 grams of high-quality protein. (For the calcium content of foods, see page 342.)

You'll need at least 60 grams of protein daily, more if there are any special problems as, for example, if the pregnancy was unplanned and you are undernourished because you were dieting before it happened, or you are an adolescent and still growing, or you have a history of previous miscarriages (some doctors recommend up to 100 grams of protein).

While you're focusing on all that food, don't forget the fluid. Drink at least eight 8-ounce glasses of water to meet your pregnancy needs. You will enjoy it more if you add some lime or lemon juice. Saccharin may be teratogenic (induce birth defects), and should be avoided. Lead is harmful to the fetus, so don't use ceramic mugs. Some leach lead, especially when filled with hot beverages such as tea or coffee, or other hot, acidic liquids such as tomato soup. Do not store heavy wines in lead crystal for the same reason. There are kits you can buy that detect lead leaching from ceramic wear, but they may miss small quantities. For more information about these kits, contact the FDA at (301) 443-4667. There is also a National Lead Information Center with a toll-free number: (800) LEAD-FYI or (800) 532-3394.

If you're a vegetarian, is it okay to eschew meat during your pregnancy? If you are a strict vegan (that is, you eat no animal foods or their derivatives and consume only fruit, nuts, seeds, legumes, and vegetables), you may safely continue your diet even after you are pregnant provided you take at least 2.2 micrograms of supplemental vitamin B_{12} per day. Unless you do, your breast-fed infant may be at risk for B_{12} deficiency. Your baby will probably weigh a little less than average at birth anyway, but should be normal in all other respects. The table on page 389 contains a list of foods from vegetarian and nonvegetarian sources that are rich in vitamin B_{12}. Many vegetarians mistakenly believe that fermented foods such as sauerkraut, sourdough bread, and pickles contain enough B_{12} to meet their needs during pregnancy. That's a myth! They are not good sources at all, for which reason they are not even listed on page 389.

Vegetarian or not, in order to meet all your vitamin and mineral needs, start taking a prenatal supplement (always with meals to ensure maximum absorption) containing zinc, iron, magnesium, vitamins A, B, and C, and folic acid *before you become pregnant*. Infants of women who take multivitamin pills containing *folic acid* at the time of conception have only half the expected or usual rate of birth defects. This vitamin is so important that the FDA has proposed making it mandatory for food manufacturers to add it to grain products in order to prevent birth defects. This important B vitamin is used to supplement enriched flours, breads, rolls, buns, corn grits, cornmeal, farina, rice, and noodles. Most prenatal supplements contain iron because it was always believed that pregnant women need amounts over and above what is present in iron-rich foods to ensure the development of healthy blood cells in the infant. We are no longer sure about that, and some doctors don't insist on additional iron except for women whose nutrition is poor or who clearly have iron-deficiency anemia. If you do not consume enough iron, either in your diet or in supplements, nature gives priority to the fetus, drawing on your iron stores and leaving you anemic. (Do not take any antacids within three hours of ingesting iron in any form, whether by supplement or in foods, because antacids interfere with its absorption.) My own recommendation at this time is for all women who are pregnant or trying to be to take 30 milligrams of supplemental iron (just to be sure) and 400 micrograms (0.4 milligrams) of folic acid—the latter to prevent abnormalities of the brain and nervous system.

It has recently been observed that diets deficient in iron may also lack zinc (found in meat, liver, seafood, eggs, and nuts). Pregnant women whose zinc intake was less than half the RDA (6 milligrams during pregnancy) are twice as likely to deliver premature or underweight babies. That's why you'll find zinc in your prenatal vitamin. But don't take more prenatal vitamins than recommended on the bottle or by your obstetrician. Too much vitamin A, for example, can result in birth defects. In any event, keep in close touch with your doctor throughout your pregnancy so that he or she can adjust your nutritional needs, which vary at different stages of your pregnancy.

The Surgeon General of the United States advises *no alcohol* for the entire forty weeks of gestation because it can cause birth defects, including fetal alcohol syndrome. Some doctors I know permit their patients to have one glass of wine a week. I am not aware of any studies proving that this small amount is harmful, but I'd go along with the Surgeon General just to be on the safe side.

For your own health and that of your baby, *tobacco,* which is not a food even when it's chewed, should be stopped. This is a good time for you to break this lethal habit—permanently. Most women are sufficiently motivated to do so when pregnant. Psychological support from your spouse, your family, your doctor, or a psychologist may be necessary if you find it hard to do on your own. I am opposed to the use of the nicotine patch or nicotine gum at this time because it exposes the fetus to a constant and committed, though possibly lower, level of nicotine.

Then there is the perennial question of *coffee*. Should pregnant women abstain completely, moderate their intake, or drink as much as they like? Caffeine, a stimulant, is present not only in coffee but also in chocolate, cocoa, colas, tea, and several "cold" remedies that you can buy without a prescription. It frequently provides a needed boost in energy, especially for mothers who must look after toddler number one while incubating toddler number two. But is it safe? Coffee-drinking mothers do tend to be more anemic, and their infants generally weigh less at birth. According to the National Institutes of Health, a limit of three 8-ounce cups of coffee per day is *not* associated with a higher risk of abortion or retardation. But that's not what Canadian researchers think. They have found that as little as ½ cup of coffee daily the month *before* becoming pregnant raised the miscarriage rate by 29 percent. Every additional cup during pregnancy was responsible for an additional 22 percent increase. I do not, at this point, know who is right, but for your own peace of mind, you had better consume as little caffeine as possible while you're pregnant! (For a list of caffeine-containing foods, see page 311.) Sexual intercourse more than once a week during the twenty-third to twenty-sixth weeks apparently also reduces the risk of preterm delivery! So if you haven't been able to reduce your coffee intake as much as you should, you might consider that protective activity—with your doctor's okay and assuming, of course, that you do not have a vaginal infection. Caffeine is also a mild diuretic, so increase your daily fluid intake from eight glasses to ten to compensate for the extra fluid loss if you insist on drinking three or more cups of coffee a day. (Remember, too, if you are breast-feeding, that caffeine makes its way into breast milk, and so the baby drinks it too!) Here's a tip for coffee addicts. An easy way to reduce your caffeine intake by half and still enjoy the taste of coffee is to prepare a fifty-fifty mix of water-processed, decaffeinated, fresh-ground coffee with regular ground coffee.

Fish is good for you, and I advise my pregnant patients to eat at least three servings a week. It's an excellent source of low-fat protein. Mind you, I worry these days about possible contamination of some fresh-water fish such as lake trout and bass by chlorinated hydrocarbon pesticides and industrial chemicals (PCBs). Some consumers can spot a bad fish every time. My wife and daughter are such experts. They never order any fish sight unseen. They look at the eyes to see if they are clear; they check out the gills to make sure they are red; and they smell it. I am no such authority and, if you're not either, ask your supplier where his or her fish come from and then check the pollution status of those waters with the local health department. Better still, call a seafood specialist at the FDA. The hot line for all fifty states and Puerto Rico is (800) FDA-4010; the Washington, D.C., metropolitan area number is (202) 205-4314. Any questions you have about buying, storing, or labeling seafood will be expertly answered.

Unfortunately, pregnant women are still often advised to remove the salt shaker from the table and to avoid salt as much as possible, especially if their feet are a little puffy. The truth is that you need salt when you're pregnant because of an increase in normal body fluid volume; the fetus requires extra salt too, as does the amniotic fluid. So unless you have heart failure, or the kind of high blood pressure that is salt dependent, or any other condition mandating salt restriction, use the amount of salt you need in cooking and at the table to make your meals tasty, and make sure you consume at least 2 grams per day. But do avoid frankly salty foods.

Any woman who develops diabetes during pregnancy (it usually occurs in the last trimester and has nothing to do with how much sugar she has been eating) must be closely monitored for the duration of the pregnancy. *Gestational diabetes,* as this disorder is called, is identical to the non–insulin-dependent diabetes that occurs in adults (see page 129) and is treated in much the same way—avoidance of simple sugars combined with exercise. Limiting weight gain is important if you are found to have a high blood sugar level during pregnancy. Check with your doctor. Even though this complication often clears up after delivery, you should have your sugar monitored regularly in the ensuing years because at least 20 percent of women who develop diabetes during pregnancy redevelop it within ten years.

As many as 92 percent of women use at least one medication during pregnancy; the average take three to five. Two-thirds of these drugs are taken in the first trimester, when the risk to the fetus is greatest; 68 percent are over the counter and thus unmonitored, while 32 percent are prescription items. Most are painkillers, antispasm medications for "indigestion," antibiotics, cough mixtures, antacids, and cold and allergy preparations. Relatively few of these drugs have been studied for their effect on the fetus. Aspirin, for example, alone or in combination, is probably the most widely taken medication in pregnancy and, although it is probably safe when used now and then, a link between frequent dosing and birth defects has not been ruled out. You are better off using Tylenol (acetaminophen), which does the job as well and may be safer. Nasal congestion is very common during pregnancy and difficult to treat. Do not use decongestants in the first trimester if your blood pressure is high; try a "dose" of chicken soup instead.

Here is the bottom line with respect to medications. Review all of them with your doctor, especially those you were taking "routinely" for whatever reason before you became pregnant, and that includes antihistamines, aspirin, and megavitamins. Don't forget to mention both prescription and over-the-counter drugs, no matter how commonplace or innocuous they appear to be. Set aside for the duration those that are not absolutely necessary. Your obstetrician can provide you with a list of drugs known to be safe and those to avoid, but it's wise to assume that every one is best left in its container until after the baby is born.

Nonpregnant women, ages twenty-five to fifty, require 150 micrograms of dietary iodine daily. The RDA during pregnancy is somewhat higher—175 micrograms a day. The richest food sources are shellfish such as clams, lobster, and oysters, a 3-ounce serving of which provides about 100 micrograms. Other saltwater fish, especially sardines, also contain lots of iodine. Pregnant women should always make certain that their salt is iodized (1 teaspoon of iodized salt contains 400 micrograms of iodine).

Then there is the matter of *constipation*. Bowel movements can slow down during pregnancy, frequently because of iron supplements, some of which are more constipating than others. A change in brand may have a salutary effect. Don't try to solve the problem with laxatives; enemas aren't good for you either, especially late in the pregnancy. You are better off managing your constipation by drinking more fluids and eating extra bran and wheat fiber.

Even though it is referred to as *morning sickness*, the nausea experienced by some women early in pregnancy can occur at any time of day. It can be so debilitating as to require hospitalization for some fifty-five thousand pregnant women every year. Some doctors believe it is nature's way of cutting your appetite so that you eat less of the foods that can harm the fetus. As proof, they point to the fact that women with morning sickness have fewer abnormal births than those who sail through the first trimester with a hearty appetite! On the other hand, submitting to your cravings may be the right thing to do, even if it means eating "junk" food. Recently, sweet lemonade and potato chips were found to minimize the symptoms of morning sickness. They provide the additional benefit of making you thirsty so that you drink more water and thus prevent fetal dehydration. If you are sick to your stomach day after day, eat small, protein-rich meals—and stay away from medication. If you're nauseated, you'll find that you can keep hot or cold drinks down more easily than those that are lukewarm. My mother (who gave birth to two healthy and quite remarkable sons—my brother, John, and me) advised my pregnant wife to prevent morning sickness by keeping salty crackers on her night table and eating one or two before getting out of bed in the morning. She (my mother, that is) tells me that it worked!

If you are constantly burping and have chronic indigestion, antacids will provide relief, but never take them with your iron supplement, whose absorption they block. Better yet, try eating smaller amounts more frequently rather than three large meals a day. Remember that the pregnant uterus pushes up on the diaphragm (the muscle that separates the chest from the abdomen), causing increased pressure on the stomach and food pipe. That familiar feeling of fullness is more pronounced when the stomach is loaded with food.

I came across an interesting explanation of why some women habitually go into labor too early and deliver babies of low birthweight, i.e., less than five and a half pounds. Labor begins when certain body chemicals called prostaglandins stimulate the uterus to contract and expel the baby. If they do so too early, the infant is born prematurely. Omega-3 fatty acids, present in deep-sea cold-water fish such as salmon, tuna, and halibut, neutralize these prostaglandins and can delay labor by an average of four days. So vulnerable women should start eating these fish at about the thirtieth week. A four-day

delay may add an additional 4 ounces to your baby's weight at birth—
which can make a difference. Remember, however, that omega-3
fatty acids in supplement form should be avoided by anyone with high
blood pressure or a bleeding or clotting disorder. Never take them on
your own: *Always check with your doctor.*

The other side of the coin is the woman whose baby is overdue, and
who is convinced her tenant is a "squatter" with no intentions of ever
leaving! There are drugs to induce labor, when necessary. But you
may want to have lunch at the Caioti Café in Los Angeles, whose
owners claim their salad dressing encourages uterine contractions. I'm
told it is attracting large numbers of overdue women who order the
salad to get things going! Although the ingredients in this dressing
have not been divulged, I suspect that the active agent is probably
balsamic vinegar. But then again it may simply be concentrated sug-
gestibility! Closer to home, my editor, who you see is very knowledgeable, swears by spaghetti and meatballs. She tells me she went into
labor right on time with both her children under its garlicky influence.
Other patients think Chinese food will do the trick—and if all else
fails, there's always a good dose of castor oil.

In recent years, in addition to the usual nutritional dos and don'ts
during pregnancy, the issue of listeriosis has been raised. This is a
food-borne illness to which persons with an impaired immune system, the elderly, and pregnant women are especially susceptible.
(The highest incidence is in newborns and persons over sixty.) If a
pregnant woman becomes infected, she may either suffer a spon-
taneous abortion or give birth to an abnormal fetus. The responsible
bacterium has been found in cheese that is mostly soft and white and
Mexican-style (such as queso blanco and queso fresco) as well as feta,
Brie, Camembert, and blue-veined cheeses like Roquefort. Hard
cheese, processed slices, cottage cheese, and yogurt have not been
implicated. You can also contract listeriosis by eating undercooked
poultry, hot dogs that haven't been thoroughly reheated, delicatessen products, and other ready-to-eat foods. In fact, the biggest threat
is from any food that has been contaminated as a result of improper
handling compounded by undercooking. So, unless you have personally prepared them, avoid frankfurters, bologna, jerky, and any
meat salads or spreads from a delicatessen. Remember, you can't tell

by just looking, smelling, or even tasting the food whether or not it is infected. To avoid listeriosis and other bacteria-borne illness, follow these guidelines:

1. Do not drink raw or unpasteurized milk, and do not eat raw fish (sushi) or very rare or undercooked meat (steak tartare).

2. Separate raw and cooked foods when shopping, preparing, cooking, or storing them. Bacteria from the juices of raw meat, poultry, or fish may contaminate a cooked food, so never transfer a food you have cooked back to the dish that held the raw food.

3. Wash all raw vegetables.

4. "Sterilize" in your dishwasher or wash very thoroughly anything used in the preparation of uncooked food—including dishes, knives, and cutting boards. Also, be sure to wash your hands with soap and water.

5. All food of animal origin including eggs should be cooked thoroughly: meat to a temperature of 160 degrees, poultry to 180 degrees, and fish to 160 degrees (or until it is white and flaky).

6. Thoroughly reheat all leftovers.

7. Pay attention to labels that say "keep refrigerated" or that specify use by a certain date.

8. Don't let cold foods sit around at room temperature for longer than two hours before eating them.

9. Use wooden rather than plastic cutting boards; the latter harbor more bacteria.

10. Discard raw eggs that have cracked shells.

In addition to all of the above, eat lots of garlic. Something in this bulb's oil prevents the growth of harmful bacteria in the intestine, notably *Listeria*!

In summary, remember that proper nutrition to ensure a successful pregnancy should ideally begin before conception. If you are "working" on a family, it's a good idea to take prenatal vitamins even before you get pregnant. Avoid fad diets and fasting while still in the planning stage so that when the "moment" occurs, your body will be ready. Good prenatal care means more than just having your obstetrician examine you. Every visit should include a discussion of your dietary needs and habits at your particular stage of pregnancy. Pages 391 and

392 contain summaries of your daily dietary goals during pregnancy whether you're omnivorous or a vegetarian.

I hope that your pregnancy is one of the most exciting and happy times of your life. The joy and anticipation of creating another life are all-consuming. The mother-child relationship begins with the infant's first movement long before birth. Eat right so that you'll end your forty-week wait with the delivery of a healthy, bouncing baby.

VITAMIN B_{12} CONTENT OF FOODS

FOOD	PORTION	VITAMIN B_{12} (mcg)	CALORIES
Beef			
ground, extra lean, broiled	3.5 ounces	2.17	256
kidney, cooked	3.5 ounces	51.30	144
liver, braised	3.5 ounces	71	161
Cheese			
cottage, lowfat, 1% fat	1 cup	1.43	164
cream cheese, lite	1 ounce	0.09	62
Edam	1 ounce	0.44	101
mozzarella, part-skim	1 ounce	0.23	72
mozzarella, whole	1 ounce	0.19	80
Swiss	1 ounce	0.48	107
Chicken breast, roasted, skinless	3.5 ounces	0.34	173
Egg	1 large	0.56	77
Egg white	1 large	0.7	17
Fish/Shellfish			
clams, cooked by moist heat	3 ounces	84	126
cod, Atlantic, cooked by dry heat	3 ounces	0.89	89
grouper, cooked by dry heat	3 ounces	0.59	100
halibut, cooked by dry heat	3 ounces	1.16	119
lobster, cooked by moist heat	3 ounces	2.64	83

VITAMIN B$_{12}$ CONTENT OF FOODS *(Continued)*

FOOD	PORTION	VITAMIN B$_{12}$ (mcg)	CALORIES
salmon, Atlantic, cooked by dry heat	3 ounces	2.6	155
tuna, canned, packed in water	3 ounces	2.54	116
Milk			
Lactaid, skim	8 ounces	0.93	86
1% fat, protein fortified	8 ounces	1.05	119
skim, protein fortified	8 ounces	1.05	100
Pork, center loin, lean, broiled	3.5 ounces	0.74	231
Soy milk	8 ounces	0	79
Yogurt			
plain lowfat, with added nonfat dry milk solids	8 ounces	1.28	144
plain nonfat, with added nonfat dry milk solids	8 ounces	1.39	127

DAILY DIETARY GOALS IN PREGNANCY

FOOD	PORTION	PROTEIN (gm)
Poultry, fish, lean beef, or eggs	4 to 6 ounces	28 to 42
Fruits	3 to 4 servings	3 to 4
Milk, nonfat, or nonfat yogurt	4 cups	32
Vegetables, cooked or uncooked	3 to 5 servings	6 to 10
Whole-grain breads, whole grains, and enriched cereals	7 or more servings	14
Desserts	limited amounts	—
Fats, monounsaturated	2 tablespoons	0
		75 +

A serving of fruit is one small fruit such as an apple or pear, ½ banana, ½ cantaloupe, or ½ grapefruit.

A serving of vegetables is approximately ½ cup cooked or 1 cup uncooked.

A serving of bread is one slice.

A serving of whole grains or cooked cereal is ½ cup.

A serving of cold, enriched cereal is ¾ cup.

Eat nonfat desserts sparingly and count your calories.

DAILY DIETARY GOALS IN PREGNANCY FOR VEGETARIANS

FOOD	PORTION	PROTEIN (gm)
Beans, legumes, tofu, or soy protein	2 to 3 servings	14 to 18
Fruits	3 to 4 servings	3 to 4
Milk, nonfat, or nonfat yogurt	4 cups	32
Vegetables, cooked or uncooked	3 to 5 servings	6 to 10
Whole-grain breads, whole grains, and enriched cereals	7 or more servings	14
Desserts	limited amounts	—
Fats, monounsaturated	2 tablespoons	0
		61 +

A serving of beans or legumes is approximately ⅔ cup cooked.
A serving of tofu is 4 ounces.
A serving of fruit is one small fruit such as an apple or pear, ½ banana, ½ cantaloupe, or ½ grapefruit.
A serving of vegetables is approximately ½ cup cooked or 1 cup uncooked.
A serving of bread is one slice.
A serving of whole grains or cooked cereal is ½ cup.
A serving of cold, enriched cereal is ¾ cup.
Eat nonfat desserts sparingly and count your calories.

PREMENSTRUAL SYNDROME (PMS)

ALL I WANT FOR CHRISTMAS

IS—CHOCOLATE!

Many healthy, happy women without a complaint in the world suddenly begin to feel miserable a few days before the onset of their period each month. They retain fluid, their clothes are tight, they become bloated, they gain weight, their ankles swell, and their breasts become tender and swollen. They may have mood swings and become depressed, anxious, nervous, or irritable. They often sleep poorly and are tired the next day; they may find it hard to concentrate and they have no energy. They suddenly crave sweets—especially chocolate—or they may lose their appetite, even develop nausea, vomiting, and diarrhea; they often ache all over. However, as soon as their period begins, miracle of miracles, all these symptoms disappear within twenty-four hours and life returns to normal—until the next month! This cyclical scenario is referred to as *premenstrual syndrome* (PMS), something almost every woman experiences at one time or another. It usually begins in the late twenties or thirties, reaches a crescendo in the forties, and continues until menopause. Fortunately, only one female in four suffers from it on a regular basis. Symptoms may be mild or severe. In the great majority, it's a hit-or-miss affair—some months are good, others are not.

The causes of PMS have never been identified, although they are clearly hormonal, not psychiatric. (The symptoms may, however, be aggravated by an underlying psychiatric disorder.) No one knows why some women are affected and not others, or why this condition varies in severity from person to person, and even in the same individual. Although the onset of symptoms—anywhere from four to fourteen days before the beginning of the next period—is associated with changes in hormonal levels in the blood, these same levels are also present at that time of the month in women without PMS. The villain is therefore something other than the usual hormonal fluctuations. There is no blood test that predicts who is vulnerable and who isn't. Race, marital status, and educational level make no difference, but women who work, use alcohol, and have had children are more likely to have PMS.

Hundreds of different PMS symptoms have been described by millions of women over the years—everything from profound fatigue to joint pains, fear of being left alone, panic attacks, lack of coordination, usually diminished but sometimes increased sex drive, depression, anger, fluid retention—and on and on. Approaches to therapy are as different as the complaints themselves. Some women are convinced that diuretics help, others deny it; evening primrose oil (a substance related to vitamin E and prostaglandin) has been reported to relieve depression and painful breasts. There are those who swear that vitamin B_6 does the trick for them; a number of women benefit from antidepressants, hormone manipulation, or herbal preparations.

Since PMS manifests physical, emotional, and behavioral symptoms (singly and in combination), it may in fact be several different entities. That would explain why a particular treatment is effective in some women and not in others. If your PMS symptoms require relief, discuss their management with your doctor, and do try all the various regimens suggested until you find one that works for *you*. But don't count on it. The only thing you can depend on is that the PMS will stop once your period begins happening—and then will cease permanently with menopause.

An especially common manifestation of PMS is an intense desire for sweets, especially chocolate. Females who are absolute paragons of dietary virtue—disciplined and weight conscious in the first half of their menstrual cycle—suddenly become chocoholics. Doctors have one reflex reaction you can usually count on. With the possible exception of sex, they believe that anything you enjoy cannot possibly be good for you! Since "normal" women do not crave chocolate, physicians assume that "giving in" to the longing for it must be harmful, and most of them advise you not to do it.

I have always believed that there is usually a method to nature's madness—that we hunger for what we need. In pregnancy, many of the unusual dietary preferences some women develop do, in fact, seem to be due to subtle deficiencies that nature is signaling them to replenish. And so it is in women with PMS who are depressed. They really do feel better after they've eaten the candy or chocolate they crave, a response that can be documented in psychological tests. Other forms of depression also respond to sweets. For example, seasonal affective disorder (SAD), which occurs mostly in the fall and winter and strikes both sexes, is associated with an intense desire for sweets. Eating them improves mood. So if your main PMS symptom is depression, surrender for those few days to your passionate yearning for chocolate (or whatever else makes you feel better) without guilt—except, of course, if you are diabetic. But remember, 1 ounce of plain chocolate contains 150 calories and a lot of fat, and there will be a day of reckoning. Once you are in control again, you'll have to go back to your regular eating pattern.

Unfortunately, some women cannot tolerate the chocolate that they crave—a real Catch-22! Too much simple sugar induces in them an overproduction of insulin, which in turn results in a sharp and rapid drop in their blood sugar level. This generates an array of hypoglycemic symptoms—sweating, palpitations, nervousness, and weakness. If you can't handle the sugar in chocolate, there are many sugar-free chocolate products in which you can wallow! These include a variety of mousses, ice creams, cocoa mixes, and milk shakes. You should also check out the new fat- and cholesterol-free brands. These products come in many forms—chocolate cake and cookies, frozen yogurt, desserts made with skim milk—all of which retain the cocoa and the chocolate taste but with far fewer calories. Eating more complex carbohydrates such as pasta, whole-grain breads, cereals, baked yams, potatoes, and brown rice will raise the blood sugar more slowly than do simple sugars, without provoking the hypoglycemia of insulin overshoot. Their beneficial effects on your PMS symptoms may not be as dramatic as that of chocolate, but they may help.

What is it about chocolate and candy that counters the depression of PMS? Doctors at the Massachusetts Institute of Technology have come up with an interesting explanation as to why some women develop a passion for chocolate and not for, say, tacos or gefilte fish. Pure carbohydrates such as chocolate and candy raise the amount of a chemical called *serotonin* in the brain. The more serotonin there is, the less likely you are to be depressed. Several antidepressant drugs (Prozac, for example) also work by increasing serotonin levels. So nature does what's practical; it stimulates your desire for sweets—a craving you can satisfy without asking your doctor for a prescription. There are other serotonin-stimulating foods that are less caloric than chocolate and are worth trying. If the serotonin theory is correct, then plums, eggplant, walnuts (which, by the way, lower cholesterol too), tomatoes, and pineapples may also lighten the depression.

Remember, too, that although chocolate eases your depression, it will have no effect on your other PMS symptoms. Strangely enough, the *bloating* of PMS is not primarily caused by fluid retention. The real problem is failure of the body to excrete enough of the salt it contains. Excessive salt causes water to accumulate in the tissues. The best way to deal with such fluid retention is to reduce your salt consumption to less than 2 grams a day. That's easily done by removing the salt shaker from the table and eliminating frankly salted foods such as pickles, bouillon, soy sauce, most fast foods, herring, and all smoked, pickled, and cured foods. (See page 247 for a list of foods high in sodium.) If you really do cut down on your salt, you may be able to drink all the water you like without feeling bloated. Some women turn to diuretics at this time to rid themselves of excess fluid. Don't depend on tea and coffee for their diuretic properties; the caffeine is apt to make you more nervous and irritable during this phase of your menstrual cycle.

Many women are convinced that their PMS symptoms are improved by extra vitamin B_6. That doesn't surprise me because B_6 is a cofactor in the synthesis of serotonin. You can either take this vitamin as a supplement or obtain it from rich food sources such as cereals fortified with B_6, fresh salmon, pork, beef, tuna, avocado, liver, and many complex carbohydrates. (For other vitamin B_6–rich foods, see page 364.) But remember that too much vitamin B_6 can cause a nerve disorder, so do not take more than 200 milligrams a day in supplement form.

In summary, controlling the symptoms of PMS is a matter of trial and error. Although there is a great deal of myth, superstition, and even stigma involved, several things are clear. The chocolate you crave really does make you feel better, and I allow my patients to have as much as they need to ease the depression of PMS. In addition, I recommend you eat complex carbohydrates instead of simple sugars whenever possible, follow a low-salt diet, and take extra vitamin B_6.

PSORIASIS

WHEN IT SNOWS

ON YOUR BLUE SERGE SUIT!

No weatherman can predict the "snowfall" on the shoulders of your blue suit or dress. If it's only a light accumulation, it's probably only dandruff. Heavier precipitation, despite the "best" antidandruff shampoo, may be due to psoriasis. That forecast is all the more likely if you also have some silvery plaques on various parts of your body.

The cause of psoriasis, which affects about 1 percent of the population in the United States, is not known. It strikes men and women equally, and inheritance is an important determinant. One-third of all persons with psoriasis have a relative who also suffers from it. Although psoriasis is not an infection in the great majority of cases, there is one form, called guttate psoriasis, in which the typical skin lesions are triggered by or at least occur following a respiratory infection, usually strep. Psoriasis is not contagious, and you won't get it from touching someone's scales. Stress sometimes seems to make it worse. Occasional cases of psoriasis have been observed at birth, and there was a report of it developing in someone age 108(!), but most cases begin in the twenties. (The average age is twenty-nine.) It is much less common among blacks than Caucasians, very low among Japanese and Eskimos, and virtually unheard of in North American and South American Indians. There is more of it in the northern climes than in the tropics. Unlike so many other skin conditions, psoriasis is not caused by overexposure to sun, whose rays, in fact, are usually beneficial. (However, in some patients with lesions in an unstable phase, of recent onset, and very "aggressive," sunlight can make matters worse.)

The "rash" of psoriasis consists of silvery, pinkish plaques of varying size that appear most frequently on the elbows, knees, scalp, legs, buttocks, the belly button, and even the external genitalia. Whether or not they are cosmetically embarrassing depends on their size, their location, and how you personally cope with them. Flaking from patches on the scalp leaves a white coating on dark clothes that looks very much like a bad case of dandruff. Psoriasis sometimes itches, but not as a rule, and it can be accompanied by joint pains—a form of arthritis that is difficult to treat.

There is no treatment that will permanently eradicate the plaques of psoriasis, but there are several measures that can provide at least temporary relief. These include a wide variety of topical steroid creams, ointments, and solutions; a number of tar products and their derivatives (arthralin); salicylic acid ointment; ultraviolet light B therapy; psoralen combined with ultraviolet A (PUVA); methotrexate (an anticancer drug); synthetic vitamin A; and even cyclosporine (an antirejection drug). People who can afford to do so avoid cold weather and head for the sun in wintertime. The most famous and most effective place to go is the Dead Sea, the lowest place in the world below sea level. The particular mix of the sun's rays there (a predominance of the UVA long waves and minimal B or burning rays) makes it virtually impossible to get a sunburn even if you're exposed to it all day!

You won't find a word about diet for psoriasis in any textbook of medicine or dermatology because, until recently, there was no known or even speculative association. However, some dermatologists are interested in the possible beneficial effect of the omega-3 fatty acids present in deep-sea cold-water fish such as tuna, halibut, and mackerel. The same properties that make these fatty acids useful in some cases of rheumatoid arthritis, asthma, and inflammatory bowel disease may account for the improvement occasionally reported in persons with psoriasis. Omega-3 fatty acids block the formation of prostaglandins and reduce the number of anti-inflammatory cells that migrate to the skin. There have been a few positive reports (but many more dissenting voices) of a favorable effect on psoriasis by either a daily 6-ounce serving of fresh fish containing the omega-3 fatty acids or daily supplements of 1 gram of ECA and 750 milligrams of DCA (the two kinds of fatty acids involved). Many dermatologists say that the amount of fish you'd have to eat to see any worthwhile results is simply too much and impractical, and that the number of capsules of the fish oil required is not well tolerated. I wouldn't have bothered even mentioning this approach except that I have occasionally seen some improvement in persons taking these capsules. I continue to recommend them to anyone made miserable by psoriasis, in whom nothing else works. Remember, however, that while eating fish is fine, the supplements should be taken only after discussion with your doctor. They must be used with caution by anyone with a bleeding disorder (they act on the blood platelets somewhat like aspirin does) or high blood pressure. Also, if you're diabetic, take no more than 2½ grams of the capsules daily.

The table on page 221 lists the best sources of omega-3 fatty acids. You're better off with the fish than with the supplements because some (not all) of the latter contain as much as 5 milligrams per capsule of cholesterol! Read the label on the bottle carefully. The natural route, that is, eating these fatty fish two or three times a week, is also a good way to replace high-fat beef, pork, and veal entrées. Remember that fish is low in total fat content and especially saturated fat. But watch out for caviar and squid; both are high in cholesterol.

RAYNAUD'S

A DISEASE AND A PHENOMENON!

THE WOMAN WHO CAME IN

FROM THE COLD

Are the pads of your fingers a little wrinkled? Do they blanch and hurt when you go out in cold weather without gloves, run your hands under cold water, hold an iced drink even on a warm summer afternoon, or grope for a TV dinner in the freezer compartment? Do they turn red, become painful and tingle, and maybe even swell a little as they warm up? If so, you are experiencing a *Raynaud's reaction* (also called "Raynaud's phenomenon"), which can occur whenever your unprotected fingertips are exposed to a drop in temperature.

A Raynaud's reaction is caused by cold-induced spasm of the small arteries (arterioles) in exposed areas of the body, such as the fingers, tip of the nose, and ears. (For some reason, the toes are almost never affected.) When these blood vessels constrict, they deliver less blood to the area in question, which turns first white, then blue. As the tissues warm up, they become red, tingle, and throb. Raynaud's reactions are usually experienced by persons with some disorder of the immune system, the best known of which are lupus, rheumatoid arthritis, and scleroderma.

Raynaud's can occur not only as a manifestation of some other disease but as an independent entity, in which case it's called Raynaud's *disease*. People with Raynaud's disease may be perfectly well in every other respect except that their fingers cannot tolerate the cold. Raynaud's disease is virtually limited to women between the ages of fifteen and forty-five.

Here's how to distinguish the *disease* from the *phenomenon*. In Raynaud's disease, both hands are usually affected, while only one is apt to be involved in the phenomenon. However, in both conditions symptoms usually start in first one digit, then two, and ultimately all five fingers become painful when exposed to lower temperatures.

If you have Raynaud's *phenomenon*, your doctor will treat the underlying condition with which it is associated. As that improves, so will your symptoms. However, the first and most effective therapy for the symptoms of *both* the disease and the phenomenon is to get out of the cold. Always wear gloves in a cool environment and ask someone to do your frozen food shopping and to serve the cold drinks at your parties.

There are several medications that can control the spasm of the small arteries in persons with Raynaud's. The most effective are the calcium channel blockers nifedipine and diltiazem. Behavioral and feedback programs may also help. Some vascular specialists say you can bring additional blood to your fingers and abort an attack by swinging your arms like a windmill as soon as your fingertips begin to blanch and become painful. I tell my own patients to dip their fingers in warm water, if it's available, or to put their hands into their armpits.

There is an interesting dietary approach to Raynaud's. In one study, the digits remained pink and warm after exposure to cold in patients with the disease (not the phenomenon) who took twelve capsules of Maxepa fish oil daily for twelve weeks. The fish oils in Maxepa capsules are of the omega-3 variety—polyunsaturated fatty acids unrelated to those in vegetable oils. They are found in deep-sea, coldwater fish, the richest sources of which are anchovy, bluefish, herring, mackerel, salmon, canned sardines, trout, tuna, and whitefish (see page 221). The omega-3 fatty acids act on the platelets in the blood and slow down the clotting process. They also cause the cells lining the interior of the blood vessels to release prostaglandins and a "relaxing factor," which help prevent the blood vessels from going into spasm.

Although it is still premature to recommend fish oil supplements to everyone with Raynaud's disease, if your symptoms are bad enough you should consider trying them. However, don't rush out to buy them (especially if it's cold outside) without first consulting your doctor. Do not take them if you have high blood pressure or any bleeding disorder, and limit the dose to 2.5 grams a day if you have diabetes. Try to get your omega-3 from the fish themselves rather than from the supplements. Four ounces of pink salmon contain the omega-3 equivalent of seven Maxepa capsules.

RECTAL ITCHING

WHEN YOU CAN'T

SCRATCH IN PUBLIC!

Like fever, pain, constipation, or diarrhea, an itch is not a disease. It's a symptom—the result of some underlying problem such as the food you're eating (perhaps an allergy to shellfish); the detergent or soap you're using; the perfume you're wearing; the bug that bit you; the medication you're taking; a disorder of the kidneys, liver, or blood; infection; or even cancer. Then again, you may simply need to bathe more often (or less frequently, if your skin is dry). If you have ever endured a really bad itch for any length of time (and itching is often chronic), you know what a nightmare it can be. Whatever the cause, it's very hard to resist scratching. Ogden Nash put it very aptly:

> There was a young belle of old Natchez
> Whose garments were always in patchez,
> When comment arose
> On the state of her clothes
> She drawled, When Ah itches, Ah scratchez!

The first thing to do about any itch, anywhere in or on your body, is to identify the cause and, if possible, eliminate it: Treat whatever underlying disease is responsible for it; stop eating the offending food;

switch medication if that's what's doing it; etc. However, until these definitive measures work, you can obtain temporary relief from a wide variety of lotions, creams, and ointments containing local anesthetics or steroids, many of which are available over the counter. There are also certain antihistamines, such as Atarax, that can ease the itch. Occasionally, the symptom is so relentless that only a powerful pain-killer will help.

This short section is devoted specifically to rectal itching (doctors call it *pruritus ani*), because it is very common and may respond to changes in your diet. There are many possible causes of itching in this area—infection, diabetes, an immunological disorder—in fact, every-thing from hemorrhoids to tiny parasites called pinworms that settle down happily in households with small children. The proper medica-tion will eradicate these little nasties. Itching and irritation from hem-orrhoids can be helped by eating fiber, which keeps the stools soft as they pass over the dilated, inflamed veins (see page 226). The veins themselves can be tied off by a rubber band, laser-beamed away, or surgically removed.

The anal area is almost always moist, and that alone may account for the chronic irritation for which there is often no other explanation. Whatever the cause of your rectal itching, you may be able to improve matters by taking the following steps: Stop eating tomatoes and other nightshade vegetables such as potatoes and eggplant and see what happens (I have several patients whose mysterious anal itches cleared up completely when they did so); hold off on your vitamin C supple-ments; discontinue beer for the duration, together with all brands of soda pop; and eliminate spicy foods and citrus juices. While you're abstaining from all of these, use one of those wonderful soothing ointments, creams, suppositories, or oral medications that can alleviate this annoying symptom.

ROSACEA

THE TRUTH WILL MAKE YOU BLUSH

Are you one of those people who can't tell a little white lie, or be the slightest bit embarrassed, without a telltale blush or flush? If so, it's probably the result of some chemical release by your body, a condition called episodic erythema, or rosacea. Emotions are not its only cause. Many people become red in the central part of the face, sometimes in the neck too, and in the V-shaped area of the chest after consuming alcohol; being exposed to ultraviolet radiation, heat, or cold; eating spicy foods; or drinking hot tea and coffee. In the latter instance, it's not the caffeine but the temperature that's doing it. If you love tea or coffee, but won't drink it because it leaves you flushed, take it cold. I promise your skin will not change color.

TINNITUS

THE RADIATOR IS *NOT* HISSING!

As we grow older, we hear less well. The first sounds to go are the high-pitched ones such as the ring of the telephone. You'll also find it difficult to make out what that lovely woman is saying to you at a noisy cocktail party. "F" sounds like "S," "V" like "B," and you may well miss "TH" entirely. Imagine ringing a doorbell on 63rd Street when you were invited to dinner on 53rd Street! Hearing aids help matters to some extent by increasing the volume of the sound, but despite all the hype advertising, they do not restore normal hearing.

In about a third of persons over sixty-five or seventy years of age, hearing loss for high-frequency sounds (presbycusis) is accompanied by noises in the head (tinnitus)—usually hissing, ringing, or buzzing. So persons with both presbycusis and tinnitus can't make out sounds that are there—and they hear others that are not!

If you develop tinnitus, first make sure that your ear canal is not plugged up with wax. You can't imagine how many cases of "deafness" and tinnitus I have cured just by removing an earful of wax! High blood pressure is another common cause of these head noises, and lowering it to normal sometimes abolishes tinnitus too. Several drugs can produce these unwanted noises, the best known of which are quinine (present in tonic water and, until recently, widely used in the treatment of nocturnal leg spasms); quinidine (commonly prescribed for the treatment of heart rhythm disorders); and aspirin and nonsteroidal anti-inflammatory drugs (NSAIDs) such as ibuprofen. Eliminating them, or reducing the dose, often miraculously cures the tinnitus! If none of the foregoing is the cause, I refer my patients to an ear specialist, who may diagnose Ménière's disease, which is characterized by dizziness, deafness, and tinnitus (see page 313). In such cases, a low-salt diet and diuretics may improve the tinnitus by reducing the swelling in the inner ear that is at least partially responsible for this disorder. Tinnitus is occasionally a reflection of a serious underlying disorder, such as vascular disease or even a brain tumor, and should always be reported to your doctor as soon as it develops.

In most cases of tinnitus, all you can really do is accept your fate stoically. I have never seen any impressive results from the medications that are sometimes prescribed—vitamins A, C, or B_{12}, nicotinic acid, antihistamines, decongestants, and tranquilizers. I sometimes recommend a masking device that produces a more pleasant sound, such as the surf, for example, to drown out the unpleasant ones originating in the head. Eventually, however, most people become accustomed to their noises and learn to live with them.

There is one popular dietary approach to tinnitus. About one third of the cases that are accompanied by deafness appear to be associated with a deficiency of zinc in the tissues of the inner ear, where it is normally abundant. It's not clear how or why this occurs, but if you have recently developed tinnitus with no other discernible cause, have your zinc levels measured. Ask your physician to draw a blood sample and to send it to a special laboratory able to analyze trace elements. Occasionally, when a zinc deficiency is corrected, by either diet or supplements, hearing and tinnitus improve.

Oysters are the richest source of zinc in food, and contain twenty times as much of this mineral, weight for weight, as does beef. (Who knows? It may improve your sex life as well as your hearing! See page 147.) Other food sources of zinc are meat, chicken, fish, milk, and milk products. (For a more detailed list of foods rich in zinc and the amount per serving, see the table on page 151.) The RDA for zinc in adults over age fifty is 15 milligrams per day for men and 12 milligrams for women. If you decide to take supplements, don't exceed the RDA dose without checking with your doctor. Very large amounts of zinc, between ten and thirty times the RDA, taken for weeks and months, have been reported to cause anemia, a decrease in the number of white blood cells, and impairment of immune function.

URINARY INFECTION
THE CRANBERRY FACTOR

You suddenly need to empty your bladder every few minutes; it burns or feels hot whenever you "go"; you may even panic at the sight of some blood on the tissue or in the bowl. There's no time to dawdle when you get the "call," because even a slight delay can leave you with soaking underpants! This constellation of symptoms, which doctors call "urgency" and "incontinence," are the hallmarks of a bladder infection.

The *kidneys* (one in each flank) make urine, which travels down the tube or *ureter* (again, one on each side) to the *urinary bladder,* where it is stored until it's time to "pee," at which point it passes out of the body through the canal called the *urethra.* Anything that interferes with the flow of urine down and out of the body can cause it to back up and stagnate in the urinary bladder. Bacteria swim up the urethra and into the bladder very easily in women because their urethra is so short. It's a little harder in men in whom the urethra is longer. An enlarged prostate predisposes men to recurrent urinary tract infection because as the gland gets bigger, it presses on the urethra and prevents them from voiding freely and easily. When the urine backs up, accumulates, and stagnates in the urinary bladder, this limpid pool of urine is a sitting duck for bacterial infection. In women, cystitis (infection of the bladder and urethra) is the most common cause of recurrent urinary infection, and is usually triggered by vigorous and frequent sexual intercourse. If you use a diaphragm and do not empty your bladder promptly after sex, you're even more vulnerable to cystitis. Sexually transmitted diseases such as gonorrhea and chlamydia can lead to direct infection of the urine in both sexes. Scar tissue from previous infections within the female pelvis (chronic pelvic inflammatory disease) can involve the ureters and interfere with the excretion of urine from the body. Postmenopausal women who are estrogen deficient have dry vaginal walls that can become irritated and infected, especially after the friction of intercourse, but such infections develop spontaneously too.

Bacteria can enter the bloodstream from a distant site of infection too—from a diseased heart valve, a boil on the skin, or an abscess in the lung. They are carried in the circulation to the kidney and so infect the urine.

Urinary tract infections are by no means limited to adults. Infants are vulnerable too. It is not easy to detect urinary discomfort, frequency, urgency, or incontinence in a baby who is still in diapers and too young to tell you what's wrong. When your child is irritable or cries for no apparent reason, you're right to think of the ears first, but also keep in mind the possibility of a urinary tract infection, especially if you did not breast-feed, or weaned him or her before three months. For some reason, such kids are more vulnerable to urinary tract infections.

The wrong diet will not cause infection of your urine, and the right one will not cure it, but there are some nutritional tips that can ease your symptoms. The key to treatment at all ages and in both sexes is drinking enough water, meaning at least eight to ten glasses daily. You don't have to be Einstein to figure out why this is so. A copious fluid intake dilutes the toxins in urine and flushes the system. However, such large amounts of liquid may not be desirable if you have heart failure or certain kidney and liver disorders. That's something you must check with your doctor. I also advise my patients with urinary tract infections to avoid alcohol, mainly because its diuretic action promotes dehydration. The more you "go," the drier you become. This sets you up for infection and enhances its chances of persisting.

Before antibiotics became available for the treatment of urinary tract infections, people turned to *cranberry juice*. We used to think that it helped because it made the urine acid, but there is more to it than that. Cranberry juice actually engulfs the infecting bacteria and prevents them from becoming attached to the lining cells of the urinary tract. Because they can't hold on, the bugs are washed away. I am not suggesting that you use cranberry juice instead of an antibiotic, but you should drink one or two 8-ounce cups in addition to whatever else has been prescribed by your doctor. After the acute attack is over, make cranberry juice part of your dietary regimen if you are prone to recurrent urinary infections. Although I recommend 1 cup every day as a preventive, as little as ½ cup may be enough, or you may need 2 cups. That's something only you can determine. However, not all cranberry drinks are created equal! Most commercial brands sold in supermarkets consist of sugar and water, to which cranberries have been added, and they are full of calories. Look for those that are sugar free. Eight ounces of a low-calorie cranberry juice cocktail will set you back only 44 calories, while the others contain almost 150! Better still, pick up a bottle of pure cranberry extract available at health food stores. Mind you, it's expensive, ranging in price anywhere from ten to seventeen dollars, but adding only 1 teaspoon to 1 cup of tea makes a delicious and healthful drink, and the same amount in an 8-ounce glass of cold seltzer creates a refreshing cranberry fizz. There are also herb teas made of a combination of pure cranberries and other herbs. You can also buy fresh cranberries by the bag (November is the best month to do so), freeze them, and use them throughout the year. One whole cup contains less than 50 calories, and you can make cranberry sauce or relish to put on your turkey or chicken, or a stew to enhance the taste of other fruits. We eat lots of cranberries at home and my wife does marvelous things with them. When she reviewed this section, she insisted that I tell you how delicious homemade bread and muffins taste when made with fresh cranberries. (Do not, however, depend on the small amount in baked goods to ease your urinary tract symptoms.)

According to folk literature and anecdotal accounts (but nothing in the medical literature that I could find), *blueberries* and *licorice* help prevent urinary tract infections. I only mention this because a urologist friend with considerable experience tells me he recommends them to his own patients and that they are pleased with the results. He says that 1 cup of blueberries a day eases his patients' symptoms. Like cranberries, blueberries are not available in most places year-round, so you've got to buy them fresh and freeze them. The licorice I refer to is the whole root, not the candy kids love. I do *not* recommend it because the glycyrrhizic acid present in the natural form causes loss of potassium and the retention of sodium. The amount required to have a positive effect on your urinary tract may very well raise your blood pressure and interfere with the action of blood pressure–lowering medication.

The bottom line for anyone with repeated urinary tract infections is to drink lots of fluid, skip the alcohol, take the right antibiotic, and make cranberries a part of your daily diet—and consult your urologist.

VAGINAL YEAST INFECTION

CANDIDLY, IT'S EITHER BUGS OR FUNGUS

Women who are diabetic, pregnant, or have been taking steroids or antibiotics are especially prone to chronic or recurring vaginal yeast infections. When the bacteria that normally inhabit the vagina are reduced in number, yeast organisms (*Candida*), usually present in small numbers, multiply and take over. The result of this overgrowth is a chronic discharge, itching, and pain. Before assuming that these symptoms are due to yeast, see your doctor to make sure that other organisms such as *Trichomonas,* chlamydia, or gonorrhea are not the cause.

Vaginal yeast infections can be treated with antifungal medications, topically or by mouth, but they tend to recur because yeast inhabits the gastrointestinal tract as well as the vagina. When a woman wipes in the wrong direction (it should always be done front to back), she reinfects her vagina with yeast from the bowel.

For years, women have been telling their doctors that yogurt effectively controls their vaginal yeast infections. Very few listened to these "anecdotal" accounts. Why, it's heresy to suggest that something from the supermarket works as well as a prescription item from the pharmacy! Happily, studies were finally done to see whether there was anything to these claims. There is! Eight ounces a day of a commercially available yogurt can either cure vaginal candidiasis or relieve its symptoms. (Most women prefer to eat it, but it has been suggested that putting live yogurt cultures directly into the vagina is equally effective.)

Yogurt works because, unlike the vaginal suppository, its lactobacillus organisms overwhelm and replace the yeast in both the vagina *and* the bowel—a double whammy. Also look at the expiration date on the container. If the yogurt is "expired," so are its organisms, and dead lactobacillus won't do you any good.

If you have chronic or recurrent vaginal yeast infection, eat 8 ounces of yogurt at least three times a week to maintain an effective level of lactobacillus. (Frozen yogurt does not have the same effect.) Make sure that the brand you've bought has *live lactobacillus* (some do not) because other organisms may not be as effective (the label should have the word "lactobacillus" or "acidophilus" or both). If you don't like the taste of plain, unflavored yogurt, you won't have any trouble finding a flavor that appeals to you. There are scores of such products on the market. If you won't eat yogurt under any circumstances, there are tablets that contain the live lactobacillus. They usually come in soft-gel capsules, each of which contains millions of active lactobacillus acidophilus, including the naturally occurring metabolic products produced by the lactobacilli. The usual dose is one capsule a day.

INDEX

ABOUT THE AUTHOR

While continuing to practice internal medicine and his subspecialty of cardiology full-time, ISADORE ROSENFELD, M.D., also teaches at Cornell University Medical College in New York, where he has recently been named the Rossi Distinguished Clinical Professor of Medicine. He is also the co-author of a textbook on cardiology for the medical profession and writes a monthly health column for *Vogue* Magazine. During his distinguished professional career, Dr. Rosenfeld has served as president of the New York County Medical Society, on various task forces of the Heart Institute of the National Institutes of Health, and was for ten years a member of the joint Russian-American Council on Sudden Death. He is perhaps best known for his weekly appearances as health adviser for eight years on the nationally syndicated TV program *Hour Magazine* and for almost four years as the medical consultant on the *CBS Morning News*. Dr. Rosenfeld is currently a member of the Practicing Physicians' Advisory Council to the U.S. Secretary of Health, an Overseer of Cornell University Medical College, a member of the Board of Visitors of the University of California School of Medicine at Davis and of the National Advisory Council of the Emory University School of Medicine, and president of the Rosenfeld Heart Foundation. He lives with his wife, Camilla, in Westchester County, New York. Their four children are married, and this book is dedicated to his first grandchild, Rebecca. His hobbies are humor, collecting wine—and writing.